PUBLIC HEALTH AND HEALTH PROMOTION

For our children
Kate, Alice, Jessica and Declan

For Baillière Tindall:

Commissioning Editor: Susan Young
Development Editor: Catherine Jackson
Project Manager: Gail Wright
Designer: Keith Kail
Illustrator: AntBits Illustration

PUBLIC HEALTH AND HEALTH PROMOTION

developing practice

Second edition of
Practising Health Promotion: Dilemmas and Challenges

Jennie Naidoo

Principal Lecturer, Health Promotion and Public Health,
University of the West of England, Bristol, UK

Jane Wills

Reader, Public Health and Health Promotion Education and Development,
London South Bank University, London, UK

Baillière Tindall

Edinburgh   London   New York   Oxford   Philadelphia   St Louis   Sydney   Toronto   2005

BAILLIÈRE TINDALL
An imprint of Elsevier Limited

First edition 1998
Second edition 2005

ISBN 0 7020 2661 1

British Library Cataloguing in Publication Data
A catalogue record for this book is available from the British Library

Library of Congress Cataloging in Publication Data
A catalog record for this book is available from the Library of Congress

Note
Knowledge and best practice in this field are constantly changing. As new research and experience broaden our knowledge, changes in practice, treatment and drug therapy may become necessary or appropriate. Readers are advised to check the most current information provided (i) on procedures featured or (ii) by the manufacturer of each product to be administered, to verify the recommended dose or formula, the method and duration of administration, and contraindications. It is the responsibility of the practitioner, relying on their own experience and knowledge of the patient, to make diagnoses, to determine dosages and the best treatment for each individual patient, and to take all appropriate safety precautions. To the fullest extent of the law, neither the publisher nor the authors assumes any liability for any injury and/or damage.

The Publisher

 your source for books, journals and multimedia in the health sciences
www.elsevierhealth.com

The publisher's policy is to use **paper manufactured from sustainable forests**

Printed in China

Contents

Acknowledgements

Thank you to Verona Bryant, Stephanie Cash, Jeremy Cole, Robert Hoskins, Deborah Loeb, Alexandra Lucas, Jo Mussen, John Quirk, Debra Salmon, Vicki Taylor, Lynne Townsend, Stephen Young, and numerous colleagues and students whose ideas have informed this book; and Elizabeth Oliver, Gess and Ed for allowing us the space and time to write.

Introduction

Public health and health promotion have very different origins and antecedents, yet increasingly in the modern world they are seen as two complementary and overlapping areas of practice. This has had the effect of broadening the scope of both disciplines. For historical reasons, public health, with its roots in public health medicine, tends to be seen as the senior partner, embodying the status and kudos of medicine and science. In government documents, public health is used as an umbrella term to encompass health promotion; however, health promotion, with its diverse origins and roots, has much to offer that is distinctive, valuable and unique. One need only think of the following principles and ways of working that derive from health promotion but are now firmly embedded in public health: involving people and communities, working across boundaries and partnership working, empowering people, and a concern with structural causes of health inequalities.

We have taken the opportunity of a second edition of our earlier text, *Practising Health Promotion: Dilemmas and Challenges*, to reflect these changes in practice and terminology by giving this book a new title. *Public Health and Health Promotion: developing practice* uses both terms because we wish to acknowledge the separate history and contribution of health promotion to the overall development and improvement in the health of the public. Tilford et al (2003) have usefully teased out the distinctions between public health and health promotion and concluded that retaining both terms, the approach adopted by the Cochrane Collaboration Health Promotion/Public Health field, is the preferred option.

Health promotion refers to efforts to prevent ill health and promote positive health. From a relatively narrow focus on changing people's behaviour, health promotion has become a broad and complex field encompassing policy change and community action. A central aim is to enable people to take control of their own health. Promoting health is now to some extent everybody's business. It is not just a concern of the NHS but also of all those involved in health and welfare work, education and environmental protection.

Public health has been traditionally associated with public health medicine and its efforts to prevent disease. It has been defined as 'the science and art of preventing disease, prolonging life and promoting health through the organised efforts of society' (Acheson 1988). Public health includes the assessment of the health of populations, formulating policies to prevent or manage health problems and significant disease conditions, the promotion of healthy environments, and societal action to invest in health-promoting living conditions.

The aim of this book is to help practitioners clarify for themselves the scope, direction and skills embodied within health promotion and public health practice. Our starting point is to acknowledge the multidisciplinary nature of health promotion and public health; however, we argue that a social structuralist model of health remains the most helpful explanatory model. Such a model recognizes the profound effects on health of social structures such as income distribution, employment opportunities and social capital, whilst still allowing scope for individual agency and empowerment.

The twenty-first century poses enormous challenges for public health including the major demographic change of ageing populations in the developed world; environmental threats and increased urbanization; anti-health economic forces of globalization such as tobacco and junk food; economic growth alongside increasing poverty and inequality; and the rise of chronic and degenerative diseases alongside a resurgence of infectious diseases. People have the right to healthy choices and governments have a responsibility to tackle those issues that impact on health. Public health needs to negotiate the line between individual freedom and social responsibility, which means engaging in public debates about evidence, risk and values. To be effective, public health needs to have the informed consent and support of the population.

In our first book, *Health Promotion: Foundations for Practice* (Naidoo & Wills 2000), we reviewed some of the knowledge and skills with which practitioners need to be familiar if they are to promote health, and looked at some examples of differing approaches to this task. This book explores further what should inform the practice of public health and health promotion. The challenge for practitioners is to embrace the health promotion principles espoused by the World Health Organization – equity, community participation, intersectoral collaboration, and primary health and social care services – with the pressures of everyday practice. Many practitioners find it difficult to incorporate such a broad approach and move 'upstream' to tackle the determinants of health. Our aim in this book is to support the efforts of practitioners to achieve this task and to become committed and skilled public health practitioners.

Practitioners need to be aware of the forces that contextualize, drive and sometimes constrain their practice. These forces or drivers of public health and health promotion practice include theoretical and conceptual frameworks that inform interventions, a developing research and evidence base, and the values that underpin and feed into the policy context. These drivers of practice are discussed in Part 1 of this book.

Practitioners also need to understand core strategies for public health and health promotion practice. These strategies inform and underpin a multitude of interventions, programmes and projects spanning priority topics, key agencies and targeted client groups. Developing an understanding of, and competence in, these strategies enables practitioners to increase the impact of their health promotion and improvement work. The core strategies that we identify and discuss in Part 2 of this book are: tackling health inequalities, participation and involvement, working in partnerships, and information, education and communication strategies.

Practitioners need to be familiar with current public health priority issues and how they are being addressed in practice. Priorities for public health and health promotion may be defined in different ways. Categories used in policy and strategy documents include social determinants of health; disease conditions, lifestyles and behaviours that constitute risk factors for disease, and vulnerable or marginalized groups of people. We address each of these four priority categories in Part 3 of this book. Each chapter in Part 3 discusses why these topic areas are priorities, and provides examples of the range of approaches used to tackle these issues. The four chapters in Part 3 are completely new for this edition.

This book uses a clear, user-friendly but challenging style that encourages readers to engage with the subject. The book is clearly structured and signposted for ease of reading and study. A checklist at the end of this introduction provides a tool for practitioners to interrogate their own practice and make links to relevant sections in the book. Each chapter starts with a few key points and an overview outlining the contents of that chapter and ends with a conclusion, further discussion questions and recommended reading. Interspersed throughout the text are a number of helpful features:

- Discussion point – to enable individual or small group discussion to clarify and consolidate understanding and learning
- Example, research or case study of practice – to demonstrate good practice developments and innovative interventions
- Practitioner talking – quotes to use as triggers to engage the reader in the topic and encourage reflection on practice
- Reflection point for individual assessment – to enable the reader to reflect and make links between their own practice and relevant theory and research.

When appropriate, feedback on these features is provided in the text.

We hope that this book will enable practitioners to develop their public health and health promotion knowledge, skills and confidence. Public health and health promotion are constantly evolving and developing, and the speed and scope of change can be daunting for practitioners. We hope that this text will go some way towards unpacking what is included in public health and health promotion and thereby enable practitioners to identify and develop their public health role.

REFERENCES

Acheson D (1988) Public health in England. Report of the committee of inquiry into the future of the public health function. London, HMSO

Naidoo J, Wills J (2000) Health promotion: foundations for practice, 2nd edn. Edinburgh, Baillière Tindall

Tilford S, Green J, Tones K (2003) Values, health promotion and public health. Leeds, Centre for Health Promotion Research, Leeds Metropolitan University

Checklist for public health and health promotion practice

Drivers of public health and health promotion	What are the key drivers for public health and health promotion? What is the relative contribution of scientific evidence versus theory and values?	Part 1
Theoretical perspectives and frameworks	What informs my understanding of public health and health promotion problems?	Chapter 1
	What is my vision for public health? What principles should underpin its practice?	Chapter 1
	Is my practice founded on a theoretical understanding?	Chapter 1
Research and evidence	Is my practice founded on research?	Chapter 2
	How robust is the research base for public health and health promotion?	Chapter 2
	Can I identify appropriate and valid sources of information/evidence to address public health questions and issues?	Chapter 3
	How do I know my practice is effective? How do I know it is acceptable or appropriate?	Chapter 3
Policy	What is the value base underpinning policies? Can I critically appraise government initiatives aimed at improving health and well-being? How can I work effectively within the existing policy framework? How am I able to influence policy?	Chapter 4
Strategies in public health and health promotion	What are the key strategies used to promote and protect the health of the public? What knowledge, skills and	Part 2

	competencies are needed to use these strategies effectively?	
Tackling health inequalities	What is the extent of avoidable health inequalities? What is the range of strategies aimed at tackling health inequalities? Is equity an underlying principle in my practice? How can I tackle inequalities, poverty and social exclusion in my practice?	Chapter 5
Engaging communities and patients	How are patients and the public engaged in service/programme design and delivery? How could I involve and support different communities in assessing their own health and well-being needs? How is information about needs disseminated and responded to?	Chapter 6
Working in partnerships	To what extent is partnership working encouraged in my practice? Do I understand and value the contributions to public health of different disciplines, practitioners and agencies? Are the skills and resources for partnership working recognized and provided in my work practice?	Chapter 7
Information, education, communication	How can I enable my clients to increase control over their health? How can I provide information for my clients? How do I know it meets clients' needs? How do I know it reaches marginalized groups?	Chapter 8
Priorities for practice	How do I know what the priorities for practice should be? What are effective strategies for addressing priorities for practice? How can my practice build on and complement strategies addressing priorities at a community or national level?	Part 3
Social determinants	To what extent, and how, does my practice reflect a social perspective	Chapter 9

of health	and understanding of the determinants of health?	
Major causes of ill health	What are the major priorities in terms of disease conditions?	Chapter 10
Lifestyles and behaviours	How can I address lifestyles and behaviours in a non victim-blaming manner? How do I know what are effective strategies for changing lifestyles?	Chapter 11
Population groups	How do I reach marginalized groups without stigmatizing them?	Chapter 12

Drivers of Public Health and Health Promotion Practice

INTRODUCTION

Public health and health promotion are undergoing a period of rapid change and transition. Changes in population demographics and the epidemiology of diseases, together with changing structures of health care delivery, including a focus on the primary care sector, have highlighted and expanded the role and potential of public health and health promotion to positively develop health. Various factors drive this process, including research evidence, government policy, public expectations and practitioner expertise. These changes lead to new challenges – of effectiveness, relevance, acceptability and appropriateness – for public health and health promotion practitioners. Practitioners need the opportunity to reflect on their role, contribution and response to these challenges of the twenty-first century. The identification of a body of knowledge, theoretical frameworks and concepts that practitioners can draw upon to develop an analytical approach to a problem is central. All practitioners are called upon to base their practice on evidence, particularly evidence generated by good quality research. In addition, practitioners' interventions need to be solidly based on ethics and consensual values. An agreed ethical and value base underpins policy making and implementation.

Part 1 explores in turn the key elements that enable practitioners to develop their public health and health promotion practice so that they can feel confident and justified in the decisions they make. Chapter 1 examines the body of theory and some of the key principles that inform public health and health promotion, and discusses why their application to practice is difficult. Chapter 2 discusses the evidence and research that informs public health and health promotion. A reliance on epidemiology leads to a focus on addressing individual behavioural risk factors for disease, whereas a broader view of research would include collective and

1

structural determinants of health. Chapter 3 discusses the current emphasis on evidence-based practice and the criteria for effectiveness that are used to evaluate interventions. Chapter 4 explores the ways in which policy is based on both research evidence and values. The impact of the policy context in the UK on practice, and the ways in which practitioners can affect policy, are also discussed.

1 Theory into practice

Key Points

- Relationship between public health and health promotion
- Professional roles
- Process and principles
- Skills for public health and health promotion practice
- Theoretical frameworks

OVERVIEW

An understanding of public health and health promotion theory is essential to informed practice. Yet identifying that body of theory is difficult and applying theory to practice is not straightforward. Many occupational groups claim a role in promoting health. Yet each may draw from a different knowledge base (biomedicine, education, psychology, social sciences, organizational development) and have a different perspective on what constitutes public health and health promotion. This chapter argues that practitioners should be aware of the values implicit in the approach they adopt. In so doing practitioners begin to clarify their view of the purpose of public health and health promotion and which strategies are suggested by different aims. Otherwise practitioners merely respond to practice imperatives and their health improvement work is limited to narrow tasks.

INTRODUCTION

> Public health is what we, as a society, do to assure the conditions for people to be healthy.
>
> (Committee for the Study of the Future of Public Health Washington 1988).

From the seventeenth to nineteenth centuries, public health was preoccupied with eliminating diseases such as bubonic plague, smallpox and cholera. With industrialization and rapid urbanization in the nineteenth century, public health work became focused on environmental issues such as clean water supplies, disposal of waste and better housing, which were the province of engineers and planners. In 1842 Chadwick wrote in the *Report on the Sanitary Condition of the Labouring Population of Great Britain* that to prevent cholera 'aid must be sought from the civil engineer, not from the physician who has done his work when he has pointed out the diseases that result from the neglect of proper administrative measures, and he has alleviated the suffering of the victim'.

The epidemiological transition during the twentieth century saw the main causes of death and disability shift from infections to chronic illnesses such as heart disease, stroke, cancers, respiratory illness and accidents where lifestyles play a causative role. Public health interventions included mass screening and vaccination and immunization programmes as well as education and advice delivered by practitioners and mass media campaigns. Public health in England can thus be divided into two periods – the Sanitary Reform period when improvements were sought through a better physical environment and the Personal Services period when the emphasis was on personal health and hygiene.

In more recent times, the political agenda in most of the Western world has been dominated by 'social responsibility' and a recognition of the links between poverty and ill health. Promoting health is now recognized as a multi-agency task. Health improvement cannot be delivered by the health service alone, but it will arise from cross-sector action on the environmental, economic and social determinants of health such as low income, housing, crime and disorder and employment.

This chapter will explore some of the complexities involved in translating modern public health into a multidisciplinary and multiprofessional area of practice. It will examine:

- the context and settings through which public health and health promotion is carried out
- the scope of modern public health
- the knowledge base of public health and health promotion
- the skills and competences of a multidisciplinary public health specialist/practitioner
- the process of modern public health
- the values and principles underpinning public health.

THE RELATIONSHIP BETWEEN PUBLIC HEALTH AND HEALTH PROMOTION

If public health is 'the science and art of preventing disease, prolonging life and promoting health through the organized efforts of society' (Acheson 1988) then health promotion would appear to be subsumed under public health. Traditionally, however, public health has meant disease prevention, an approach demanding a knowledge of medical conditions and an ability to assess and monitor disease trends. In many Western countries therefore public health has been a specialty of medicine. More recently, the term 'New Public Health' has been used to reflect a broader, social view of public health.

Health promotion was defined in the Ottawa Charter (WHO 1986) as being centrally concerned with empowering people to take greater control over their health and thus includes a range of strategies to strengthen communities, develop supportive environments and inform and educate about health issues. Health promotion has not become a profession with regulated entry and a licence to practise although there have been health promotion specialists and departments since the 1980s. Perhaps because of this, much effort has been expended in trying to define health promotion. This discussion is evidenced in debates about terminology and at least 25 published models of health promotion. In many countries health promotion is well established as a field of study and area of activity with a clear ideology deriving from the World Health Organization's principles of 1984 (WHO 1984). Despite this, the robustness of health promotion is still questioned and it is widely perceived as a-theoretical and a loose confederation of practice (McQueen 2000).

Table 1.1 highlights some of the differences between health promotion and public health medicine. It is apparent that they are two very different disciplines drawing on different bodies of theory, strategies and values as observed by Webster and French:

> The public health and health promotion professions embody – and tolerate – conflicting ideas of why and how health should and could be improved. The meaning of public health and health promotion are themselves contested and open to misunderstandings. The origins of these conflicts lie in the contested nature of health itself, of the causes of ill health, of the methods for reducing health and promoting well-being and fundamentally, in the motivation for such interventions.
>
> (2002, p. 11).

Reflection point

What does improving health mean to you?

Modern public health includes both public health medicine and health promotion, and thus has a huge remit and a multidisciplinary knowledge base.

Actions to improve health take different forms. If the reduction or absence of disease is the principal aim; health improvement centres around preventive medicine and influencing or persuading people to

Table 1.1 Public health and health promotion

	Public health medicine	Health promotion
Focus	Disease prevention, monitoring and management	Protection and promotion of health
Knowledge base	Biomedicine Epidemiology Health economics	Sociology, social policy, education, psychology
Core tasks	■ Research into the aetiology, incidence and prevalence of diseases ■ Surveillance and assessment of population health ■ Managing outbreaks of communicable disease (and non-biological hazards) ■ Planning, monitoring and evaluating screening and immunization programmes ■ Planning programmes and services to improve health-care provision	■ Developing policies to protect and promote health in different settings ■ Education and information for health and behaviour change ■ Working with communities to identify and meet needs ■ Organizational development
Areas of practice	Health sector	All sectors where people 'work, live and play'
Process	Top down: collecting information and policy development	Bottom up: collaboration and partnerships, capacity building of communities and individuals
Values	Authority, expertise, adherence	Collaboration, partnership, advocacy, mediation, enablement

adopt healthier lifestyles. Health may be viewed more broadly as a way in which people can begin to achieve their potential; health improvement then centres around community development and involvement. Health may be seen as socially determined and a fundamental right; health improvement then centres on addressing the root causes of ill health in the physical, social and economic environment through developing integrated health strategies tackling areas such as housing, employment and nutrition.

The key elements of modern public health are seen to be:

- having a population perspective
- recognizing the role of governments in tackling underlying socio-economic causes of ill health
- working in partnership with local communities to ensure their involvement in all stages of service development and planning
- working in partnerships with other agencies and the public to develop health improvement strategies
- developing the capacity of communities, professionals and organizations to work in this way.

Saving Lives: Our Healthier Nation (DOH 1999a, 10.2) signals this change in focus:

'Our new approach to better health comprises:
- reorienting local services – including the NHS – to give a high priority to health improvement
- local partnerships for health, where organizations and people work together to improve health overall.'

Modern public health therefore incorporates many of the activities, strategies and principles of health promotion. Multidisciplinary public health has become a widely accepted term to describe the range of professions and fields that will make up the public health and health improvement field and to overcome the distinction between medically qualified public health specialists and the non-medically qualified. In an early study of multidisciplinary public health, Levenson et al (1997) suggest, however, that the term not only describes the breadth of activities and the range of professionals contributing to public health but also the methodologies encompassed by this broader public health task. The disciplines underpinning public health have different philosophies and forms of enquiry that inform different kinds of interventions to promote health, and disciplinary battles continue to rage over the relative contribution of biomedicine, epidemiology and the social sciences to our understanding of ill health. The challenge for modern public health then is to move beyond public health medicine and to acknowledge the role of health promotion in the overall task of health improvement.

PROFESSIONAL ROLES

Promoting health has become 'everybody's business'. Many practitioners now have public health or health promotion identified as an aspect of their role. There is also a body of professionals who are deemed 'specialists' by virtue of their training, functions and experience. For the past 50 years in the UK specialist public health practice was the province of doctors who chose this medical specialty although this is now open to those who are not medically qualified. Health promotion was a clearly defined function within the NHS and open to people from diverse backgrounds. Recently, the task of national health improvement has come to be seen as multidisciplinary and including:

- those who lead and influence public health strategy (specialists) e.g. directors of public health
- those whose work contributes directly to health improvement (practitioners) e.g. public health nurses, midwives
- those whose practice should be informed by health improvement principles e.g. social workers, teachers (DoH 2001a).

Example

Professional roles and health improvement

'health visitors will lead public health practice and agree local health plans'
(DoH 1999b, 11.17).

'we expect health visitors to . . . work with local communities to help them to identify and tackle their own health needs such as measures to combat the social isolation of elderly people or the development of local accident prevention schemes'
(DoH 1999b, 10.18).

'the school nursing team will provide a range of health improvement activities . . . immunization and vaccination, support and counselling to promote positive mental health in young people, providing advice on relationships and sex education'
(DoH 1999b, 11.19).

'Pharmacies provide a non-stigmatizing, one-stop shop that attract a clientele that other professions find it difficult to reach. Pharmacists are an under-exploited resource that we need to use to deliver a broader public health agenda'
(Buckland 2001, p. 727).

'The average GP fulfils several useful public health functions in the following areas: infectious diseases . . . media "scares" (when) GPs provide the patient with a balanced view of this information . . . involvement in planning . . . screening . . . immunization . . . acting as a link in a chain of communication between agencies'
(McCalister 2003, pp. 141–148).

'Environmental health officers (EHOs) play a key role in public health within local government . . . no other professionals have such wide ranging involvement in so many health issues. . . . As such, they seem ideally placed to lead local government in its new role to promote the economic, social and environmental wellbeing of local communities'
(Brown 2002, Issue 8).

Many professional groups have integrated health promotion into their practice. It has been claimed enthusiastically, particularly by nurses. *Project 2000*, a major review of the professional education and training of all branches of nursing in the 1980s (UKCC 1986) reflected a shift to a more holistic view of health. There was recognition of the need to move away from a single practitioner–single patient approach to one of greater partnership with clients and more work in and with communities. Yet this shift in focus has not been easy to put into practice. For most practitioners, such activities are additional to their primary role which remains individual client care. Inclusion of community activities into a practitioner's remit poses an additional burden of work and extra time, resulting in it becoming 'bolted on' rather than integral to their way of working. Many health visitors, for example, struggle to release time from caseload work and routine assessment to focus on community-based activities. It is not surprising then that nurses frequently regard communication skills and the quality of the nurse–patient relationship as their most significant contribution to health promotion (Gott and O'Brien 1990). The nursing process itself still encourages nurses to identify individual problems and therefore the ability to understand health as an interrelationship between social and political factors as well as biomedical and psychological factors is rare: ' "facilitate", "enable" and "empower" is being interpreted in practice as communicating to people what their risks of specific diseases are, then further communicating what people should do to reduce these' (Gott and O'Brien 1990, p. 14).

How practitioners interpret their health improvement role will depend on many factors including their professional training, their role in the organization, their personal experience, interests and social and political perspective. Environmental Health Officers (EHOs), for example, work directly within communities and as such, seem ideally placed to lead local government in its role to promote health. In practice, the spectrum of activity for EHOs is limited by their statutory duties under the Environmental Protection Act 1990 which enables action to be enforced where there is risk of disease. Work pressures and statutory duties mean EHOs spend their time on population protection and enforcement work and do not have the available time or resources to work proactively with communities. The examples of nurses and EHOs demonstrate how difficult it is to prioritize public health, even though practitioners may be very positive about their role and potential. By making public health everybody's business, there is a danger that it becomes nobody's responsibility.

> **R eflection point**
>
> How do you think your professional group interprets their health promotion and public health role?

THE SCOPE OF MODERN PUBLIC HEALTH

The purpose of modern public health is to protect and promote health by:

- improving people's life circumstances (e.g. housing, employment, education, environment)
- improving people's lifestyles
- improving health services
- protecting the public from communicable diseases and environmental hazards

■ developing the capacity of individuals and communities to protect their health.

One way of articulating a profession is by defining its field of activities and functions. What does someone do when they are promoting the public health? The Health Visitor and School Nurse Development Programme (DoH 2001b) suggests that a health visitor may be engaged with health prevention with families, running and supporting groups, developing community-based health projects and developing public health strategy.

These areas thus incorporate activities traditionally viewed as within the remit of both 'health promotion' and 'public health medicine'. Modern public health acknowledges the importance of living conditions in improving health yet targets are set to improve health that focus almost exclusively on health risks (coronary heart disease, accidents, cancer) (see Ch. 10). Measuring such disease trends places a premium on data analysis and statistics. At the same time, action on health inequalities, the physical and social regeneration of neighbourhoods, the development of healthy public policy for food, transport and the workplace and the modernization of services all place a premium on public involvement and participation, collaboration across sectors and professions and community development. Modern public health thus embodies conflicting ideas about why and how health can be improved. A practitioner quoted in a review of the public health function in Scotland reflects the ambiguities of modern public health:

I find the concept of 'the public health function' a difficult one to get my head around. Many years ago we moved beyond the traditional concept of public health towards 'the new public health'. This brought a change of focus, with new dimensions such as 'Healthy Cities' ways of working, and led us towards valuing the contribution of other disciplines working together to achieve improvements in the health of the public. Alongside this in recent years we have seen the drawing in of public health expertise (or perhaps more accurately public health medicine expertise) into NHS matters, particularly in relation to the service commissioning process. There are a lot of different views of what the public health function is, and what it should be doing. There are some views that the public health effort has 'lost its way'.

(Anderson & Croucher 2001)

The task of health improvement is potentially overwhelming. The determinants of health are far wider than can be tackled by any one profession. It is therefore not surprising that many groups find themselves confused by how they can re-orient to a public health role.

SKILLS AND COMPETENCES FOR PUBLIC HEALTH AND HEALTH PROMOTION

As we have seen, an increasing range of practitioners see themselves as promoting health. What then are the skills that are necessary? There will be some practitioners who believe that modern public health is an additional role but more likely it is seen as another way of describing what

Discussion point

What are the central tasks for developing the nation's health? How do public health and health promotion differ from other forms of health and social care?

they already do. Anti-intellectualism is prevalent in many occupations, with practitioners valuing their client relationship and 'good old-fashioned caring' above macro level social change.

Many occupations including health promotion and multidisciplinary public health try to characterize their professional activity in terms of competencies or standards for practice. Occupational standards help to define professional activity and these were developed for Health Promotion and Care in 1998. What is surprising is that many of the skills identified are generic and apply to all health and welfare work, e.g. communication, planning, networking, management of change and using research evidence. Standards for public health specialists and practitioners have also been developed that relate to key functions and the competencies that need to be evidenced to show achievement. For example to demonstrate competence in surveillance and assessment of population health, a specialist would need to have undertaken needs assessments using appropriate epidemiological and/or other approaches (see www.skillsforhealth.org.uk). Core skills that public health specialists additionally need to demonstrate competence in are strategic leadership, research and development, and ethical management.

The concept of competence has aroused much controversy. It can be seen as narrow and mechanistic, focusing on task and not enabling practitioners to acquire the value base essential for critical practice. All practitioners need to be not just technicians but reflective practitioners with a professional literacy. Competencies cannot cover all types of activities nor the personal processes entailed in health improvement. In specifying a range of activities in which the practitioner must perform, the role of theory and understanding is diminished. 'Knowing' becomes merely preparation for 'doing' with no requirement to reflect on theoretical bases or make sense of working practice.

Discussion point

Consider the task of health improvement. What do multidisciplinary public health practitioners need to be able to do?

Example

The functions of public health practice (Skills for Health 2001)

- Surveillance and assessment of the population's health and well-being, e.g. undertaking needs assessments, analysing routinely collected data, monitoring and controlling communicable disease outbreaks.
- Promoting and protecting the populations health and well-being, e.g. monitoring and evaluating the implementation of a screening programme, setting up smoking cessation groups.
- Developing quality and risk management within an evaluative culture, e.g. using research evidence to inform decision making about interventions.
- Collaborative working for health and well-being, e.g. developing local partnerships.
- Reducing inequalities through the development of policies, strategies and service, e.g. analyse local data on access to and uptake of primary care services.
- Developing and implementing policy and strategy, e.g. carrying out a Health Impact Assessment on a proposed planning decision.
- Working with and for communities, e.g. mapping local organizations and holding a community planning event.

REFLECTIVE PRACTICE

The professional education of many practitioners, particularly in health and education, has been dominated in recent years by the work of Schon and the concept of the 'reflective practitioner'. Schon (1983) characterizes professional practice as the high ground of research and theory and a swampy lowland that is the messy, confusing problems of everyday practice. He likens many practitioners to the jazz musician or cook who is highly skilled at what they do and because of their experience is able to improvise but who may not know or understand the theoretical basis of musical syncopation or the emulsification of fats. Schon argues that through reflection-in-action a practitioner learns the tricks of the trade and what works in practice. This personal or experiential knowing is an essential part of a practitioner's understanding. Schon also says, however, that practitioners need to be able to reflect *on* action and to remove themselves from the swamp of practice and take a broad view. The reflective practitioner is able to integrate these two aspects. The reflective practitioner uses theory, understanding how it may help in their practice and how their experience can become part of a wider theoretical understanding. 'Those responsible for health promotion should be able to describe the philosophical aspects of what they are trying to do, and some guiding principles, as well as the values and ethics involved' (Evans et al 1994, p. 10).

Through this process, links are made between experience and theory and practice. Kolb (1984) argued that if we are to learn effectively, experience

---

Discussion point	Think of an action which you have taken recently, or a programme that you have been part of, about which you felt uncertain or confused. Figure 1.1 shows a cycle of questions to encourage you to reflect on this experience and identify any learning points from it and how other learning can help you to make sense of it.

Figure 1.1 The cycle of reflection

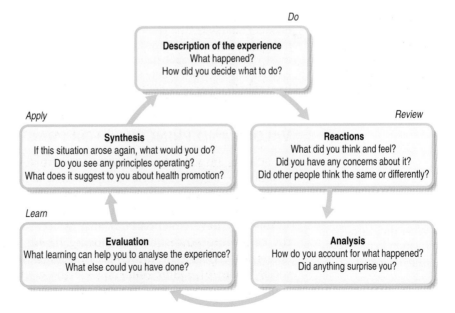

needs to be carefully and systematically reflected upon. Practitioners and students in classroom situations who focus on an 'experience' or a situation about which they felt uncomfortable may begin to understand the ways in which their knowledge was inadequate for the situation. Through sharing that information they can discover how others experience in a different way something they may have taken for granted. Through analysing or interpreting the issue or situation they can abstract general principles from it. By drawing on theoretical frameworks they can see what further knowledge may be required, and then apply this back to their practice, perhaps trying out new ideas or doing things a different way. The whole process is a cycle of practice–theory–practice or PRAXIS.

Schon (1983) argues that "technical rationality" dominates professional thinking. But it is important that practitioners think about *why* things are done in the way they are, *how* they could be done differently and *what* they are trying to achieve. Practitioners may believe they can apply their professional knowledge to select the best method for their purposes. But the problems of the real world (and the practice of public health and health promotion is no exception) do not present as neatly parcelled issues. When practitioners decide the form of their health improvement activity they are also choosing to frame the issue in a particular way which may mean reconciling, integrating or choosing among different interpretations and approaches. The action they take reflects particular aims and values – particular beliefs about health, about the influences on people's health and about the role of the practitioner. In the following example, reflection has facilitated development.

Example

Many local projects are funded from pots of money allocated for specific programmes such as Sure Start or New Deal for Communities. Practitioners have to submit bids with a project proposal. One such bid allocated for regeneration was for Community Food Workers to act as local nutrition educators. The lead practitioner comments 'The community kitchens were poorly attended. I was led by the money. The idea of consultation was alien to my professional culture. The most I had done was a patient satisfaction survey. I now see that if we had worked with the community they would have owned the projects and may even have chosen other priorities.'

VALUES AND PRINCIPLES FOR PRACTICE

All actions are value-based in the sense that we have a view about the desirability, worth or merit of a particular action. In relation to practice therefore, values are concerned with what multidisciplinary public health wants to achieve and how it will act to reach those goals.

You may have couched your answer according to what you regard as the central purpose such as reducing health inequalities or improving access to services. The principles that guide your practice may then be social justice or equity. You may see the central purpose as preventing avoidable diseases. A guiding principle may then be one of effectiveness and getting the most from available resources. Alternatively you may have

Reflection point

What do you value in relation to health improvement?

couched your answer according to the process of health improvement such as recognizing different understandings of health and the perspective of clients or building confidence and skills for people to take control of their lives. The principles guiding your practice may then be empowerment and participation. Every activity then reflects an underlying ideology or set of values. Seedhouse (1997) argues that community development, for example, reflects values of egalitarianism and social democracy while biomedicine reflects values of prudence and conservatism. The key issue is whether there should be some congruence between ends and means such that activities should encourage participation, be based on need and seek to establish a fair distribution of health, health care and resources.

Values thus determine the way in which the world is seen and the selection of activities and priorities and how strategies are implemented. A King's Fund Project on public health and public values (New 1999) identified the following values as having major implications for policy making:

- Fairness and equality – understanding these values is key to developing strategies to tackle health inequalities and poverty.

- Efficiency and health – these values relate to the effectiveness of public health policy in terms of favouring the least costly option and/or maximizing health gains.

- Autonomy and security – these values need to be considered when public health measures involve restrictions on individual liberty or require allocation of responsibilities for risk.

- Democracy – this value underpins the authority of the state to engage in any public policy, including public health.

Discussion point	The World Health Organization outlined a set of guiding principles for health promotion as part of its commitment to Health for All (WHO 1985):

- equity
- empowerment
- community participation
- multisectoral collaboration
- emphasis on primary health care.

What kind of tasks or services would be developed by adherence to these principles?

Are these appropriate principles to guide your work?

What other principles guide your work?

Are the principles you came up with distinctive and specific to health work or are they more general notions such as 'respect' or 'enhancing the quality of life'?

One of the characteristics of a profession as opposed to an occupation is said to be the way in which expertise is applied and what influences the way practitioners carry out their role. To work in a health promoting way means:

- **A focus on health not illness** – working with the well not just the sick, enhancing well-being not merely reducing or alleviating illness.

- **Empowering clients** – enabling individuals and groups to have a say in how their health is to be promoted and recognizing the value of their perspective; supporting people to acquire the skills and confidence to take greater control of their own health.
- **Recognizing that health is multidimensional** – mental, social, emotional, spiritual and sexual needs are as important as physical ones and the whole person and their needs must be taken into account.
- **Acknowledging that health is influenced by factors outside individual control** – trying to address the root causes of ill health and not 'blaming the victim'.

Another characteristic of a profession is that there is a code of conduct, the purpose of which is to persuade the public that the occupation can be trusted and acts with integrity. Codes of conduct derive from the values which underpin that profession. Traditionally a doctor's duties to their patients are outlined as doing good (beneficence), not doing harm (non-maleficence), being fair and equitable (justice) and respecting autonomy (Beauchamp and Childress 1995). Many professions attempt to establish a commonality of purpose through subscription to a shared set of values and principles.

Example

'promoting the independence of service users while protecting them as far as possible from harm' (General Social Care Council, 2002).

Health promotion (SHEPS 1997) principle of practice (I): 'adequate needs assessment and/or consultation with the client, target group or community'

Public health specialists (Faculty of Public Health 2001)
'practise good standards of public health
make sure individuals and communities are not put at risk
work within the limits of professional competence'

Professional practice frequently involves ethical dilemmas where central tenets such as a respect for autonomy conflict with the desire for equity or a professional value in minimizing risk and providing protection. For example, sexual health workers are frequently confronted with the ethics of testing for HIV status and how they present the benefits of doing this to their clients.

Modern public health, as all health care, is about making decisions and choosing between alternative actions. In making those decisions we may draw upon:

Reflection point

Which of these is most influential in guiding your practice?

- personal preference based on principles and values
- past practice and precedent
- professional judgement
- views of users, clients and the public
- available resources
- evidence of effectiveness from sound, rigorous research
- theoretical frameworks.

PUBLIC HEALTH AND HEALTH PROMOTION THEORY IN PRACTICE

Within the planning and development of strategy and programmes, the explicit use of theory is not common despite Kurt Lewin's oft quoted statement that 'There is nothing as practical as a good theory'. The reality is that for most practitioners theory is unrealistic and inapplicable in the face of the stark realities of day-to-day practice. Many practitioners adopt a pragmatic or common-sense approach.

Discussion point

What is the common sense that underpins public health and health promotion?

'Practitioners just need to find the best ways of getting the message across'

'Middle class people are more educated and understand how to look after themselves'

'We need to understand peoples' attitudes so we can challenge their negative beliefs'.

But as Thompson points out: 'common sense is ideological – it serves to reinforce traditional values and the inequalities associated with these. It is based on implicit assumptions and if we rely on common sense to guide our thoughts, we are not in a position to question those assumptions' (Thompson 1995, p. 28).

It is often assumed, for example, that there is a healthy way of living and practitioners focus on the individual or individuals with the aim of changing their behaviour to this end. As discussed in Chapter 5, the 'healthier choice' is not available to all. Thus people may be blamed for health behaviours over which they do not have control. The simple equation that knowledge + attitudes = behaviour has also formed the basis of much health education work, yet the provision of information alone is unlikely to change behaviour. The giving of information can reinforce the expert status of the practitioner and fail to provide for the active participation of clients in an education process which addresses issues of concern to them. Middle class, educated people are often seen as 'easier' clients and so are targeted more (yet need it least). When practitioners do not derive their practice from a theoretical framework, the practice wisdom regarded as 'common sense' tends to reinforce simplistic assumptions which serve to reinforce inequalities.

Reflection point

What traditional values and associated inequalities do you think are exemplified in the above quotations?

Theory is perceived by many practitioners to be book learning. Many practitioners value received wisdom – 'we do it like this' – and learning on the job over an intellectual understanding of the practice process. To know 'how to' is more important than to 'know why'. This issue has been vehemently debated in recent years by those involved in professional education. Nurse educators have expressed concern that less time is spent on the wards and in hands-on work and more emphasis is being placed on research-based knowledge. Those involved in teacher education have expressed equal concern about the reverse situation – that more time is to be spent in classrooms and less on the theoretical underpinning of education! The apparent reluctance to use theoretical models for practice has led to long debates in many health and social care fields about a theory–practice gap and its implications for service provision and programmes.

Consider the following opposing viewpoints on the importance of theory. Which comes closest to your own view? What further arguments could you use to support this view? (You might want to debate this with a colleague.)

A. Theory isn't important. Accounts of interventions show little evidence of them having been based on theory. Promoting health is just common sense and experience. The skills gained in previous training are quite adequate for this role. We just need to find out the best way of getting through to people. All this high flown stuff is unrealistic.

B. It's important that our work does derive from a sound knowledge base and a logic for the intervention. We need to be able to see why we do it the way we do and to be able to explain this to others who may have a different view. Understanding theory helps to clarify purpose and effectiveness and makes it less likely to suffer contradictions.

In the complex and evolving field of public health and health promotion an understanding of theory assumes great importance:

- It gives a common method and language through which to conduct a more thorough and informed debate (Caplan 1993, p. 156).
- It gives credibility to practice and gives the practitioner the confidence to justify their choice of action when confronted with differing interpretations by colleagues, managers or politicians.
- It allows us to make conscious decisions rather than take shots in the dark (Jones and Walker 1997, p. 71).
- It provides explanations which are based on empirical reality and a tool for more logical and coherent practice.

The attempt to conceptualize health improvement beyond a set of activities, competencies or skills raises questions about the status of public health and health promotion as a field of study. What knowledge do practitioners draw on to practise?

Mr Jones is 76 and has leg ulcers. He is in the early stages of Alzheimer's disease and lives alone since the death of his wife in the previous year. The District Nurse visits Mr Jones daily to dress his leg and draws upon her technical knowledge to do so, regarding herself as a competent practitioner. She is aware that she must include Mr Jones' health needs in her nursing assessment.

- How does the District Nurse begin?
- What factors will influence how she 'frames' the health promotion aspects of her work?

The District Nurse might regard health promotion as integral to her care of Mr Jones or she might regard it as an additional task to be 'bolted on' to her essential work of monitoring his disease status. She might see her role as enabling Mr Jones to keep himself safe and in good health, or as preventing harm or disease from befalling him. Whichever role she prioritizes will affect her activities. If her priority is safety and good health she might advise Mr Jones about a healthy diet and home safety precautions and spend considerable time talking to Mr Jones in order to enhance his capacities. She might enlist the services of voluntary and self-help organizations and try to broaden Mr Jones' social contacts. If her priority is to prevent disease or harm, she might focus on providing support for Mr Jones by liaising with Social Services to provide Meals on Wheels or day care and refer him to the occupational health service to assess his home for cooking and bathing aids.

This example illustrates how practitioners work in different paradigms. A paradigm can be defined as 'a way of knowing' and thereby interpreting a field of study characterized by particular beliefs and values, by particular theories and ways of problem solving and by particular methods and tools that are used in practice. The paradigm within which many practitioners work is that of Western science which has a mechanistic view of the body and views health as the antithesis of disease. Within this paradigm there are several theories or sets of propositions that explain or predict events such as theories about behaviour change or risk factors for disease. Practitioners may work in different paradigms, drawing upon different theories, and this will depend on their role, their professional background and training and their personal beliefs and interests.

Example	An occupational health nurse set up a workplace health and activity programme. Based on her common-sense belief that everyone wants to protect their health, the programme combined an educational input stressing the risks to health from lack of exercise and excessive weight. Opportunities for change were provided through a programme of exercises, monitoring of exercise recovery rates and food diaries. She also persuaded the company to pay employees half time rates for attending the programme. The programme was quite successful but many employees did not participate, some dropped out and few managed to maintain an activity programme for themselves.
Using theory to inform practice	When planning a subsequent programme, the occupational health nurse drew particularly on social cognitive theory and the concept of value expectancy which states that people are likely to take some action if they believe the action will be effective and if they value the action's results (Ajzen 1988). The occupational health nurse thus realized that a vague promise of better health in the future didn't mean as much to the employees as it did to her in her professional role. Through informal discussions she learned that the participants' values related to 'feeling more attractive', 'wearing different clothes', 'being able to take part in sports and exercise'. Social cognitive theory also helped her to understand the importance of boosting participants' confidence in their ability to take up and maintain an exercise programme. This resulted in her introducing smaller targeted group sessions which combined exercise and discussion of health related topics (adapted from Hochbaum 1992).

In the example above, the practitioner drew on theories from social psychology and used them as a tool to help her question her purpose and consider the factors influencing uptake of the intervention. Theory helped her to understand the variables affecting behaviour and provided insight into the strategies most likely to effect change. A reflective practitioner is constantly examining practice and adapting what to do in the light of experience. Without a theoretical base, however, they are merely a technician.

There are many different theories derived from different disciplines that practitioners may draw upon:

- How people learn.
- How diseases are caused and how they may be prevented.
- How people make decisions and change their behaviour.
- How society is organized and how social structures influence health.
- How messages are communicated and can be targeted to particular groups.
- How organizations change their focus and ways of working.

These theories derive from many different disciplines. Rawson (2002) has described health promotion as a 'borrowed discipline' importing theories from other bodies of knowledge such as sociology and psychology. Alternatively public health and health promotion can be seen as disciplines in their own right with discrete bodies of knowledge and distinct theories, perspectives and methods.

Example

Modern public health – is it multidisciplinary?

Consider the ways in which the disciplines outlined below contribute to health improvement. How, for example, would each discipline contribute to an HIV/AIDS prevention strategy?

Psychology

Psychology helps us to understand and explain human behaviour essential to health and the ways in which individuals make health-related decisions about, for example, taking up exercise, using a condom or changing drinking patterns. Psychological theories of mass communication in the 1960s, which assumed a direct link between knowledge, attitudes and behaviour, are still widely adhered to despite the ineffectiveness of programmes based on this premise. Psychology explores lay and professional health conceptualizations and the ways this might affect decision making.

Sociology

In analysing how society is organized and the social processes within it, we can examine the social role of medicine and how health and illness have come to be defined. An analysis of power and control and an understanding of the relationship between social structures and individual action helps us to consider how changes to promote health might come about. An analysis of the way in which society is stratified helps practitioners to consider how individual behaviour is constrained and influenced and how socio-economic status, gender and ethnicity influence health status.

Epidemiology

Epidemiology contributes understanding about the aetiology of disease and the effectiveness of preventive medicine. Epidemiology is based on a medical science model, although increasingly there have been calls to establish a social epidemiology of health. The study of risk factors for disease and health should, it is argued, go beyond traditional lifestyle or medical factors, to embrace factors such as degree of social networks and isolation and socially produced stress.

See Bunton & Macdonald (2002), Naidoo & Wills (2001)

Theories are organised sets of knowledge that help to analyse, predict or explain a particular phenomenon. A theory may explain:

- The factors influencing a phenomenon, e.g. why some parents refuse immunization for their children.
- The relationship between these factors, e.g. whether this is related to levels of knowledge and perceptions of risk; attitudes to interventions; beliefs about disease; levels of media attention; social norms.
- The conditions under which these relationships occur, e.g. do immunization rates fall when there is media attention to risk; in particular seasons; in particular social groups?

Modern public health is a complex field drawing on a range of disciplines. Inevitably then its theoretical base is equally diverse:

- Theories that explain individual health behaviour, e.g. the Health Belief model.
- Theories that explain change in communities, e.g. the Diffusion of Innovation.
- Theories that explain how communities can be mobilized for action, e.g. Achieving Better Community Development.
- Theories that guide the use of communication strategies, e.g. social marketing.
- Theories that explain changes in organizations, e.g. Force Field Theory.

Theory can help at different stages of programme development from initial conceptual thinking through design to evaluation (see Figure 1.2). Theoretical frameworks illustrate the key assumptions about how the programme will achieve the desired outcomes. Many practitioners, however, have only vague ideas about how and why a programme may work and any theory is implicit. Yet theory enables the practitioner to identify the issue, think through alternative strategies having identified the factors influencing the issue, identify the interventions most likely to be effective, and the factors that need to be taken into consideration during implementation and evaluation.

The wide choice of interventions that might be used to promote health involving a range of practitioners and professionals in different settings makes it difficult to see what knowledge base might be used to guide practice. Practitioners are often eclectic and use different models reflecting the way in which they frame the issue. Theories of behaviour change for example, have been widely adopted and have diffused into the design of health promotion interventions, reflecting the view that individuals are responsible for their own health.

Psychological theories such as the Health Belief Model (Becker 1974), the Theory of Reasoned Action (Ajzen & Fishbein 1980), Social Learning Theory (Bandura 1977) and the Transtheoretical Model of Change (Prochaska & DiClemente 1984) have dominated the field of health promotion as practitioners try to understand how to motivate and maintain behaviour change. Three sets of beliefs have emerged as important in determining behaviour or health change:

Figure 1.2 The role of theory in programme planning (from Nutbeam D & Harris E 2004 Theory in a Nutshell, 2nd edn. Sydney, McGraw-Hill. © McGraw-Hill Australia Pty Ltd)

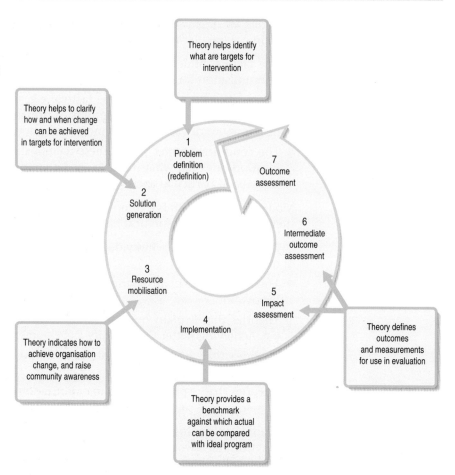

- Perceived benefits versus the costs associated with change
- Perceptions about the attitudes of others to the behaviour
- Self-efficacy or the belief in one's ability to achieve the change.

Individuals and population groups differ in their perception of the need for change and its benefits and this understanding has been critical in the adoption of more targeted and client led approaches. Learning theory seeks to explain how behaviour is maintained. The likelihood of an individual behaving in a particular way (e.g. quitting smoking) tends to increase when that behaviour is followed by positive reinforcement (e.g. sweeter breath). A person's motivation to change will depend in part on how desirable are the reinforcing factors.

The theories described above focus on understanding how individuals can modify their health risks. A key element of modern public health is the capacity of communities to identify and act collectively on issues affecting their health. Many practitioners have been influenced by Freire (1972) whose liberation education model provided both a philosophy of education and development and a practical method of getting people actively involved, breaking through apathy, and a way of developing a critical awareness of the causes of problems. Arnstein's ladder of involvement (1969) has also been influential in encouraging practitioners to review community levels of participation in decision making (see Ch. 7). Increasingly, the policy focus has been on describing a 'competent' or healthy community as a way of helping us to understand how to create safer and more productive communities that can implement local actions.

As Nutbeam & Harris (2004, p. 38) observe 'unlike the theories and models of health behaviour, community mobilisation does not lend itself so comfortably to highly structured study and comprehensive theory development'. Much of the understanding about community action derives from practitioner experience and observation and much of the theoretical development focuses on identifying the process of capacity building and its elements driven by a desire to develop indicators to measure change.

Organizational contexts also play a part in achieving health improvement. Management theory has developed particularly in relation to understanding how to improve organizational performance but it also illuminates the process of change. Understanding why change occurs and the political, economic, societal and technological factors that operate on organizations and affect their development helps to remind practitioners to take account of the internal and external environment (Senior 1997). The 1990s in the UK saw, for example, a Labour administration after 18 years, low inflation, a commitment to low personal taxation and demoralized trade unions. The White Paper on the NHS introduced early in the new government (1997) stated that the status quo for the NHS was not an option and the modernization agenda has entailed torrents of change. Understanding the psychological process entailed in change is crucial to its implementation whether it be shifting the practice role of a health visitor, developing a health promoting school or being part of a new Primary Care Trust. Resistance to change is normal according to Lewin's Force Field Theory (1951). During any period of change, there will be pressure to change and to maintain the status quo and a balance needs to be found. If the pressure to change is too great then resistance sets in.

These different theoretical frameworks derive from different disciplines and traditions and all provide the constructs in which the myriad tasks of public health and health promotion may be understood. In addition there are numerous models of health promotion that emerged during the 1980s in an attempt to define and clarify practice. Such models help to:

- conceptualize or map the field of health promotion
- interrogate and analyse existing practice
- plan and chart the possibilities for interventions.

Beattie's model for example (1996, p. 140) is useful for 'charting and selecting the particular mix of approaches that make up a programme or project and also in exploring and reviewing the ethical and political tensions within an intervention in terms of the balance of social values it encompasses'. The model shows how health promotion is embedded in the socio-cultural and political framework. It is not a technical activity in which practitioners merely choose the best strategy for improved health. The field of health promotion clearly reflects the tension between different value positions about power, knowledge, responsibility and autonomy. Health promotion models are discussed in detail in our first book *Health Promotion: Foundations for Practice* (Naidoo & Wills 2000).

CONCLUSION

It is difficult to draw boundaries around public health and health promotion and agree who is promoting health and protecting the public and what sorts of activities this entails. Attempts to specify core competencies and skills of public health specialists and practitioners reflect a professional strategy to safeguard a specific role and identity along with associated benefits, both economic and psychological. However such attempts also risk causing division, hierarchy and competition amongst the many different practitioners who need to work collaboratively in order to gain maximum benefits for public health. Health promotion is a central aspect of public health activity that needs to be recognized and valued, instead of being assumed to be a common-sense, bolt-on task for all health practitioners. It would be easy to be side tracked into defining and defending professional roles and competencies. Perhaps the most important aspect is to reflect on what we are doing in the name of health improvement and what it is we are trying to improve (Wills & Woodhead 2004). Many authors despair of this debate:

> There is a danger that obsessive concern with the meaning of 'health' can paralyse our activity and create sectarian divides between workers who should be cooperating. There will always be a wide range of activities that everyone agrees to be health promoting. We should get on with these tasks without waiting for agreement on all matters.
>
> (Kemm and Close 1995, p. 23)

As you will see in Part 2, it is not as simple as just getting on with it. Public health and health promotion have a close, but at times uneasy, relationship, mainly because public health medicine has traditionally been the 'senior partner', accorded a greater status and authority than health promotion. Modern public health seeks to integrate both health promotion and public health medicine into a new multidisciplinary endeavour. Inevitably, different practitioners will have different views on the purpose of public health and health promotion and the best methods to achieve health improvement. A public health consultant may prioritize the uptake of available screening and immunization programmes locally, whereas a health promotion specialist may prioritize community development activities focusing on identifying local needs and empowering communities to address these needs. Differing roles, professional backgrounds and funding constraints as much as ideology will influence the way in which a practitioner defines the purpose of public health. Our position is that public health and health promotion need to be based on sound theoretical underpinnings and adhere to certain core principles. In the rest of this book we explore how these principles might be put into practice and the sorts of dilemmas this throws up. It is from these dilemmas and trying to apply theory to practice that practitioners can learn and contribute to a developing field.

FURTHER DISCUSSION

- A reflective practitioner is one who is capable of improving practice by 'asking difficult questions and being sceptical of practices taken for granted' (Fitzgerald 1994, p. 75). In what ways are you incorporating reflective practice into your work?
- Consider a health improvement intervention with which you have been involved. What theoretical assumptions underpinned this activity? How would it be influenced by a consideration of other theoretical perspectives?

Recommended reading

- Adams L, Amos M, Munro J (2002) Promoting health: politics and practice. London, Sage.
  An accessible discussion of health promotion theory and its application to practice.
- Bunton R, Macdonald G (eds) (2002) Health promotion: disciplines and diversity, 2nd edn. London, Routledge.
  An important book which traces the theoretical roots of health promotion in disciplines such as psychology, sociology, education, politics, genetics and epidemiology.
- Griffiths S, Hunter D J (eds) (1999) Perspectives in public health. Abingdon, Radcliffe Medical Press.
  An edited text that provides an overview of multidisciplinary new public health, encompassing a range of topics and professions and based on diverse theoretical frameworks.
- Scriven A, Orme J (eds) (2001) Health promotion: professional perspectives. Buckingham, Open University.
- Watterson A (ed) (2003) Public health in practice. Basingstoke, Palgrave/Macmillan.
  These two texts examine the public health and health promotion roles of a range of professionals and explore the organizational and policy contexts and disciplinary approaches that influence practice.

REFERENCES

Acheson D (1988) The future of public health in England. London, HMSO

Ajzen I, Fishbein M (1980) Understanding attitudes and predicting social behaviour. Englewood Cliffs, Prentice Hall

Anderson D, Croucher K (1999) Overview of the written evidence received as part of the review of the Public Health Function in Scotland. Edinburgh, Scottish Office

Arnstein S (1969) Eight rungs on the ladder of citizen participation. In: Cahn S E, Passelt B A (eds) Citizen participation: effecting community change. New York, Praeger

Bandura A (1977) Social learning theory. Englewood Cliffs, Prentice Hall

Beattie A (1996) The health promoting school: from idea to action. In: Scriven A, Orme J (eds) Health promotion: professional perspectives. Basingstoke, Macmillan

Beauchamp T L, Childress, J F (1995) Principles of biomedical ethics. Oxford, Oxford University Press

Becker M H (1974) The health belief model and personal behaviour. Thorofare, NJ, Slack

Brown S (2002) Countless opportunities. Health Development Today April/May

Buckland Y (2001) Health promotion – moving beyond leaflets. Pharmaceutical Journal 266(7149): 727

Bunton R, Macdonald G (eds) (2002) Health promotion: disciplines and diversity, 2nd edn. London, Routledge

Caplan R (1993) The importance of social theory for health promotion: from description to reflexivity. Health Promotion International 8(2): 147–157

Committee for the Study of the Future of Public Health (1988) The future of public health. Division of Health Care Services/Institute of Medicine, Washington, National Academy Press

Department of Health (DoH) (1997) The new NHS: modern, dependable. London, The Stationery Office

Department of Health (DoH) (1999a) Saving lives: our healthier nation. London, The Stationery Office

Department of Health (DoH) (1999b) Making a difference: strengthening the nursing, midwifery and health visiting contribution to health and health care. London, DoH

Department of Health (2001a) The report of the Chief Medical Officer's project to strengthen the public health function. London, DoH

Department of Health (2001b) Health Visitor practice development resource pack. London, DoH

Evans D, Head M J, Speller V (1994) Good practice in health promotion: assuring quality in health promotion. London, Health Education Authority

Faculty of Public Health (2001) Good public health practice – general professional expectations of public health physicians and specialists in public health. London, Faculty of Public Health Medicine

Freire P (1972) Pedagogy of the oppressed. Harmondsworth, Penguin

General Social Care Council (2002) Codes of practice for social care workers and employers. London, General Social Care Council

Gott M, O'Brien M (1990) The role of the nurse in health promotion: policies, perspectives and practice. Maidenhead, Department of Health/Open University

Hochbaum G M (1992) The role and uses of theory in health education practice. Health Education Quarterly, 19(3).

Jones I, Walker D (1997) The role of theory in public health. In: Scally G (ed) Progress in public health. London, FT Healthcare

Kemm J, Close A (1995) Health promotion: theory and practice. Basingstoke, Macmillan

Kolb D A (1984) Experiential learning – experience as the source of learning and development. New Jersey, Prentice Hall

Levenson R, Joule N, Russell J (1997) Developing public health in the NHS – the multidisciplinary contribution. London, King's Fund

Lewin (1951) Field theory in social science. London, Harper

McCalister P (2003) The role of primary care in public health: a GP perspective. In: Watterson A (ed) Public health in practice. Basingstoke, Palgrave/Macmillan, pp 132–158

McQueen D V (2000) Perspectives on health promotion: theory, evidence, practice and the emergence of complexity. Health Promotion International 15(2): 95–97

Naidoo J, Wills J (2000) Health promotion: Foundations for practice, 2nd edn. London, Baillière Tindall

Naidoo J, Wills J (eds) (2001) Health studies: an introduction. Basingstoke, Macmillan/Palgrave

New B (1999) Public health and public values, London, King's Fund

Nutbeam D, Harris E (2004) Theory in a nutshell: a guide to health promotion theory. London, McGraw Hill

Prochaska J O, DiClemente C (1984) The transtheoretical approach: crossing traditional foundations of change. Harnewood, Il, Don Jones/Irwin

Rawson D (2002) The growth of health promotion theory and its rational reconstruction: lessons from the philosophy of science. In: Bunton R, Macdonald G (eds) Health promotion: disciplines and diversity, 2nd edn. London, Routledge

Schon D (1983) The reflective practitioner. London, Temple Smith

Seedhouse D (1997) Health promotion: philosophy, prejudice and practice. Chichester, Wiley

Senior R (1997) Organizational change. London, Pitman

Skills for Health (2001) National standards for specialist practice in public health. Bristol, Skills for Health

Thompson N (1995) Theory and practice in health and social welfare. Maidenhead, Open University Press

UKCC (1986) Project 2000: a new preparation for practice. United Kingdom Central Council for Nursing, Midwifery and Health Visiting, London

Webster C, French J (2002) The cycle of conflict. In: Adams L, Amos M, Munro J (eds) Promoting health: politics and practice. London, Sage

WHO (1984) Health promotion: a discussion document on concepts and principles. Geneva, WHO

WHO (1985) Targets for health for all. Copenhagen, World Health Organization

WHO (1986) Ottawa charter for health promotion. Copenhagen, World Health Organization

Wills J, Woodhead D (2004) The glue that binds – articulating values in multidisciplinary public health. Critical Public Health 14(1): 7–15

2

Research for public health and health promotion

OVERVIEW

Research is a link between theory and practice. It should, and does, inform practice but using such knowledge and applying it can be difficult. The greater emphasis on accountability in the NHS has led to calls for practice to become more evidence based and, therefore, for practitioners to develop skills in research. This chapter looks at the nature of the research that informs public health and health promotion. It argues that research for public health and health promotion should provide the tools for tackling the social causes of ill health and disease. This suggests the need for research methods that are participative, involving researchers and researched working together, and which explore lay people's knowledge and understanding of their own health. The chapter concludes by looking at the ways in which practitioners can become researchers themselves as well as active and critical consumers of research.

INTRODUCTION

In Chapter 1 we discussed the importance of practitioners becoming critical and self aware. A reflective practitioner will be looking closely at their professional practice, asking 'what is the best way of doing this?', or 'why do we do it this way?'. It may be that a practitioner acts on the basis of tradition or an intuitive 'knowing in action' which derives from experience (Schon 1983) but a reflective practitioner will wish to inform their decision.

The shift from an occupation to a profession which has taken place in nursing and multidisciplinary public health, is characterized by an increased focus on research as the profession attempts to establish its own body of knowledge. There is considerable pressure for all health and social care practitioners to be research based and be aware of studies relevant to their practice. Practitioners may be aware that research forms the base of their practice but could not pinpoint any specific findings. This may be because practitioners are not aware of the relevant research journals or they may not have access to specialist sources of information or the opportunity to keep up to date with research. The weight of new information, even though it may be more readily available through the internet, means practitioners may suffer from information overload and be unable to sift out the useful and relevant. Other reasons why practitioners do not use research are to do with the skills and confidence of practitioners themselves in assessing the quality and relevance of published papers. They may also be sceptical of the value of research because it is difficult to institute any change in their practice.

Example

The following practitioners, when asked to identify research that had made an impact on them, were all able to cite a particular study:

Paula, a nurse

'Marmot et al's (1991) research into social status, empowerment and health made me realize how important it is for people to feel in control of their lives and exercise autonomy. Instead of going in and telling people what to do, I now make time to find out their priorities and preference, and work together with them to achieve their goals.'

Penny, a health visitor

'Putnam's research (Putnam et al 1993) about social capital was an eye opener for me. The fact that improving community relationships and trust had a direct and positive effect on life expectancy and infant mortality, meant I could justify working with communities and this could become a legitimate part of my work.'

Peter, a health promotion specialist

'I remember reading the official mortality and morbidity statistics about continuing social class inequalities (Drever & Whitehead 1997), and how this was linked to social class differences in smoking and diet. It made me think twice about the need to target and prioritize messages about healthy lifestyles, and also consider how to promote healthier lifestyles to people whose living conditions make it difficult for them to change.'

Pat, a teacher and counsellor

'Research – I think it was Walker (1997) – into how young people learn about sex from talking to each other was important to me. Apart from it ringing true – after all, that's how I learnt about sex when I was a teenager – it made me think about developing peer education programmes about personal relationships, instead of giving the usual "I'm the expert, here's the information" talk about sex and personal relationships.'

Few practitioners see research as an integral component of their practice. It is seen as 'out there', separate from the knowledge base that informs practice, which is often received wisdom passed on from practitioner to student.

A practitioner may, however, have a whole host of questions relating to their practice. The Macmillan nurse may want to know why women choose not to come for mammography screening. The health promotion specialist may want to know whether a safety education programme for young children has made any difference to the accident rate. A midwife might want to find out the needs of prospective fathers from the antenatal services. If we see research as providing the information on which to plan and carry out interventions, then research ceases to be seen as a remote activity but becomes an extension of everyday work.

This chapter aims to help you reflect on what distinguishes research in public health and health promotion. It looks at the social context in which research for public health and health promotion takes place and the kind of information that informs practice. It is not a tool kit to make you a better researcher. Some excellent texts are recommended at the end of the chapter which can provide guided tours of research methods and the fine-tuning in using particular methods. Above all, being a researcher involves doing research and 'getting your hands dirty'; it cannot be learnt from a book.

WHAT IS RESEARCH?

Health improvement is based on theories about what influences people's health and what then constitutes an effective intervention or strategy to improve health. Such theories are based on research. The term 'research' may be used to describe any systematic information-gathering activity which is used to describe, explain or explore an issue in order to generate new knowledge.

Research is:

- the investigation of the real world
- informed by values about the issue under investigation
- follows agreed practices and ethical guidelines
- is guided by theory and assumptions about the presumed relations between different phenomena
- asks meaningful questions
- is systematic and rigorous.

There are several ways in which research informs public health and health promotion and contributes to its development. It may help, for example, to determine priorities for action from a seemingly endless list of possibilities. Epidemiological research or a needs assessment exercise may be the starting point for deciding which issues should be tackled. Evaluative research may determine the effectiveness or acceptability of particular interventions. A research audit may examine which resources and systems are in place for the purpose of improving the performance of an organization or project. Research can also support, challenge or generate new theory. The studies cited by the practitioners in the Example above are all examples of research which contributes to the body of knowledge informing public health and health promotion.

Research has achieved a much higher profile in health organizations in recent years. Policy and service provision is expected to be based on research and practitioners are being exhorted to base their practice on evidence derived from rigorous research. Professional judgement and the preferences of users and clients may also influence decision making but the cultural shift to evidence-based health care that is explored further in Chapter 3 represents a major challenge for practitioners. A large body of research for public health and health promotion derives from public health medicine and epidemiology. Epidemiology has been described as 'completing the clinical picture' (Last 1994, p. 119). It is concerned with the pattern of diseases in a population. By discovering those groups with high rates of disease and those with low rates it is possible to identify the distinctive features of each group in terms of their environment or lifestyle and which might be associated with their likelihood of disease.

Discussion point

What do you think distinguishes research from everyday finding out about things that interest you?

Example

Methods used by
epidemiologists

1. Cross-sectional studies to determine prevalence or patterns of conditions or behaviours in populations or groups at one point in time – e.g. *Health Survey for England: the Health of Minority Ethnic Groups* (Erens et al 2001) interviewed minority ethnic groups about a range of health issues (alcohol, smoking, physical activity, diet, use of health services, self-reported health status) and took objective health measurements such as blood samples to compare with the general population.
2. Case-control studies to investigate the causes of a condition by comparing a group with the condition with a control group – e.g. an investigation into exposure to radon in Cornwall (Darby et al 1998).
3. Cohort or longitudinal studies to observe a group over time to see if there is any association between particular behaviours or characteristics and patterns of disease – e.g. the Whitehall 2 study of 10 000 civil servants looks at different employment grades and their incidence of ill health (Brunner 1996).
4. Randomized control trial which compares a group which experiences an intervention with a similar control group which does not – e.g. Stanford Heart Disease Prevention Programme 1972–80 looked at the risk factors for coronary heart disease among three communities in the USA. One community received intensive health education through the mass media and one-to-one advice; one community received a mass media campaign; the third control group received no intervention (Maccoby et al 1977).

The investigation of health problems in populations has been a key function for public health. Epidemiology is a population science basic to public health medicine. Its techniques in examining the patterns of disease problems within and between populations and in looking for the causes of disease have been widely applied. For example, the Whitehall study has, since its inception in 1978, reminded practitioners of the influence of social factors as risk factors for coronary heart disease (Brunner 1996). The Nurses Health Study (Grodstein et al 1996) is a large cohort study that began in 1976 and has monitored the mortality and morbidity of over 120 000 female nurses aged 30–55. This study found a marked decrease in coronary heart disease among women who took hormone therapy.

Example

The uses of
epidemiology

- **To observe the effects of social factors on health** – e.g. linking the rise in the number of cars on the road with the incidence of asthma.
- **To provide a 'map' of the distribution and size of health problems in the population** – e.g. infant mortality being distributed unequally among social classes.
- **To estimate the risks to an individual of suffering disease** – e.g. the risks of a woman becoming infected with HIV from having unprotected sex with a male partner who is HIV-positive.
- **To assess the operation of services and the extent to which they meet the population's needs** – e.g. the take-up rate for the breast cancer screening programme and the effect on breast cancer incidence and outcomes.

Source: adapted from Ashton (1994)

Epidemiology is thus undoubtedly useful. But it should not be thought of as providing the only information required. Its findings, as with all research, need to be interpreted within the specific theoretical framework in which it is grounded. The particular use of theory will depend on the paradigm or school of thought in which the researcher is working. When we look at the different methodologies used in research we are also looking at different disciplines – either an attempt to explain phenomena following the procedures of natural science or an attempt to understand the world from the point of view of the people in it. Epidemiology reflects the dominance of the medical science paradigm. This approach seeks to identify the risk factors of disease and is informed by a belief that research needs to be objective and scientific.

POSITIVIST AND INTERPRETIVE PARADIGMS

Knowledge is determined by the context in which a question is framed and the methods used to obtain data, analyse and interpret it. The same topic can thus be investigated from different angles. The dominant research tradition in health and social care derives from a positivist approach which uses the methods and principles of the natural sciences. It claims that there are phenomena or 'facts' which are real and can be studied. However, this claim for objective neutrality has been questioned – all knowledge production is influenced by values, ideologies and funders' agendas.

In apparent contrast, the interpretive tradition aims to explore and describe the meaning of phenomena as experienced and perceived by the individual. The tradition derives from the concern of social sciences to understand the subjective meaning of human experience.

Positivism is associated with quantitative research methods – the gathering of 'hard' data which can be quantified in some way. Quantitative research attempts to measure aspects of a situation and to explain any differences in these variables between groups or over time. Quantitative research tests a hypothesis which is a suggested explanation of why differences occur. The experiment is the main method. In experimental studies one aspect in two matched groups is varied to see if it makes any difference to the result. Any difference can then be attributed to that variable. Controlled trials in which participants are randomly allocated to the control or experimental group are used to assess the effectiveness of interventions. In research involving people and their lives, it is impossible to control for all the factors which may influence outcomes. There may also be ethical concerns about withholding a potentially beneficial intervention from one group of participants. There is further discussion about the role of randomized controlled trials and their contribution to understanding the effectiveness of interventions in Chapter 3.

Example

A randomized controlled trial of methods to promote physical activity in primary care

The Newcastle Exercise project recruited 523 adult participants aged 40–60 and of similar demographic and behavioural backgrounds from general practice lists. They were randomized to 4 intervention groups or control comprising:

1. Brief motivational interviewing
2. Intensive motivational interviewing
3. Brief motivational interviewing plus financial incentive (vouchers to an exercise facility)
4. Intensive motivational interviewing plus financial incentive.

At 12 weeks all 4 groups had improved physical activity levels compared to the control group. The highest proportion of participants with improved levels was group 3. At one year, the increases in physical activity had not been maintained regardless of the intensity of the intervention.

Source: Harland et al (1999)

The interpretive tradition is associated with qualitative research methods which are more about 'coming to know' the ways in which an issue is perceived by the people whom it affects. Thoughts, feelings and meanings are real phenomena which can be studied by the researcher. Through methods such as interviews, observation and case studies the researcher can come to understand the perspective of the participants. In contrast to quantitative methods, there is no assumption about what are the important issues which are then confirmed or disproved. Instead qualitative methods are inductive. Plausible explanations for people's views and experiences are induced from the mass of data these methods can generate. This approach has also been called 'grounded theory' (Glaser & Strauss 1986) because the theory is grounded in and emerges from real life experience.

If we use the example of research into sexual health we can see how different paradigms or schools of thought determine what is to be studied. Most research into the spread of HIV/AIDS has been concerned with discovering the incidence, prevalence and distribution of HIV in the population over time. By comparing the proportion of infected people engaging in different risk activities, attempts are made to correlate risk of infection with behaviour. This knowledge can be used in the targeting and design of health education messages. Epidemiologists can also evaluate the effectiveness of health promotion activities by charting rates of HIV infection against interventions.

Gary Dowsett, who designed research programmes for the WHO Global Programme on AIDS, commented on the need for more close-focus research which looks at contexts and social situations in which people make sexual decisions:

Discussion point

What contribution do you think qualitative research could make to HIV prevention?

> Utilizing precious research resources to maximize the measurement of HIV infection and AIDS in any one country will not greatly enhance the prevention and care/support response. A less exact and more general idea of HIV/AIDS prevalence/incidence will, when coupled with well-theorized understanding of sexual and drug use cultures or contexts, offer far more useful starting points for action than all the surveillance data in the world.

(Dowsett 1995, p. 28)

Quantitative and qualitative research derive from different epistemological perspectives or views about the nature of knowledge and so are often presented as diametrically opposed. Table 2.1 summarizes the two philosophically divergent positions.

Table 2.1 Quantitative and qualitative research

	Quantitative	Qualitative
Paradigm	Positivism	Interpretive/naturalistic
Epistemological base	Science	Humanities
	Knowledge is part of an objective reality separate from individuals	Knowledge is based on how individuals perceive experiences through 'individual lenses'
Researcher's role	Objectivity and detachment	Subjectivity and engagement
Aim	To progress towards the truth and verify knowledge	To understand multiple realities
Purpose	To understand causality	To interpret and reveal complexity
Methodology	To isolate and study discrete variables e.g. experimental study	To understand the issue in context e.g. ethnography, phenomenology
Methods	Less detailed information from larger number of participants e.g. questionnaire	More detailed information from smaller number of participants
	To measure size of an effect	To measure why effects occurred
	Uses standardized measuring instruments	Uses a variety of methods e.g. interviewing, focus groups to find out participants' reality, concepts and meanings
Values	Validity, reliability	Validity, trustworthiness, credibility, confirmability, transparency
Presentation	Analysis of numbers and systematic quantification and analysis	Analysis of words and meanings e.g. thematic content analysis, discourse analysis
Contribution to theory	Falsification (to disprove hypothesis) and test theory	To build theory e.g. grounded theory emerges from the data
	Deductive	Inductive
	Generalization	Understanding complexity

In recent years this apparent divide between these research traditions has been disputed. As Watterson & Watterson (2003, p. 26) point out, 'Public health methods are essentially eclectic'. Most health issues are so complex that different methods are suitable for different tasks and one method may illuminate or inform another.

Those using quantitative methods are often advised that good practice is to inform their study with exploratory qualitative research. Different methods can, in addition, tap multiple realities and thus arrive at more valid findings. Triangulation refers to the use of multiple methods as a means of increasing validity. 'Triangulation in surveying is a method of finding out where something is by getting a fix from two or more places. Analogously, Denzin (1988) suggested that this might be done in social research by using multiple methods, investigators or theories' (Robson 2002, p. 290).

Despite such arguments about interdependence, we claim that there remains an epistemological divide. Qualitative research is often seen as subjective and lacking rigour because the researcher does not just observe but is directly involved with the subjects of the study. Bias can be minimized by acknowledging the researcher's perspective and being open about all aspects of the process (transparency). Findings are not seen to be generalizable as samples are usually too small and unrepresentative to be statistically significant. Yet enough should be known about the sample being studied to be able to judge the extent to which the findings are applicable elsewhere (transferability). Because qualitative research does not require any particular statistical expertise, it is often assumed that anyone with a modicum of interpersonal skills can do it. Qualitative research is no less rigorous than quantitative research and needs to meet additional criteria to ensure it is of high quality.

WHAT COUNTS AS RESEARCH?

Discussion point

Why do a high proportion of women stop breastfeeding within two weeks of their return home after delivery?

Consider the following two research studies and decide which of the two studies is more likely to get research funding and why.

Which of the two studies is more likely to get published in a nursing, midwifery or medical journal?

Study 1

A cohort study to compare breastfeeding rates at two and four months after delivery in women discharged 48 hours after delivery and women discharged more than 72 hours after delivery. Using a statistical package, the effect of support on the maternity ward by length of time breastfeeding, was analysed.

Study 2

An ethnographic study using participant observation in which the midwife's interaction with breastfeeding mothers was observed and their conversations with them about breastfeeding were noted in field notes. Mothers' perceptions of the support received were collected by phone interview at two and six weeks.

Although this is a very simple example, you probably concluded immediately that the first study would be more likely to get funding and to be published. Researchers seeking funding often find that there is a methodological status hierarchy whereby qualitative research is deemed less legitimate than quantitative biomedical or epidemiological research (Pope & Mays 1993). When seeking to get work published, the format many journals require – of hypothesis or question, method, results and discussion – reflects the type of research which will be deemed acceptable.

In recent years there has been a significant emphasis on monitoring and evaluation. This concern with outcome measures and quantitative data is at odds with the focus of health promotion on subjective health (Macdonald & Davies 1998). The shift towards consumerism and accountability in the NHS has served to increase interest in qualitative research which gives people a voice. Nevertheless quantitative research still enjoys a higher status and credibility than the qualitative work that informs much health promotion. Most Research and Development strategies do not explicitly include health promotion as a category and health promotion is interpreted within the dominant preventive medical framework; in other words, epidemiological studies of particular diseases, studies on individual lifestyle determinants or the prevention of specific conditions through screening, surveillance or immunization. In line with the agenda of evidence-based practice, the criteria for research projects in the NHS do not cater for exploratory projects but focus on reviewing effectiveness. The tradition of high status quantitative research presents a dilemma for practitioners who are caught between emulating quantitative research or promoting qualitative research with all the problems of credibility and authority this entails.

The definition of the issue to be studied, the research design, the methods used to carry out the research, the interpretation of the results and the dissemination of findings all reflect the way in which health improvement is perceived. So when we think about research for health improvement we need to think about what sort of information we need and what paradigm we are working in.

RESEARCH FOR HEALTH IMPROVEMENT

Scott-Samuel (1989) has argued that what health promotion requires is a social epidemiology which is:

- subjective
- collective
- participative and non-expertist.

The principles of the World Health Organization Health For All strategy (WHO 1985) acknowledge that health is a relative concept to which people attach different meanings. Lay views of health and illness must be taken into account when trying to promote health. The WHO defines health promotion as enabling people to increase control over their health and the factors influencing their health. This demands research which enables the subjects of any study to be active participants in it and for the research to achieve change for that community.

Reflection point

Can you think of an example of research relating to issues of interest or significance to a particular group which has not been taken up or funded?

Lay knowledge

Epidemiology, upon which public health knowledge has depended, rests upon the concept of disease. It tends to focus on the causes and risks of dying or becoming ill. What is lacking is an understanding of the subjective experience of health and illness. Medicine depends on the ability to diagnose – that there is some sign and indication of pathology which takes precedence over the individual experience of ill health or disease. Yet the current commitment of the NHS to identifying population and community needs demands a form of inquiry which describes health as ordinary people perceive it. The WHO recognized this many years ago when they stated that 'more emphasis should be laid on qualitative methods of observation, namely, those that allow lay people to define a problem and its solution from their own viewpoint' (WHO 1986, p. 121). Research that provided more insight into meanings and socio-cultural contexts might help illuminate the conundrum for health promotion about the lack of relationship between people's knowledge, attitudes and behaviour.

Research has shown that people have their own lay epidemiology and understanding of the causes of ill health which is influenced by:

- beliefs about 'candidacy' (the image of the kind of person who suffers from, for example, heart disease)
- beliefs about luck and fate in relation to illness
- how social networks develop and affirm ideas about 'candidacy'
- beliefs about the life cycle and personal assessments of what it means to be healthy at different ages.

The ways in which researchers find out about people's ways of seeing and talking about illness vary from the large-scale survey (Blaxter 1990) to studies from an ethnographic or biographical perspective. Cornwell's (1984) ground-breaking case study of a group of families in the East End of London gives not only a fascinating insight into the ideas and concepts about health, illness and health services but also shows how health is integral to people's lives. Cornwell states that her study 'has more in common with social anthropology than with other disciplines in the social sciences, in so far as the emphasis in social anthropology is all the time on the whole and on the links between apparently discrete areas of social life' (Cornwell 1984, p. 1).

Hilary Graham's studies of the lives of working-class women uses data from open-ended accounts recorded by researchers and the personal views of women recorded in letters, diaries and pictures. This commentary on how women represent themselves and make sense of their lives is presented in contrast to official and survey data which tends to 'exclude and misrepresent those most affected by disadvantage and discrimination' (Graham 1993, p. 34). Williams & Popay (1994, p. 122) suggest that lay knowledge represents a challenge to medicine 'because it means taking subjectivity seriously rather than seeing it as an impediment to understanding'. One of the claims of scientific knowledge is that it is objective and impartial. Lay knowledge represents another way of knowing. Although unrepresentative in a statistical sense, studies of lay beliefs do

Discussion point

Take a health issue with which you are familiar. How might lay concepts of health and illness help to develop culturally appropriate practice around this issue?

draw upon ideas that are general and shared. They thus present other discourses which need to be acknowledged and which compete with and contest the truth-claims of scientific knowledge.

Williams & Popay also see lay knowledge as representing a political challenge to the power of experts to determine the way in which issues for policy are defined. Increasingly, organizations providing services are recognizing their responsibility to involve the people who use them (see Ch. 6). In the case of young people, it is now recognized that only by listening to their views about their own health and what they see influencing it can appropriate strategies be developed. Harden & Oliver (2001, p. 132) show how issues can be seen very differently when the adult or professional agenda is not prioritized; 'The problem of young carers has attracted the attention of the authorities who have considered it in terms of interference with young people's school work and social life. Seen from the families' point of view, however, the primary problem is lack of support for the sick and disabled parent.'

One of the challenges facing public health and health promotion research is to discover what people mean by health or well-being. Most attempts to tap into this area have focused on defining indicators of well-being, the best known being the Nottingham Health Profile. The questions used to form the basis of this assessment are, however, generally couched in negative terms focusing on the absence of symptoms, e.g. 'Have you felt tired this week?' Antonovsky (1993) has highlighted some of the limitations of the 'pathogenic' paradigm which looks for the causes of disease. He argues that the focus on eliminating disease has led to the identification of risk groups and ignored those aspects which enable some people to cope with disease. Antonovsky calls instead for a 'salutogenic' model of health which would seek to identify 'symptoms of wellness', helping us to understand why some people cope and others do not, why some consider themselves to be healthy in spite of chronic illness and indeed why some who are disadvantaged do very well.

Participative research

One of the core principles of health promotion, according to the World Health Organization (WHO 1986), is that people have a right and duty to participate in the planning of their health care. If research forms the basis for this, then people also have a right to be active and equal participants in that research process and its dissemination. Research from whatever paradigm is often seen as 'expert' knowledge. It is often produced by and for other experts and can be intimidating and inaccessible to the lay person.

Research typically involves an expert researcher and passive subjects. Empowering research attempts to shift the balance of power by acknowledging and valuing the participants in such a way that they are actively involved rather than 'subjects'. This can easily become a principle to be espoused through the use of ethical principles of procedure or non-directive, qualitative methods. There is a growing recognition that members of the public could and should be involved in health research; in helping to set the research agenda, helping to get research funded, designing and conducting the research perhaps by formulating questions, designing

---

D iscussion point

How would using a 'salutogenic' model of health affect the kind of research carried out around specific issues, e.g. smoking or population groups such as older people?

questionnaires or conducting interviews. The level of involvement of lay people may vary from acceptance of researchers' proposals to a situation where lay people generate knowledge of the problem through their own methods of observation (Baxter et al 2001, see www.conres.co.uk)

Example	In the late 1980s 334 women attending the Bristol Cancer Help Centre took part in a clinical trial comparing their treatment which combined complementary therapies and traditional chemotherapy and radiography with the conventional treatment of women at the Royal Marsden Hospital and two district general hospitals. All the women were aged less than 70 and had a single invasive primary cancer of the breast. The study appeared to show that women with breast cancer in the control group who were free of metastases at the time of the study were nearly three times as likely to survive as women in the Bristol group; in other words women would be better off receiving conventional treatment. Almost inevitably a study which produced such clear findings on an issue of great concern meant that the research design was heavily scrutinized and called into question (Bagenal et al 1990).
Bristol Cancer Help Centre	

The Bristol trial is cited as an example of research in which the participants had no control and the women ended up publically objecting to its design and findings. They felt that it supported a dominant medical agenda and reflected the scepticism with which complementary therapies are viewed. The women at Bristol Cancer Help Centre felt strongly that a clinical trial was inappropriate to evaluate its work and that their health experience was not taken into account.

Williams & Popay (1994) have shown how research can be used by communities in this way to attract attention to a health issue of concern. They describe the way in which the people of Camelford in Cornwall systematically gathered evidence of the effects on health from their contaminated water supply. Their experience is an illustration of the way in which vested interests can control research findings and how this can be challenged by people becoming active researchers themselves.

Example	In 1988 a lorry accidentally tipped 20 tonnes of aluminium sulfate into the treated water supply of the people of Camelford in North Cornwall. Local people organized themselves and carefully monitored the health effects of the incident. Their evidence was presented to an independent expert group set up by the Department of Health. The Clayton Committee refuted the local evidence claiming that it had not been collected in a systematic manner and was not representative of the whole population. The report concluded that 'in our view it is not possible to attribute the very real current health complaints to the toxic effects of the incident inasmuch as they are the consequence of the sustained anxiety naturally felt by many people'.
Camelford and 'lay epidemiology'	

Although the people of Camelford knew they were experiencing ill health, their evidence was put down to hysteria fanned by the media. It was not given credence when compared to the technical, toxicological and clinical measurements of a panel of scientific experts (Williams & Popay 1994).

Example

Participatory
appraisal

Participatory appraisal (PA) is a way of engaging lay people in identifying issues and problems to investigate (see Ch. 6). It is a quick method of appraising community needs using local knowledge and uses a wide variety of tools that do not rely on literacy skills. Residents and workers in a foyer for young homeless in East London were trained in PA methods to investigate the health needs of young people and what needed changing about the foyer service. The researchers found the techniques which included visualization, spider diagrams and ranking exercises, allowed young people who would not normally come forward to have a voice. The residents were helped to think through problems and solutions to their anxieties over safety and experiences of isolation.

Source: Fildes et al (2001)

Participative research involves working in partnership with the subjects of the research. Research should be seen as an exchange – those who take part should get something from the exchange. Involving participants in the research design and planning can involve complex negotiations and slow down the progress of a project. It may be difficult to get people interested and approaches may need to be made through voluntary organizations or user groups. Groups of people, such as older people, may be targeted using agency records. Some people may be identified because they are key informants or through a snowballing process whereby participants are identified by other recruits. Giving control over the findings can be similarly time-consuming and dispiriting if it is perceived that the research is not of direct benefit.

Discussion point

Should 'consumers' be paid to take part in research? If so how much?

Social research

Social research is the term used here to describe research which seeks to explore the context in which health decisions are made and the mechanisms which link socio-economic status to health.

For the 18 years of Conservative administration, the Department of Health acknowledged that there are significant social variations in health but refused to acknowledge the relationship between income and health. The focus of research was into sociobehavioural factors and studies of the factors influencing access to and uptake of health and social care (DoH 1995). A review of the evidence linking inequalities with health was one of the first tasks of the Labour government in 1997, culminating in the Acheson Report (1998).

As the official neglect of health inequalities research under the Conservative government shows, research is a powerful tool which takes place in a political context. The political acceptability of research findings is often more important than its quality in determining the profile and level of publicity of research. Despite the UK Labour government's commitment to addressing health inequalities it has emphasized the importance of wealth creation rather than distribution and has refused to give any commitment to income redistribution. The evidence and arguments put forward by Wilkinson (1996, 1997) about relative inequality and its impact on health are acknowledged in the White Paper *Saving Lives: Our Healthier Nation* (DoH 1999) but appear to have had little impact – as Moran & Simpkin (2000, p. 103) remark 'a sharp reminder of the limitations of joined up government when health priorities conflict with others'.

The health impact of housing, and in particular the link between damp housing and respiratory disease, had been largely ignored until a study by Hunt and others in 1986. Hunt suggests that there were two reasons for this:

- The unfashionable nature of the topic and its potentially political implications
- The way in which the topic was fragmented among different professional groups (allergies from mould being the province of doctors, Environmental Health being concerned with dampness, the identification of mould being done by building surveyors).

The ill health of people living in damp housing was thus seen as the consequence of poverty and individual behaviour such as smoking and boiling nappies and potatoes rather than as a consequence of mould in the air and on the walls which Hunt's study confirmed as a major cause of ill health.

Source: Hunt (1993).

The practitioner–researcher

The utilization of research depends on effective dissemination. Practitioners have access to a large volume of research, evidence and guidance through electronic databases, evidence syntheses and journals. Unless the recommendations arising from these studies are incorporated into practice then such research initiatives are wasted. Practitioners need to become critical consumers of research, knowing the research in their area and being able to evaluate it with confidence (see Ch. 3 on evidence-based practice). Merely knowing about research findings is rarely, however, sufficient to change practice. The diffusion and adoption of innovation takes years not months. Often it requires practitioners to change long-held patterns of behaviour – at what point should research be used to justify a change in practice?

Examples from midwifery and health visiting might include the change in advice to parents about the sleeping position of babies who should not be laid down on their fronts; or the abandonment of enemas and pubic shaving during delivery; or the introduction of postnatal support.

Research can challenge taken for granted assumptions and therefore being research-minded is a crucial part of reflective practice. But it is also important to be critical: how does one decide which evidence is sufficiently convincing to influence practice? Because this is difficult, and because knowledge is never a given but is always changing, practitioners often resort to their 'knowing-in-action' and ignore new findings. There may also be a delay in the diffusion and adoption of interventions because they are not widely known. The publication of effectiveness reviews and meta-analyses (see Ch. 3) may help to diffuse knowledge but they need to be more user-friendly and adopt wider criteria than the randomized controlled trial as the 'gold standard' if they are to help practitioners directly.

Most training courses for health and social care practitioners now include research awareness and skills and alert students to ways in which research studies can lack rigour. Common problems include making claims that are not substantiated by the data, or claiming findings from exploratory studies can be generalized, or providing selective data to support a particular point of view. It is also important to be able to identify when research has been conducted rigorously. For quantitative research, rigour is achieved through representative samples which ensures that findings can be generalized. Statistical manipulation of the data must be appropriate for the kind and quality of data obtained. For qualitative research, rigour is achieved through being systematic and open in the methods used and applying critical reflection to the research process. Rigorous qualitative research achieves relatability; or the discovery of insights which can be used in similar situations.

In the following chapter we look at the very strict criteria which are used to classify studies of effective public health and health promotion interventions. For practitioners, reading about research is a key component of developing research expertise both substantively and practically. Making a reasoned judgement about the value of a research study takes skill and practice but analysing strengths and weaknesses in the work of others helps practitioners in the design of their own studies.

Published papers are usually refereed by external reviewers in the field but this does not guarantee that the research is trustworthy. There is also a mass of needs assessment and evaluation studies which practitioners carry out routinely but which are not published and so remain invisible. It is important that practitioners do share their findings and experiences by bringing them into the public domain through reports, articles and conference papers. In this way the body of knowledge and theory about the relatively new field of health improvement can be developed.

A practitioner–researcher is someone who, in addition to their work, carries out systematic enquiry relevant to their work. Apart from the few posts which are designated as having these joint roles, for the majority, doing research is an additional responsibility. Practitioners, with their knowledge, contacts and position within an organization are in a valuable position to carry out research, but carrying out research as a practitioner does have particular difficulties (NHS Centre for Reviews and Dissemination 1999):

- lack of time
- lack of funding
- lack of expertise in research design and methods
- lack of confidence
- lack of credibility within the organization that small-scale research could offer anything more than existing knowledge
- research not being perceived as relevant or a priority for the setting in which it would take place
- the need to negotiate with other staff or clients
- ethical considerations about the ways in which research can impact on those involved.

As well as being a critical consumer of research, there is an increasing emphasis on practitioners being accountable for their practice and therefore engaging in reviews of its effectiveness. They are called upon to demonstrate the health gain from any intervention and to base decision making on research.

CONCLUSION

Public health and health promotion have inherited a positivist tradition which has tended to mystify research and made it seem remote and difficult. Practitioners view research as a separate activity which they tend not to get involved with or use as a tool to improve practice. Yet the principles of research are ones that all practitioners can use – being aware of the way in which an issue is being defined and the philosophical principles which underpin the approach to its study, the need to reflect on theory and the ability to scrutinize and analyse available information. This practice of enquiry is an addition to the kind of knowing that an experienced practitioner already has and it is a 'means of organizing common sense and intuitive problem-solving so as to guard against some of their shortcomings' (Robson 1993, p. 461).

In addition to the argument that research is a tool for practice there is also the view that research activity should promote the values and principles of public health and health promotion. Hence the calls for research to go beyond the scientific paradigm and embrace participative research directed towards the social determinants of health and qualitative research which seeks to understand people's health experience.

FURTHER DISCUSSION

- To what extent can public health and health promotion research be translated into action and policy?
- What importance do you give to research in your work? Should your practice be more research linked? If so, how could you do this?

Recommended reading

- Bowling A (2002) Research methods in health: investigating health and health services, 2nd edn. Maidenhead, Open University.
  A comprehensive introduction to research methods.
- McConway, K (ed) (1994) Studying health and disease. Maidenhead, Open University Press.
- Unwin N, Carr S, Leeson J with Pless-Mulloli T (1996) Public health and epidemiology. Buckingham, Open University Press.
  Two textbooks which provide an introduction to the kinds of health data that are collected and how they might be analysed.
- Popay J, Williams G (eds) (1994) Researching the people's health. London, Routledge.
  An interesting collection of contributions from social researchers which looks at the relationship between lay knowledge and expert knowledge.

REFERENCES

Acheson D (1998) Independent inquiry into inequalities in health. London, The Stationery Office

Antonovsky A (1993) The sense of coherence as a determinant of health. In: Beattie A, Gott M,

Jones L, Sidell M (eds) Health and wellbeing: a reader. Basingstoke, MacMillan/Open University

Ashton J (ed) (1994) The epidemiological imagination. Buckingham, Open University Press

Bagenal F S, Easton D F, Harris E, Chilvers C E D, McElwain T J (1990) Survival of patients with breast cancer attending Bristol Cancer Help Centre. Lancet 336: 606–610

Baxter L, Thorne L, Mitchell A (2001) Small voices, big noises. Exeter, Washington Singer

Blaxter M (1990) Health and lifestyles. London, Tavistock

Brunner E (1996) The social and biological basis of cardiovascular disease in office workers. In: Blane D, Brunner E, Wilkinson R (eds) Health and social organization: towards a health policy for the 21st century. London, Routledge

Cornwell J (1984) Hard earned lives: accounts of health and illness from East London. London, Tavistock

Darby S, Whitley E, Silcocks P et al (1998) Risk of lung cancer associated with residential radon exposure in south-west England: a case control study. British Journal of Cancer 78(3): 394–408

Denzin N (1988) The research act: a theoretical introduction to sociological methods, 3rd edn. New Jersey, Prentice Hall

Department of Health (DoH) (1995) Variations in health: what can the Department of Health and the NHS do? London, HMSO

Department of Health (DoH) (1999) Saving lives: our healthier nation. London, The Stationery Office

Dowsett G (1995) Focus on HIV/AIDS research. Healthlines 28, December

Drever F, Whitehead M (eds) (1997) Health inequalities. London, The Stationery Office

Erens B, Primatesta P, Prior G (2001) Health survey for England: the health of minority ethnic groups 1999, Vol. I Findings, Vol. 2 Methodology and Documentation. London, National Centre for Social Research, Department of Epidemiology and Public Health at the Royal Free and University College Medical School/The Stationery Office

Fildes J, Smith P, White L, Lorentzon M, Wills J (2001) Health needs assessment of residents living in and using a foyer. London, King's Fund

Glaser B, Strauss A (1986) The discovery of grounded theory: strategies for qualitative research. Chicago, Aldine

Graham H (1993) Hardship and health in women's lives. Hemel Hempstead, Harvester Wheatsheaf

Grodstein F, Stampfer M, Manson J, Colditz G, Willett W, Tosner B, Speizer F, Henekens D (1996) Postmenopausal estrogen and progestin use and the risk of cardiovascular disease. New England Journal of Medicine 335: 453–461

Harden A and Oliver S (2001) Who's listening? Systematically reviewing for ethics and empowerment. In: Oliver S, Peersman G (eds) Using research for effective health promotion. Maidenhead, Open University Press

Harland J, White M, Drinkwater C, Chinn D, Garr L, Howel D (1999) A randomized controlled trial to promote physical activity in primary care. British Medical Journal 319: 828–832

Hunt S M (1993) The relationship between research and policy: translating knowledge into action. In: Davies J K, Kelly M (eds) Healthy cities: research and practice. London, Routledge

Last J (1994) The uses of epidemiology. In: Ashton J (ed) The epidemiological imagination. Maidenhead, Open University Press

Maccoby N, Farquhar J W, Wood P D et al (1977) Reducing the risk of cardiovascular disease: effects of a community based campaign on knowledge and behavior. Journal of Community Health 3, 100–114

Macdonald G, Davies J K (1998) Reflection and vision: proving and improving the promotion of health. In: Macdonald G, Davies J K (eds) Quality, evidence and effectiveness in health promotion. London, Routledge

Marmot M G, Davey Smith G, Stansfield S A et al (1991) Health inequalities among British civil servants: the Whitehall 2 study. Lancet 337: 1387–1393.

Moran G, Simpkin M (2000) Social exclusion and health. In: Percy-Smith J (ed) Policy responses to social exclusion: towards inclusion. Maidenhead Open University Press

NHS Centre for Reviews and Dissemination (1999) Getting evidence into practice. Effective Health Care 5(1)

Pope C, Mays N (1993) Opening the black box: an encounter in the corridors of health services research. British Medical Journal 306: 315–318

Putnam R D, Leonardi R, Nanetti R Y (1993) Making democracy work: civic traditions in modern Italy. Princeton, NJ, Princeton University Press

Robson C (2002) Real world research: a resource for social scientists and practitioner–researchers, 2nd edn. Oxford, Blackwell

Schon D (1983) The reflective practitioner. London, Temple Smith

Scott-Samuel A (1989) Building the new public health: a public health alliance and a new social epidemiology. In: Martin C J, McQueen D V (eds) Readings for a new public health. Edinburgh, Edinburgh University Press

Walker B M (1997) You learn it from your mates, don't you? Youth and Policy 57: 44–54

Watterson A, Watterson J (2003) Public health research tools. In: Watterson A (ed) Public health in practice. Basingstoke, Palgrave, pp 24–51

World Health Organization (WHO) (1985) Health for all in Europe by the year 2000. Copenhagen, WHO

World Health Organization (WHO) (1986) Lifestyles and health. Social Science 22: 117–124

Wilkinson R (1996) Unhealthy societies: the affliction of inequality. London, Routledge

Wilkinson R (1997) Health inequalities: relative or absolute material standards. British Medical Journal 314, 591–595

Williams G, Popay J (1994) Lay knowledge and the privilege of experience. In: Gabe J, Kelleher D, Williams G (eds) Challenging medicine. London, Routledge

3 Evidence-based practice

Key Points

- Defining evidence-based practice in public health and health promotion
- What constitutes evidence
- Skills for evidence-based practice
  - finding the evidence
  - appraising the evidence
  - synthesizing the evidence
  - applying the evidence to practice
- Limitations to evidence-based practice
- Using evidence-based practice to determine cost effectiveness
- Developing an evidence-based culture in public health and health promotion
- Putting evidence into practice
- Dilemmas about becoming an evidence-based practitioner

OVERVIEW

Evidence-based practice and policy have become the new mantra in health care. Yet there is no clear consensus about what defines evidence, or how it should be used to drive changes in practice or policy. The traditional 'hierarchy of evidence' has very clear limitations when used to evaluate practice in areas such as policy change, community development or individual empowerment. This chapter outlines current thinking about evidence, the reasons for pursuing evidence-based practice and policy, and the skills practitioners need to acquire in order to become evidence based. Evidence-based policy and practice are similar in many ways. Both are activities which take place in a complex context where other factors, such as custom, acceptability or ideology, may be more important than evidence in determining outcomes. This chapter focuses on evidence-based practice and the challenges this poses for practitioners. Many of the issues relating to evidence-based policy are discussed in Chapter 4 on policy. Specific dilemmas which arise when applying evidence-based practice to broad public health and health promotion goals are identified and discussed. This chapter concludes that evidence-based practice in health promotion and public health needs to go beyond the scientific medical model of evidence to include qualitative methodologies, process evaluation, and practitioners' and users' views. Evidence-based practice is a useful tool in the public health and health promotion kitbag, but it is not the only or overriding criterion of what is effective, ethical and sound good practice.

INTRODUCTION

Reflection point

Think of an area of your practice where you have changed what you do. Has this change been brought about by:
- policy and/or management imperatives
- colleagues' advice
- technological advances
- cost
- evidence-based practice recommendations
- your own assessment and reflection
- users' requests and feedback.

Evidence-based practice (EBP) is just one among many drivers of practice. Other factors which affect current practice are tradition, management directives concerning policy targets, peer learning and networking, and service users' views. Muir Gray (2001) argues that most health-care decisions are opinion based and driven principally by values and resources.

EBP is unique in that it claims to provide an objective and rational basis for practice by evaluating available evidence about what works to determine current and future practice. It was first applied to medicine, when Sackett defined it as: 'The conscientious, explicit and judicious use of current best evidence in making decisions about individual patients based on skills which allow the doctor to evaluate both personal experience and external evidence in a systematic and objective manner' (Sackett et al 1996, p. 71). As such, it is clearly differentiated from:

- tradition ('this is what we've always done')
- practical experience and wisdom ('in my experience, this approach is the most effective one')
- values ('this is what we should do')
- economic considerations ('this is what we can afford').

Enthusiasts claim that EBP is superior because it is more objective and trawls through more sources of evidence than are usually available to any one individual or organization.

EBP has become increasingly popular for several reasons. EBP offers the promise of maximizing expenditure by directing it to the most effective strategies and interventions. The exponential rise of information technology and almost instant access to a multitude of sources of information makes EBP a more realistic possibility. It can be difficult for individual practitioners to know what is happening in the research world and EBP can offer an already synthesized and aggregated overview of the most up to date research findings for the busy practitioner.

The opportunities for EBP include:

- current policy environment that values evidence
- links between service providers and universities to offer guidance and support
- new systems of clinical governance, audit and accountability that offer rigour and consistency in assessing outcomes

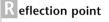

R eflection point

What are the opportunities and barriers for EBP in your organization?

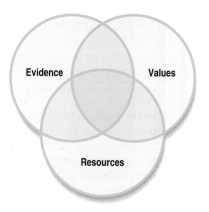

Figure 3.1 Evidence-based practice
Source: Muir Gray (2001)

Evidence   Values

Resources

- education and training that prepares practitioners to be reflective and to use and evaluate EBP
- multiprofessional working that encourages collective debate and consensus regarding EBP.

Barriers to EBP include:

- reliance on dominant positivist scientific model of evidence that may undervalue alternative sources of evidence
- increased workload and expectations with limited time for reflection
- limited research data in non-medical, non-pharmacological areas
- patchy access to information services
- critical appraisal skills shortage.

EBP has been seized upon as a tool that leads to rational and effective practice. Professionals and policy makers have their own agendas, and practice may be determined by factors such as protectionism, self-interest or ideological commitments. EBP offers the attraction of being above these concerns and offering definitive answers as to what constitutes best practice. A 'gold standard' of evidence has been established that privileges systematic reviews of randomized controlled trials. Traditional approaches to evaluating the effectiveness of health improvement programmes and interventions have answered very narrow questions about health and health outcomes, e.g. do hip protectors reduce fractures from falls? As we have seen in our earlier book *Health Promotion: Foundations for Practice* (Naidoo & Wills 2000), and as we shall discuss further in Part 3 of this book, health outcomes are influenced by complex and interrelated factors. These include social, economic and environmental factors, as well as specific health-related behaviours, interacting with psychological, genetic and biological factors. In order to understand 'what works', it is often necessary to gather qualitative and context-specific types of information or evidence.

Chapter 2 discussed how qualitative research is often denigrated as being 'soft', biased and not generalizable. However there are accepted standards for rigour in qualitative research, and finding out about people's perceptions, beliefs and attitudes is crucial to successful health promotion and public health interventions. Investigating the complex processes involved in health improvement programmes, or measuring a range of effects including people's views, provides vital knowledge for practitioners. Such evidence may not conform to the scientific model, but does offer a more realistic and useful assessment of how in practice interventions lead to outcomes (Pawson & Tilley 1997).

Example

Are role model programmes effective in behaviour modification? 'Scared Straight' is a programme in the USA that brings at-risk or already delinquent children, mainly boys, into prison to meet 'lifers'. Inmates, the lifers themselves, the juvenile participants, their parents, prison governors, teachers and the general public were very positive about the programme in all studies, concluding that it should be continued. However in a systematic review, seven good quality randomized control trials showed that the programme increased delinquency rates among the treatment group (Petrosino et al 2000 cited by Macintyre & Cummins 2001). Participants may not tell the same story as the outcome

E *continued*

evaluation for many reasons, but their views on the process are valid and important data in their own right. Participants' views on the appropriateness and accessibility of the programme are essential in deciding whether or not to adopt programmes. The ideal programme will be both effective in terms of achieving desired outcomes, and acceptable to participants.

As Davies et al (2000, p. 23) observe 'There is a tendency to think of evidence as something that is only generated by major pieces of research. In any policy area there is a great deal of critical evidence held in the minds of both front-line staff in departments, agencies and local authorities and those to whom the policy is directed.' This broader range of evidence from government advisers, experts and users needs to be included in decision making about health improvement. This more inclusive approach to evidence is advocated by many commentators and forums. For example, the 51st World Health Assembly urged all member states to 'adopt an evidence-based approach to health promotion policy and practice, using the full range of quantitative and qualitative methodologies' (WHA 1998).

WHAT DOES IT MEAN TO BE EVIDENCE BASED?

R eflection point

What does it mean to be evidence based?

For the health practitioner, becoming evidence based means building your practice on strategies which research has demonstrated are the most effective means for achieving stated aims. In theory, this would mean swapping uncertainties and traditional practices for specified techniques and strategies in the knowledge that they would lead to certain outcomes. In reality, there is never such absolute certainty, and research is not always totally reliable and valid, even if it is available for the particular issue of concern. So evidence-based practice is a journey towards more reliable and effective practice, and one that involves the practitioner becoming open-minded and flexible. To become evidence based, one has to be willing to change one's practice. This refers to organizations as well as individuals or professions. Individual practitioner attempts to become more evidence based may flounder due to organizations' entrenched practices and inability to change.

Being an evidence-based practitioner involves the systematic appraisal of the best available evidence. To do this you will need critical problem-solving skills so that you are clear about:

- what it is you need to know
- what would constitute 'doing the right things right' (Muir Gray 2001), e.g.:
  - that the intervention is effective?
  - that it is acceptable?
  - that it is equitable?
  - that it is done consistently and safely?
  - that it is cost effective?
- how you will find the best evidence
- how you will assess the quality of that evidence
- whether the evidence is applicable to the population and context in which you are working.

Many public health and health promotion interventions have been introduced without good evidence that their outcomes meet stated objectives. For example, breakfast clubs in schools have been widely introduced and promoted as part of a drive to improve healthy eating and to tackle inequalities in child health. Evaluation shows that they provide children with a nutritional start to the day, can therefore improve concentration and performance, and promote social interaction. However there is only limited evidence of their effectiveness in promoting healthy eating amongst children, or of their ability to target the most disadvantaged children (HDA 2001).

It is this uncertainty that has led the Health Development Agency (HDA) in England and the lead agencies for health promotion in the other UK countries to produce evidence-based briefings that appraise current evidence of effective interventions in a digestible form for practitioners. Evidence-based briefings select recent, good quality, systematic reviews and meta-analyses and synthesize the results. They are an important tool in the development of an evidence base for health promotion activities. HDA publications to date include evidence briefings on prevention of obesity, diet, physical activity, prevention of accidental injury, HIV prevention, teenage pregnancy and parenthood and breastfeeding promotion. Further details of publications may be obtained by visiting the HDA website at www.hda.nhs.uk/evidence.

There have been moves towards making professional practice more evidence based. One key strategy is the use of clinical guidelines. Clinical guidelines are a top-down strategy to make practice more in line with available evidence of what works and to ensure comparable standards and reduce variations in practice. Clinical guidelines translate evidence into recommendations for clinical practice and appropriate health care that can be implemented in a variety of settings. Recommendations are graded according to the strength of the evidence and their feasibility. So recommendations supported by consistent findings from randomized controlled trials that use available techniques and expertise would be graded more highly than recommendations supported by expert panel consensus that rely on scarce expertise and resources. There are now several websites that provide clinical guidelines based on evidence (see Box 3.1)

Box 3.1 Websites that provide clinical guidelines

- www.nice.org.uk   *National Institute for Clinical Excellence* is a UK government sponsored organization that collates and disseminates evidence on effectiveness and cost-effectiveness
- www.sign.ac.uk   *Scottish Intercollegiate Guidelines Network*
- www.health.gov.au/nhmrc/publications/cphome.htm   *Australian National Health and Medical Research Council*
- www.cma.ca/cpgs/index   *Canadian Medical Association Clinical Practice Guidelines*
- www.nzgg.org.nz   *New Zealand Guidelines Group*
- www.guideline.gov/index   *United States National Guidelines Clearing House*

Health promotion and public health practitioners face particular diffi-culties in becoming more evidence based. These include:

- the complexities of searching for primary studies which are sparse
- assessing evidence from non-randomized studies (including qualitative research)
- finding evidence relating to process and how an intervention works
- synthesizing evidence from different study designs
- transferability of results to other contexts which differ from those used in the original research.

SKILLS FOR EVIDENCE-BASED PRACTICE

Adopting an evidence-based approach mimics the process of primary research:

- identifying an answerable problem
- searching for potential evidence
- data extraction
- critical appraisal
- synthesis.

Being evidence based means having both the knowledge and the confi-dence to tackle issues effectively. To become an evidence-based practi-tioner means adopting a critical view with regards to research and evidence, and being willing to change your practice if the evidence sug-gests this is worthwhile. The practitioner who seeks to become evidence based needs to acquire the knowledge and skills to find out and access, critically appraise, and synthesize and apply relevant evidence. Evidence includes research as well as more anecdotal and developmental accounts linking inputs to outputs.

Being evidence based includes the ability to separate evidence from other drivers of practice including politics, custom and ethical considera-tions. Above all, being evidence based requires an open and critical mind to reflect on your own knowledge about an issue, and assess competing claims of knowledge.

The 'certainty continuum' (Ellison et al 2001 and at http://hivsa.ioe. ac.uk/hivsa/) describes the on-going search for evidence to inform practice:

1. Unsubstantiated certainty – confidence without knowledge

2. Unease – lack of confidence as lack of knowledge is recognized

3. Reflection – assess existing level of knowledge

4. Acknowledge knowledge gap – the lack of evidence to support practice

5. Search for evidence – is there available evidence?

6. Evidence-based certainty – practice now based on knowledge and evidence.

ASKING THE RIGHT QUESTION

Being clear about what you need to know is a vital first step. It is this process that starts the search for relevant evidence and the process of

A smoking cessation coordinator is concerned at the rising rates of smoking among young women. The coordinator wants to extend the service to young people who wish to quit. The coordinator thinks that a cessation group could be established in one of the local secondary schools but is not sure how to proceed or whether the accepted model of cessation would work with young people. What does she need to know?

appraisal. Asking the right question means finding a balance between being too specific (asking a question that is unlikely ever to have been researched), and being too vague (asking a question that will produce a mass of research studies, many of which will be inapplicable to the context and circumstances you are interested in).

In the above example, the coordinator will be interested in those factors that facilitate young people to quit and the factors that might act as barriers. The coordinator will search for research on smoking cessation in schools and will want to assess its effectiveness in getting young women to quit, its efficiency in relation to other methods such as health education, and its acceptability to young women. If insufficient research is available, they may look at other research on young peoples' attitudes to quitting and cessation studies in other settings.

WHAT COUNTS AS EVIDENCE?

Evidence may be of many different types, ranging from systematic reviews and meta-analyses, to collective consensual views, to individual experiences and reflections. All types of evidence have their uses. EBP traditionally reifies science above experience but as we have seen in Chapter 1, experiential reflection is an important part of informed practice. Similarly, the expertise of users is vital to developing acceptable interventions. Most EBP relies on:

- written accounts of primary research in refereed academic and professional journals
- academic and professional texts (reviewed)
- independently published reports
- unpublished reports and conference papers and presentations (grey literature).

Evidence may be defined as data demonstrating that a certain input leads to a certain output. However the use of evidence to inform practice is broader than this, and encompasses:

- information about an intervention's effectiveness in meeting its goals
- information about how transferable this intervention is thought to be (to other settings and populations)
- information about the intervention's positive and negative effects
- information about the intervention's economic impact
- information about barriers to implementing the intervention (SAJPM 2000, p. 36 cited in McQueen 2001).

The scientific medical model has gained dominance in the debate about defining evidence. This model states that evidence is best determined through the use of scientific methodologies which prioritize quantitative objective fact finding. The use of scientific models of evidence leads to a search for specific inputs causing specific outputs, regardless of intervening or contextual factors such as socio-economic status, beliefs or a supportive environment. Such intervening factors, which mediate and moderate the effect of inputs, are viewed as 'confounding variables' and study designs try to eliminate their effect. The randomized controlled trial (RCT), using the experimental method, is viewed as the most robust and useful method for achieving results which qualify as evidence and is viewed as the 'gold standard'. The criteria relevant for RCTs include:

- The intervention is experimental, with a control group which does not experience the intervention.
- There is random allocation of individuals to the experimental or control group.
- Allocation is double-blind; that is, neither patients nor practitioners know which group is the experimental or control group.
- There is baseline assessment of patients to ensure the experimental and control groups do not differ in any significant ways.
- There is full follow up of all patients.
- Assessment of outcomes is objective and unbiased.
- Analysis is based on initial group allocation.
- The likelihood of findings arising by chance is assessed.
- The power of the study to detect a worthwhile effect is assessed.

D iscussion point

What drawbacks, if any, can you identify regarding the use of this rigorous methodology?

The RCT methodology is appropriate for the analysis of alternative treatments or therapies for medical conditions affecting individual patients. Even in these cases, RCTs cannot take account of significant differences in practitioner input, such as level of enthusiasm, technical skills or knowledge. There may also be ethical concerns if one treatment looks markedly better or worse than another at an early stage. For interventions that are group or population based, it becomes very difficult if not impossible to adopt an RCT methodology. Groups differ according to geography, demographic and socio-economic factors, so finding a true control group is very difficult. It is impossible to isolate groups so there may be 'leakage' of relevant variables (such as information) from one group to another.

There is now a well established 'hierarchy of evidence' which grades research findings according to how valid and reliable the research methodology is deemed to be. Valid means that appropriate methods to answer the question are selected and correctly performed, and therefore the results are generalizable to other populations. Reliable means that the research methodology is transparent and unbiased and could be replicated, with the same results, by other researchers.

Box 3.2 The hierarchy of evidence

The hierarchy goes from the most reliable evidence (Type 1) to the least reliable evidence (Type 5).

Type 1 evidence: Systematic reviews and meta-analyses including two or more randomized controlled trials.

Type 2 evidence: Well designed randomized controlled trial, e.g. prospective experimental trial of treatment where subjects are randomly assigned to the experimental or control group.

Type 3 evidence: Well designed controlled trial without randomization, e.g. retrospective study comparing a control and intervention group.

Type 4 evidence: Well designed observational studies, e.g. case studies.

Type 5 evidence: Expert opinion, expert panels, views of service users and carers.

Reflection point

How appropriate is
the hierarchy of
evidence for public
health and health
promotion?

The hierarchy of evidence has evolved in the context of individual care and treatment carried out within one disciplinary paradigm – scientific medicine. Public health and health promotion, which focus on communities and populations, provide a very different subject for research. They are multidisciplinary bodies of knowledge, and the evidence they draw upon is correspondingly varied. To focus on the use of scientific experimental evaluation would ignore a large, important and expanding body of evidence about community focused health promotion and public health. The use of evidence within health promotion has been likened to the judicial notion of evidence, which is typically a mixture of witness accounts, expert testimony and forensic science (McQueen 2001). Using this concept of evidence, individual stories which relate processes, interpretations and outcomes are as valid as scientific trials which seek to determine the effect of single causal factors.

This more inclusive notion of evidence, with its combination of accounts which vary in terms of what they construct as the truth, seems more appropriate to public health and health promotion. A more inclusive concept of evidence enables the measurement and validation of a range of concepts and meanings relating to health and well-being, including people's subjective assessment of their health and contributing factors. It also enables multidisciplinary practice through the recognition of different concepts and methodologies. The scientific model of evidence could even be viewed as disabling multidisciplinary practice through its prioritization of scientific evidence and its discounting of other forms of evidence. Using a more inclusive notion of evidence does not mean abandoning the concept of methodological rigour and quality. As we saw in Chapter 2, research studies that use qualitative methodologies may still be assessed for rigour.

Desirable methodological characteristics of research into effectiveness include:

Discussion point

What criteria of
methodological valid-
ity (aspects of
research design which
would lead you to be
confident that the
results are meaningful
and generalizable to
other populations)
would you stipulate if
you were conducting
a review of the effec-
tiveness of health pro-
motion interventions
to initiate and main-
tain breastfeeding?

- The intervention is described in sufficient detail so that it could be replicated by others.
- The target audience is fully described.
- The size and effect of non-respondents is included.
- There are clear outcomes or health status measurements.
- These outcomes are compared to baseline measurements undertaken before the intervention.

FINDING THE EVIDENCE

The key to EBP is that evidence is collected systematically. This means that a full search of all available sources of information is undertaken, and full details are given of how the search has been conducted. This includes citing:

- key words
- databases that have been accessed
- criteria used to include or exclude research studies.

Systematic reviews, for example, typically exclude large numbers of studies that fail to meet their criteria for rigour. Such criteria include full details of non-respondents, before and after measurements, and the use of a control group. Searches for evidence are also usually only undertaken for English language materials and are often confined to research carried out in developed Western countries. It has been claimed that this omission leads to systematic bias and lack of relevance for developing countries (McQueen 2001).

The internet has greatly expanded the amount of information that can be accessed, and it is easy to waste time collecting information which is not relevant. In order to avoid this, systematic searches should be:

- explicit – use key terms, record your search, ensure it is transparent so others can assess its value and it can be repeated
- appropriate – look where the evidence is likely to be
- sensitive – collecting all the information which is relevant to your question
- specific – collecting only information that is relevant to your question
- comprehensive – include all available information.

There are a number of valuable sources of evidence that can be used to guide practice. Bibliographic databases such as Medline or Cinahl gather together articles and give short extracts. Databases such as these, however, only hold a small proportion of relevant literature. Other databases are more like libraries of information and vary in how they define 'evidence' and range from a traditional restricted single-disciplinary view (e.g. the Cochrane Collaboration) to a more inclusive and multidisciplinary view (e.g. the Health Development Agency).

Box 3.3 Sources of evidence

- *Campbell Collaboration* http://www.campbellcollaboration.org   An international collaboration which produces systematic reviews of studies researching the effectiveness of social and behavioural interventions.
- *Cochrane Collaboration* http://www.cochrane.org/   An international collaboration which produces systematic reviews of the effects of health care interventions. The collaboration covers a wide range of health care topics. There is health promotion and public health field http://www.vichealth.vic.gov.au/cochrane that seeks to provide evidence to guide practice in health promotion and public health. This field explicitly encourages collaboration and wide participation as well as the minimization of bias and ensuring quality.
- *Health Development Agency* http://www.hda-online.org.uk/evidence or www.hda.nhs.uk   A national database of evidence about what works to improve people's health and reduce health inequalities. The database includes systematic and other reviews of effectiveness and evidence-based briefing documents for practitioners and policy makers. A wide range of topics is included. Evidence Briefings synthesize research evidence whilst Effective Action Briefings focus on guidance on how to get evidence into practice. Databases also exist for the national health promotion agencies in Wales www.hpw.wales.gov.uk/research and Scotland www.hebs.scot.nhs.uk/research.

Box 3.3 *Continued*

- *The UK National Electronic Library for Health* www.nelh.nhs.uk A national database containing summaries of the best available evidence.
- *UK Economic and Social Research Council Evidence Network* A UK network reviewing research into social, community and policy interventions.
- *Effectiveness Matters* www.york.ac.uk/crd Provides summaries about research evidence
- *National Institute for Clinical Evidence* (NICE) www.nice.org.uk NICE is a UK organization that collates and disseminates evidence on effectiveness and cost-effectiveness.

Discussion point

What is helpful or unhelpful about these collections?

Systematic searches involve a number of stages. These are:

- Identifying sources of information, sweeping as widely as possible at the start in order not to exclude any relevant studies.
- Using a protocol to plan your approach so that your search is transparent and can be reproduced by others. Protocols typically include a number of stages starting with the best available evidence and moving towards less reliable evidence. For example, a search might start with meta-analyses, then move to systematic reviews of RCTs, then move to single RCTs, then on to cohort studies and so on.
- Doing the search, using relevant terms and combinations of terms including abbreviations and filters. The ways in which words are linked together to search is called Boolean logic.
- Searching for quality, or narrowing the search by excluding the least useful sources. This may involve restricting the search to high quality studies or restricting the search by specifying time limits or certain combinations of terms.

In addition to the online databases listed in Box 3.3, there are many other means of searching sources of evidence. These include:

- searching online databases of unappraised primary research
- online searching of relevant websites for unpublished articles and information
- library searches of indexed and non-indexed sources
- manual searching of academic and professional journals
- manual searching of theses and independently published reports
- contacting dedicated information clearing houses and acknowledged experts.

All searches need to be systematically carried out, using consistent keywords or phrases, and these need to be made transparent in order for others to gauge their suitability and comprehensiveness.

Example

Searching for evidence about 'fat' camps

Obesity in children is a recognized and increasing problem. While there is considerable research into predisposing factors, most interventions that aim to control and reduce weight gain are poorly evaluated. In the USA residential weight-loss 'fat' camps have been introduced. In order to ascertain whether to introduce 'fat' camps to the UK evidence is needed on:

E *continued*

- their effectiveness in reducing weight in children
- their efficiency in relation to other family-centred methods
- their acceptability to children and parents
- the factors that influence their success.

One of the main problems in searching for evidence is being too broad in the search of online databases. A search using the keywords 'child' and 'obesity' would be likely to yield an excessive amount of 'hits'. Successful searching systematically limits and combines key terms and may use exclusion criteria such as English language and a year period. A search revealed the following published papers:

Gately P J, Cooke C B, Butterly R J, Knight C, Carrol S (2000) The acute effects of an 8 week diet, exercise and educational camp program on obese children. *Paediatric Exercise Science* 12: 413–423.

Gately P J, Cooke C B, Butterly R J, Mackieth P, Carroll S (2000) The effects of a children's summer camp programme on weight loss with a 10 month follow up. *International Journal of Obesity* 24: 1445–1452.

Payne J, Capra C, Hickman I (2002) Residential camps as a setting for nutrition education of Australian girls. *Australian and New Zealand Journal of Public Health* 26: 383–388.

The Cochrane library may yield a systematic review – in this case there is a recent review on interventions for preventing obesity in children but it does not refer to fat camps (Campbell et al 2004). A hand search of journals might include the *International Journal of Human Nutrition and Dietetics* or the *International Journal of Obesity*. A web search using a search engine such as 'Google' for key experts in this example, provided a link to Carnegie International Camp – Britain's first international weight loss summer camp.

(With thanks to Alexandra Lucas)

APPRAISING THE EVIDENCE

Not all evidence is useful for planning public health and health promotion activities. Some interventions have not been evaluated in a rigorous way and so it is difficult to know if they are worth employing elsewhere. Assessing the value of evidence is a skilled task and is termed critical appraisal. Traditionally critical appraisal in EBP determines the quality of the research study. Assessing the validity and reliability of research is used when deciding whether or not the findings are generalizable and can be applied elsewhere.

Appraising the evidence can seem a daunting prospect when there are so many sources of evidence available in various formats. It is important to obtain the relevant information from research reports:

- identification (title, date, publishers, funding)
- the population, settings and activities (what, how, where, when and with whom was the intervention carried out?)
- the outcomes
- data collection and analysis techniques.

Critical appraisal for public health and health promotion may be defined as the systematic and structured evaluation of the relevance of a study. Its purpose is 'to find in the evidence anything of value that will help you make a better decision' (Hill et al 2001, p. 86). Four key questions are:

- What did the research set out to find? (Are there specified aims or questions?)
- What methods were used? (Were the methods right for the question? Were the methods carried out correctly?)
- What were the findings? (Are the findings reported in full? Can you trust them?)
- What does it mean? (Are the findings relevant to your problem? Are they applicable to your setting?) (Source: Hill et al 2001, p. 86)

Discussion point

How do you decide the relevance of identified information?

There is a large body of literature on critical appraisal skills as well as several useful guides (e.g. CASP – for details see Further Reading at the end of this chapter.) Critical appraisal guides provide questions that enable the appraiser to assess the methodological rigour of different types of research study. Questions are grouped under three main headings:

- Are the results of the study valid?
- What are the main results?
- Will the results help locally?

Critical appraisal therefore seeks to identify useful, rigorous, high quality research and exclude irrelevant or flawed research. This is a question of degree, for it is usually possible to identify flaws in published research studies and ways in which the context of the research and one's own practice differ. Critical appraisal is then a pragmatic process whereby research is screened so that only studies that reach a certain standard of rigour and relevance are taken into account.

Cummins and Macintyre (2002) refer to 'factoids' – assumptions that get reported and repeated so often that they become accepted. They describe the way in which food deserts (areas of deprivation where families have difficulty accessing affordable, healthy food) have become an accepted part of policy because they fit with the prevailing ideological approach, although there is little evidence to support their existence.

SYNTHESIZING THE EVIDENCE

Systematic reviews and meta-analyses are both forms of secondary research that take primary research studies as their object of study. Systematic reviews and meta-analyses combine the results of two or more RCTs and are widely viewed as constituting the most robust available evidence. Systematic reviews identify relevant studies, assess their methodological rigour and quality, and synthesize the results. Meta-analyses identify relevant primary research studies and then aggregate the results, giving a quantitative estimate of the overall effect. Systematic reviews and meta-analyses set out methodological criteria that are used to include or exclude research studies.

Despite the widespread and recognized value of qualitative studies, the criteria for inclusion within systematic reviews of health promotion have tended to be similar to those used by evidence-based medicine, with a dominance of experimental studies. Inclusion tends to be based on the quality of the study rather than the quality of the intervention. Their use for public health and health promotion practitioners and policy makers can be limited because, as Tilford (2000) notes, reviews give insufficient information about the process of implementing an intervention and often focus on a narrow range of outcomes rather than the complexity of the programmes with which practitioners are engaged.

A systematic review should:

- specify the inclusion and exclusion criteria
- describe and use comprehensive and systematic search methods to locate all relevant studies
- assess the validity of primary studies in ways which can be replicated
- explore the consensus and variation between the findings of different studies
- synthesize primary studies.

The Cochrane Library is expanding the reviews relating to public health and health promotion. Those relating to cardiovascular health for example currently include reviews on dietary modification, smoking cessation, physical activity promotion, weight reduction and compression stockings for airline passengers.

Techniques for the synthesis of qualitative research studies do exist and are developing rapidly. Meta-ethnography is the term used to describe the systematic synthesis of qualitative research studies (Noblit & Hare 1988). Meta-ethnography provides an interpretive synthesis rather than the aggregative, quantitative synthesis of meta-analysis. Meta-ethnography identifies, codes and summarizes themes from the literature until saturation point is reached, and further integration of themes is considered invalid. Attempts are made to preserve individual observations and nuances. Meta-ethnography has been used to systematically review evidence about patient and lay perspectives (Campbell et al 2003) and its use is expanding.

USING EVIDENCE-BASED PRACTICE TO DETERMINE COST-EFFECTIVENESS

In any discussion about effectiveness, the issue of resources is likely to crop up. Real life decisions take place within an economic context, being made with reference to costs and competing claims. It is not enough simply to argue that an intervention is effective; it also has to be cost-effective (the optimum means of producing given outcomes at least cost). The expanding field of health economics addresses these issues and seeks to provide rational tools for evaluating interventions by comparing costs with benefits. Traditionally this has taken the form of costs and benefits per individual patient, and the field of public health and health promotion, with its emphasis on social costs and benefits, has been neglected. There are now moves to address this deficit and define new constructs and frameworks which focus on public health in its broadest sense (Powell 2003).

Economic evaluation examines whether limited resources are used in the best possible way. The most rigorous economic evaluations examine both costs and consequences for two or more alternatives (one of which may be the existing status quo). There are five main types of economic evaluation (Donaldson et al 2002, Sefton et al 2002):

1. Cost-minimization analysis – used when there is strong evidence that two or more interventions are equally effective. This technique compares the costs to determine the least cost alternative.

2. Cost-effectiveness analysis – investigates the best way of achieving a single objective (e.g. life years gained, improved social capital) through measuring costs and benefits to arrive at a measure of cost per unit of benefit. The least cost intervention is then determined and prioritized.

3. Cost-consequences analysis – similar to cost-effectiveness analysis but used to evaluate interventions with more than one outcome.

4. Cost-utility analysis – measures the effects of an intervention in terms of utilities (e.g. the quality adjusted life year, or QALY), focusing on minimizing costs or maximizing benefits.

5. Cost-benefit analysis – examines the costs and benefits, expressed in monetary terms, of an intervention in order to determine its desirability. A desirable intervention is one where benefits exceed costs.

Example	Smoking cessation interventions are very cost-effective. Overall the cost per life year gained for smoking cessation interventions is tiny, at £212–£873. This compares very favourably with the National Institute of Clinical Excellence benchmark of acceptable cost-effectiveness, which is £30,000 per life year saved. Campaigns with a high level of awareness and penetration, such as the annual No Smoking Day media campaign, are even more cost-effective. Almost one million people have stopped smoking because of No Smoking Day since it first began in 1984. The estimated cost-effectiveness of No Smoking Day is around £21 per life year saved. Campaigns that target groups with high smoking prevalence may also be more cost-effective than general population campaigns. A campaign targeted at London's Turkish community, who have above average smoking rates, estimated the cost-effectiveness of this intervention was £105 (range £33–£391) per life year gained.
Cost-effectiveness of smoking cessation interventions	
	Sources: Parrot et al (1998), Stevens et al (2002), www.new.nosmokingday.org.uk

WIDENING THE EVIDENCE BASE

Reviews of evidence privilege certain forms of knowledge and information over others. However, to achieve practical results, practitioners and users need to be persuaded that the outcomes they value will be affected by an intervention. This means incorporating their views in the evidence base.

There are a number of ways in which practitioner and user views can feed into this process, including inputs into research design (see Example: Smoking in pregnancy) and representation on committees and bodies that construct and use evidence. For example, 'Consumers in NHS Research' is a committee of the NHS Executive that examines the ways in which research is prioritized, commissioned, undertaken and disseminated. Research into user views can be systematically reviewed and synthesized using the technique of meta-ethnography (Noblit & Hare 1988).

Discussion point
How can expert, practitioner and user views be incorporated into evidence-informed decision making?

Example

Smoking in
pregnancy

A systematic review reported increases in birthweight and a reduction in still-births following smoking cessation in pregnancy programmes. A letter to the author of the review commented on: 'the need for trials to address broader out-come measures such as the impact on other family members, the benefits to women's health, whether non-smoking is sustained, the impact of failing to stop smoking, stress levels, the emotional impact of having a low birthweight baby after taking part in a strategy to stop smoking and self-esteem.' Oliver (2001) reports that as a result, the revised review incorporated observational and qual-itative research, and small-scale consultations with health promotion practition-ers and health service users, which broadened the content of the work and influenced the criteria by which the effectiveness of programmes was judged. To be persuasive in changing practice, evidence on programme effects and out-comes needs to be acceptable and relevant to those delivering and receiving such programmes.

Source: Oliver (2001)

Discussion point

What, if any, prob-lems can you foresee in becoming an evidence-based practitioner?

PUTTING EVIDENCE INTO PRACTICE: ISSUES AND DILEMMAS

Although evidence-based public health and health promotion is often portrayed as the key to effective professional practice, there remain sig-nificant questions and dilemmas for practitioners seeking to incorporate evidence into their everyday practice. Common dilemmas for practition-ers include:

- how much evidence is required before introducing an intervention
- whether or not the research describes situations which are comparable to their own (including comparable caseloads or communities, organi-zations, staff and resources)
- whether or not the evidence includes the views of all relevant stake-holders
- what to do when the evidence goes counter to personal intuition or judgement
- whether evidence can ever claim to be objective or neutral.

Some of these dilemmas are discussed in greater detail below.

Is the evidence comparing like with like?

It is often assumed that evidence is comparing like with like but in reality this is unlikely to be the case. In real life, interventions, even if they are following the same design or protocol, tend to vary depending on the context in which they are implemented.

Discussion point

What factors might account for the differ-ent outcomes of studies examining the same intervention?

Contextual factors, such as the enthusiasm or commitment of organi-zations and practitioners, population characteristics, e.g social stability and cohesion, and geographical factors, e.g. declining or renewing areas, will all have a significant impact on outcomes. The criteria used to appraise evidence refer to the research rather than the intervention. This means that key aspects of the intervention may vary widely from study to study and yet not be identified as necessary for successful outcomes.

For example, research into the effectiveness of brief interventions on alcohol did not use a uniform definition of brief intervention. Brief interventions ranged from a single five-minute discussion with a GP to regular sessions of structured interventions by GPs over six months (Heather 1995 cited in Speller et al 1997). This example demonstrates the importance of investigating processes as well as outcomes in order to identify factors leading to success. This in turn makes the case for including different kinds of evidence, qualitative as well as quantitative. A useful framework is the realistic evaluation framework proposed by Pawson & Tilley (1997). Realistic evaluation recognizes that key features of an intervention relate to the specific context which needs to be taken into account. A mechanism is only causal if it leads to an outcome within a context. The context therefore needs to be identified and evaluated as well as the intervention.

Whose definitions count?

Discussion point

How might the following view the nature of the evidence for funding a community safety programme: policy maker; health promotion/public health practitioner; local population; academic researcher?

In any public health or health promotion intervention there are a number of stakeholders who will hold very different ideas of what counts as a successful outcome, or what constitutes evidence.

Views will vary significantly and cannot be accurately predicted, although it is known that factors such as occupation, socio-economic status, disciplinary background, and ideological and political beliefs will all have an impact. In order to support partnership working, different concepts of evidence need to be recognized and valued. Lay beliefs regarding evidence may be unscientific according to an epidemiological framework, but they are a valid point of view. If the recipient of a service does not value the outcome, there is little point in continuing the service. Equally, if partners include people with a background in social sciences who are constantly being told by medical scientists that their view of evidence and effective practice is misinformed, misguided or just wrong, they are unlikely to form an effective partnership. Evidence-based public health and health promotion needs to seek to embrace inclusive definitions of success that relate to the values and views of all stakeholders.

What if the evidence goes against my better judgement?

Finding and appraising evidence is a skilled task, and the findings may go counter to one's better judgement, intuition or custom. Midwives used to advise parents to put babies to sleep in the prone (tummy down) position because it seemed plausible that this was similar to the recovery position. Research has since shown that this sleeping position is associated with increased risk of sudden infant death syndrome. This research led to a major public media campaign to change practice called 'back to sleep'. This is an example where the evidence was sufficient to prompt practitioners and the public to change their custom and practice. Failure to change is attributed to lack of knowledge or appreciation of the strength of the evidence.

The government advice to use the triple vaccine for measles, mumps and rubella is founded on strong research evidence, yet many parents reject this vaccine and opt for single vaccines, even if they have to pay. The reason for this rejection of expert advice appears to lie in the many factors which impact on a parent's decision to actively treat their child. Giving a child a vaccination which might have harmful effects may be viewed as more unacceptable than taking no action and the child contracting the disease. The difference would seem to lie in the action/omission dichotomy, whereby an action is seen as more blameworthy than an omission. A parent's decision on what is best for their child takes into account factors that are invisible in large trials of treatments. So an individual child's risk of an adverse reaction to MMR might be assessed using previous history of allergic reactions, any unusual syndromes, or the reactions and behaviour of siblings. The undoubted benefits to the population of adequate levels of MMR vaccination do not apply to each individual. In addition, the severe effects of contracting measles, mumps or rubella are often downplayed because they are so infrequently seen nowadays. Parents who reject the triple vaccine would undoubtedly argue they are making a better judgement, based on their knowledge of individual circumstances, than the blanket advice of health professionals to accept the MMR vaccination.

Is evidence objective and neutral?

Social scientists accept that some degree of bias and subjectivity is inherent in qualitative research, but argue that this does not invalidate findings. As we saw in the previous chapter, they propose instead that transparency and reflexivity, documented as part of the research process, assist readers and researchers in determining the validity, rigour or robustness of the research. However, in traditional quantitative research fields claims are still made regarding the objectivity of quantitative methods, such as randomized controlled trials. Often the assumption is that, because these methods involve counting real phenomena – a process that can be verified – they are more objective, reliable and therefore 'better' or more 'desirable' than qualitative methods.

A more realistic view is that all research involves both the 'facts' and the theoretical frameworks that determine which facts count, and how they are interpreted. This stance may be termed the inclusive approach to research and evidence. Subjectivity is a matter of degree, not an either/or phenomenon. Denying subjectivity is no more realistic than accepting its inevitability and then seeking ways to allow for its effects. And even though quantitative research claims to be objective, commentators agree that there is no such thing as complete objectivity, and that pre-existing values and beliefs exert a powerful influence when conducting or interpreting research (Kaptchuk 2003). Although evidence may never be completely objective or neutral, it is still important to assess its validity, reliability and robustness according to appropriate criteria. The subjectivity involved in a researcher's decisions about which studies to include and exclude in a systematic review can, for example, be limited by using more than one researcher and a common data extraction form.

Reflection point

What are the organi-
zational and profes-
sional opportunities
and barriers to
implementing
evidence-based
approaches in public
health and health
promotion?

How can practice change in the light of evidence?

A number of recent initiatives are helping to facilitate access to evidence, for example, the evidence briefings of the Health Development Agency and the Effectiveness Matters bulletins from the NHS Centre for Reviews and Dissemination (NHSCRD). Easier access to evidence is just one hurdle to be overcome if practice is to change and become more evidence based. Changing practice involves commitment and resources as well as evidence. Practitioners need to be persuaded of the evidence but also to believe they can change their practice in the recommended ways, and that their clients will find this acceptable. Any change in practice is disruptive and likely, at least in the short term, to be resource-intensive. For many practitioners, operating within severe constraints and with large caseloads, this poses an additional barrier. However, as EBP becomes more embedded and applied to a variety of disciplines and practices, organizations and practitioners will become more used to adapting practice to conform to evidence. Critical appraisal skills and adaptiveness will become part and parcel of every practitioner's repertoire.

CONCLUSION

There has been some resistance to applying the principles of EBP to health promotion and public health. Part of this is due to the medical scientific origins of evidence-based medicine and the way in which quantitative methodologies have been privileged over qualitative methodologies. Health promotion and public health are multidisciplinary and recognize the validity of differing types of evidence including context-specific and subjective views. Their multidisciplinary nature leads to complexity and uncertainty in the search for evidence, as different disciplines have their own rules of evidence, and attempting to consolidate these differences into an over-arching holistic body of evidence is a challenging, if not daunting, prospect (McQueen 2001).

One means of consolidating available evidence would be to use the hierarchy of evidence that privileges the RCT as providing the best evidence. However there is on-going debate about whether or not RCTs should remain the 'gold standard' for public health and health promotion interventions. Proponents of the RCT argue that they are feasible in the area of health promotion and do provide the best available evidence on which to base practice (Oakley 1998). Critics respond by arguing that RCTs are inappropriate for population-based, multicomponent interventions where there may be a considerable time lag between the interventions and the outcomes (Nutbeam 1998). There is also a strong argument that, in line with underlying health promotion and public health values of equity, participation and autonomy, the views of practitioners and users deserve to be valued as a source of evidence in their own right.

The most useful stance for practitioners to take appears to be the inclusive concept of evidence that acknowledges and values a range of different kinds of evidence including RCTs, qualitative process research, and user views and accounts. Adopting the inclusive concept of evidence facilitates the involvement of different partners, including the public, and seeks to persuade people to implement interventions because they lead to valued outcomes. There is an important role here for the evidence-based practitioner to liaise between clients and the research community. Practitioners can disseminate to clients and communities knowledge and skills about the evidence gathering process as well as the evidence itself, and feed back lay concerns to researchers, organizations and colleagues. In order to undertake this role, practitioners need to be confident about their critical appraisal skills. The move to evidence-based, or evidence-informed, practice is already well under way, and offers practitioners the prospect of greater confidence and effectiveness. For clients, it offers the prospect of interventions based on the best available knowledge and evidence, rather than the preoccupations or biases of individual practitioners. However, evidence will only ever be one of several drivers of practice. The role of ethics, ideology, theory and resources as independent drivers of practice will remain, alongside evidence.

FURTHER DISCUSSION

- What are the opportunities and barriers to your profession becoming more evidence based?
- What would you include as evidence in relation to health promotion and public health interventions, and why?
- How important do you think evidence is as a driver of public health and health promotion practice? And how important do you think it should be?

Recommended reading

- Craig J V, Smyth R L (2002) Evidence based practice manual for nurses. Edinburgh, Churchill Livingstone
  An accessible and easy to follow guide to becoming an evidence-based practitioner.
- Davies H T O, Nutley S M, Smith P C (2000) What works? Evidence-based policy and practice in public services. Bristol, The Policy Press
  This readable and comprehensive book provides a useful analysis of the theoretical context in which evidence-based policy and practice are promoted. It also goes on to consider how evidence-based policy and practice are being created and disseminated in different health and welfare fields including health and social care, transport, education, housing, urban renewal and criminal justice.
- Effectiveness Matters. Available from NHS Centre for Reviews and Dissemination, University of York, York YO1 5DD or http://www.york.ac.uk/inst/crd
  Regular summaries of published research on single topics with emphasis on presenting clear messages on effectiveness.
- Oliver S, Peersman G (eds) (1997) Using research for effective health promotion. Maidenhead, Open University Press
  A comprehensive and readable edited book that guides the reader through the processes involved in appraising research. The problems

and dilemmas of using research and evidence in the field of health promotion are debated.

■ Sefton T, Byford S, McDaid D, Hills J, Knapp M (2002) Making the most of it: economic evaluation in the social welfare field. York, Joseph Rowntree Foundation

An interesting and readable introduction to economic evaluation in the social welfare field. Different ways of conducting economic evaluations are outlined and illustrated using relevant case-studies including community development.

■ www.casp.org.uk

The website for the Critical Appraisal Skills Programme provides checklists for how to evaluate different kinds of research studies.

REFERENCES

Campbell R, Pound P, Pope C et al (2003) Evaluating meta-ethnography: a synthesis of qualitative research on lay experiences of diabetes and diabetes care. Social Science and Medicine 56(4): 671–684

Campbell K, Waters E, O'Meara S et al (2004) Interventions for preventing obesity in children (Cochrane Review). In: Cochrane Library issue 1

Cummins S, Macintyre S (2002) 'Food deserts' – evidence and assumption in policy making. British Medical Journal 325: 436–438

Davies H T O, Nutley S M, Smith P C (2000) What works? Evidence-based policy and practice in public services. Bristol, The Policy Press

Donaldson C, Mugford M, Vale L (2002) Evidence based health economics. London, BMJ Books

Ellison G T H, Wiggins M, Stewart R et al (2001) The HIVSA training manual. London: Social Science Research Unit, Institute of Education http://hivsa.ioe.ac.uk/hivsa/

Health Development Agency (2001) Coronary heart disease: guidance for implementing the preventive aspects of the National Service Framework. London, HDA

Heather N (1995) Interpreting the evidence on brief interventions for excessive drinkers: the need for caution. Alcohol and Alcoholism 30: 287–296

Hill A, Brice A, Enock K (2001) Appraising research evidence. In: Pencheon D, Guest C, Melzer D, Muir Gray J A (eds) Oxford handbook of public health practice. Oxford, Oxford University Press

Kaptchuk T J (2003) Effect of interpretive bias on research evidence. British Medical Journal 326: 1453–1455

Macintyre S, Cummins S (2001) Good intentions and received wisdom are not enough. Conference speech Evidence into Practice: Challenges and Opportunities for UK Public Health, April 2001, London, King's Fund/ Health Development Agency. Available at www.hda.nhs.uk/evidence/key. html#eip

McQueen D (2001) Strengthening the evidence base for health promotion. Health Promotion International 16(3): 261–268

Muir Gray J A (2001) Evidence based healthcare: how to make policy and management decisions, 2nd edn. Edinburgh, Churchill Livingstone

Naidoo J, Wills J (2000) Health promotion: foundations for practice, 2nd edn. London, Baillière Tindall

Noblit G W, Hare R D (1988) Meta-ethnography: synthesizing qualitative studies. Newbury Park, CA, Sage

Nutbeam D (1998) Evaluating health promotion: progress, problems and solutions. Health Promotion International 23: 27–44

Oakley A (1998) Experimentation and social interventions: a forgotten but important history. British Medical Journal 317: 1239–1242

Oliver S (2001) Making research more useful: integrating different perspectives and different methods. In: Oliver S, Peersman G (eds) Using research for effective health promotion. Buckingham, Open University

Parrot S, Godfrey C, Raw M et al (1998) Guidance for commissioners on the cost-effectiveness of smoking cessation interventions. Thorax 53 Supplement 5 Part 2: S1–38

Pawson R, Tilley N (1997) Realistic evaluation. London, Sage

Petrosino A, Turpin-Petrosino C, Finckenauer J O (2000) Programs can have harmful effects!: lessons from experiments of programs such as scared straight. Crime & Delinquency 46(1): 354–379

Powell J (2003) Health economics and public health. In: Orme J, Powell J, Taylor P, Harrison T, Grey M (eds) Public health for the 21st century: new perspectives on policy, participation and practice. Maidenhead, Open University Press/McGraw-Hill Education

Sackett D L, Rosenberg W M, Gray J A et al (1996) Evidence-based medicine: what it is and what it isn't. British Medical Journal 150: 1249–1255

Sefton T, Byford S, McDaid D et al (2002) Making the most of it: economic evaluation in the social welfare field. York, Joseph Rowntree Foundation

Speller V, Learmonth A, Harrison D (1997) The search for evidence of effective health promotion. British Medical Journal 315: 361–363

Stevens W, Thorogood M, Kayikki S (2002) Cost effectiveness of a community anti-smoking campaign targeted at a high risk group in London. Health Promotion International 17(1): 43–50

Supplement to American Journal of Preventive Medicine (SAJPM) (2000) Introducing the guide to community preventive services: methods, first recommendations and expert commentary. American Journal of Preventive Medicine 18: 35–43

Tilford S (2000) Evidence based health promotion. Health Education Research 15(6): 659–663

World Health Assembly (WHA) (1998) Resolution WHA 51.12 on Health Promotion. Agenda Item 20, 16 May 1998, Geneva, WHO

4 The policy context

OVERVIEW

The previous chapter has shown how influential the available evidence is in affecting practice. Values and the policy context affect practice in an equally profound way. Although policy may sound remote from practitioners' daily concerns, policies formulated at national, regional and local levels have a major impact in determining practitioners' priorities and ways of working. For example, many practitioners are aware of targets they need to meet, duties to work in certain ways, e.g. involving other agencies and the public as partners, and general principles of transparency and accountability. These issues have all been highlighted by policy making and implementation. Policy formation is a complex process affected by many different factors including political ideology and stakeholders' agendas. Policy implementation is often thought of as an unproblematic administrative matter. However this is not the case. Policy implementation is affected by frontline workers' values and practices, and the same policy is often implemented in diverse ways with a variety of different outcomes. This chapter discusses the range of values underpinning policy formation and implementation, the policy process and key stakeholders, and some of the resulting dilemmas that affect practitioners.

INTRODUCTION

'Policy' is a vague term used in different ways to describe the direction of an organization, a decision to act on a particular problem, or a set of guiding principles directed towards specific goals (Titmuss 1974). The concept of policy therefore operates at different levels, describing both a specific input on a specific topic, and the general values and ethos (the policy context) that inform specific goals and targets. The policy context includes values that are broadly consensual, such as democracy, and also values that are contested, such as managerialism versus professionalism. The policy context is therefore dynamic, charting public debates and the views of different lobbying and interest groups. Traditionally public health policies related to medical policies of disease surveillance and control. The programme of pre-school childhood immunizations and vaccinations and cervical and breast cancer screening programmes are examples of traditional public health policies. The World Health Organization (WHO 1988) defined the main aim of healthy public policy as 'to create a supportive environment to enable people to lead healthy lives'. Most policy areas thus have implications for health. This is a reflection of the many different and complex factors that influence health and illness. Policy areas that impact on health include education, employment, neighbourhood renewal and regeneration, transport, food and housing. At the international level, policies on an equally broad range of topics have a profound impact on health.

Example	The legal and policy frameworks relating to patents and intellectual copyright coupled with policies determining how money is allocated to research and development have led to significant inequalities in health on an international scale. Most funding for new drugs is undertaken with the lucrative markets of the developed world in mind, leading to a proliferation of drugs for conditions which are not life threatening. For example, up to ten viagra substitutes for erectile dysfunction are currently being developed. Meanwhile, life-threatening illnesses, such as AIDS, sleeping sickness and Chagas disease, which affect millions in the developing world, are neglected. People suffering from these neglected diseases are denied access to drugs due to their unaffordable price, and opportunities to develop effective drugs for such diseases are ignored because pharmaceutical companies do not see such activities as sufficiently profitable. This failure of markets and public policies has been highlighted by the World Health Organization and non-governmental agencies such as Médécins Sans Frontières and Oxfam, who are seeking to develop research and development policies that will channel funding into the creation of effective drugs for neglected diseases.
Drugs development and health inequalities	
	Source: Médécins Sans Frontières Access to Essential Medicines Campaign & the Drugs for Neglected Diseases Working Group (2001)

The policy context and broad macroeconomic, environmental and demographic changes are major drivers of public health and health promotion. Practitioners tend to see public policy as beyond their remit, but policy exerts a powerful influence on practice. Changes in national policies directly affect practice and may signal changes in smaller organizations and groups. For example, the 1999 Macpherson Inquiry into the racist murder of British teenager Stephen Lawrence, which highlighted the extent of institutional racism within the Metropolitan police force, caused a number of organizations to examine their own policies and practice and, where necessary, to take action to avoid institutional racism.

Practitioners have to meet specified targets or requirements which have been identified in policy documents, e.g. to reduce waiting times in hospitals, or the requirement on health trusts and boards to work in partnership with local authorities. In some cases, this may mean diverting resources from established and effective practices, or innovative but well thought out strategies, to meet the new targets or goals. In other cases the direction of an organization may be changed because of a new priority. For example, newly created Primary Care Trusts (PCTs) in England now have a duty to oversee public health.

As we outlined in our first book Health Promotion: Foundations for Practice (Naidoo & Wills 2000, Ch. 7) the policy process is shaped by

- ideological beliefs and values
- economic considerations
- political acceptability
- evidence-based research about 'what works'.

Policies are also formed in an arena of multiple interests where stake-holders exert influence and help to shape policy. A stakeholder can be defined as any group or individual that can affect or is affected by the achievement of an organization's purpose.

In the UK opportunities for practitioners to influence policy have increased as a response to the government pledge for more open govern-ment. Consultation is invited on public health policies and strategies. For example, public consultation on the strategy for tackling inequalities in health has resulted in a number of suggestions including getting feedback from practitioners on a variety of issues. These issues include 'what more could be done at local level to improve the responsiveness of NHS primary care services and contribute to the health inequalities targets' (DoH 2001a, p. 39).

Policies are also informed by rational economic and evidence-based prin-ciples. For example, the recent Wanless Review (2002) on funding the NHS outlined three possible future scenarios. The third scenario, the 'fully engaged' model, posits services and a population which is informed and enthusiastic about protecting and promoting its health, and where research is productive in identifying effective communication and implementation of messages. Crucially, this fully engaged model is proposed within the Review as the most effective and lowest cost scenario in the long term. Within this scenario, public health investment is sound economic good sense, because better health leads to more productive employees and a stronger economy.

There have been calls for policy to be based on sound evidence about what works (Cm 4310 1999). However there is a lack of evidence about effective public health and health promotion interventions (Macintyre et al 2001). For example, there is a solid research basis about the existence of inequalities in health, but very little research into comparing the effec-tiveness of different kinds of intervention aimed at tackling inequalities in health. A UK review of evidence-based health policy reported that only 4% of public health research focused on interventions, of which only 10%, or 0.4% of the total, focused on the outcomes of interventions (Milward et al, 2001). In part, this is due to a traditional model of evidence based on individual cases and randomized controlled trials (see Ch. 3). This model is inappropriate for macro policies that are targeted at popu-lations or communities. The evaluation of such policies is complicated because finding control populations that are not exposed to policy is dif-ficult. Evidence-based policy is still in its infancy, due to competing influ-ences and the lack of appropriate evidence.

As we have seen in earlier chapters, practitioners need a solid base on which to practise. The drive to evidence-based practice, quality standards and theory driven interventions should make practitioners feel competent and secure. Yet many feel buffeted by policy initiatives and constant change. Policy takes place in a political arena, and many practitioners feel politics is removed from their core concerns. This may mean they do not engage with the political debates and feel policy makers are divorced from the reality of service delivery. People responsible for implementing policy may not be enthusiastic, and their frontline decisions may be crucial in dissipating the intended effect of policy. Conversely, enthusiastic and committed practi-tioners who feel they have had a valued input into policy formation can play a key role in achieving the intended outcomes of policies. To have a

D iscussion point

What opportunities are there for practitioners to influence policy?

R eflection point

Do you regard yourself as a political practitioner?

voice and be able to impact on policy making and implementation, practitioners need to be familiar with, and able to understand, health policy – its origins, its goals, the process and its effects, both intended and unintended.

UNDERSTANDING THE POLICY PROCESS

Policy making has been defined as 'the process by which governments translate their political vision into programmes and actions to deliver "outcomes" – desired changes in the real world' (Cabinet Office, 1999). National governments set the fundamental policy direction while locally, policies develop incrementally. Walt (1994) identifies four phases in policy making that occur whatever the level, whether national or local, and also shape any policy analysis:

1. *Problem identification and issue recognition.* Why issues get onto the policy agenda; which issues do not get addressed.
2. *Policy formulation.* The goals of the policy; different options are identified and analysed; costs and benefits of alternative policies are weighed up; determining who formulates policy; how and where the initiative comes from.
3. *Policy implementation.* How policies are implemented; what resources are available; how implementation is enforced.
4. *Policy evaluation.* How progress is reviewed; setting up monitoring systems; how and when adaptations are made.

There is an assumption that policy is the result of rational decision making in which choices are evaluated and a solution is chosen to achieve objectives. Yet this rational process rarely takes place. As Simon (1958) argued, real world decision makers are not 'maximizers' who select the best possible course of action but 'satisfiers' who look for the course of action that is good enough for the problem at hand. Sutton (1999) also refers to other models of policy making:

- The incrementalist model, where policies which represent the least possible change are preferred, and policy is a series of small steps which do not fundamentally challenge the status quo.
- The mixed-scanning model, which represents a middle position where a broad view of possibilities is considered before focusing on a small number of options for more investigation.

None of these models describes the policy making process accurately, although each model refers to elements of the process. Policy making mixes the scientific and the pragmatic; the broad vision with the narrow. The degree to which each element contributes to policy making differs according to the general political environment and the specifics of the policy under consideration.

Policy development

To understand the policy process it is important to be familiar with the structure of government. There is a complex process for the development of national policy in England due to the country's constitutional evolution as a democracy. At the national level, a new policy is signalled by the publication of a Green Paper for public consultation and discussion. After consultation and amendment, a White Paper, which is the government's plans for legislation, is published. The policy then enters the parliamentary or legislative process, when the bill is scrutinized and amended by first the House of Commons and then the House of Lords. If the bill is not thrown out at any stage, it goes on to receive the royal assent, and the bill becomes an Act of Parliament. The policy has now become legislation, which agencies are legally bound to follow. This process is illustrated in detail in Figure 4.1.

Figure 4.1 The policy process
Source: Blakemore K (2003) Social policy: an introduction, 2nd edn. Reproduced by permission of Open University Press

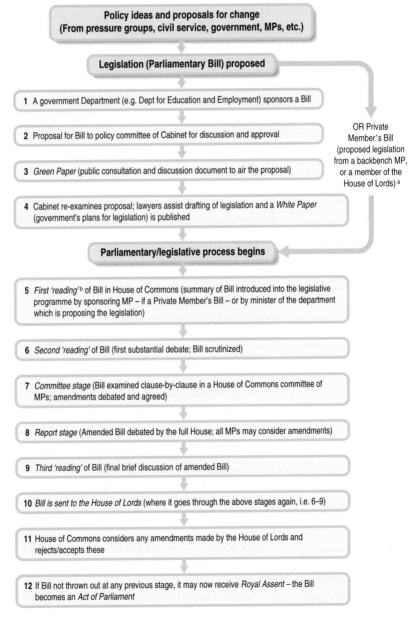

Policy ideas and proposals for change
(From pressure groups, civil service, government, MPs, etc.)

Legislation (Parliamentary Bill) proposed

1 A government Department (e.g. Dept for Education and Employment) sponsors a Bill

2 Proposal for Bill to policy committee of Cabinet for discussion and approval

3 *Green Paper* (public consultation and discussion document to air the proposal)

4 Cabinet re-examines proposal; lawyers assist drafting of legislation and a *White Paper* (government's plans for legislation) is published

OR Private Member's Bill (proposed legislation from a backbench MP, or a member of the House of Lords) [a]

Parliamentary/legislative process begins

5 *First 'reading'* [b] of Bill in House of Commons (summary of Bill introduced into the legislative programme by sponsoring MP – if a Private Member's Bill – or by minister of the department which is proposing the legislation)

6 *Second 'reading'* of Bill (first substantial debate; Bill scrutinized)

7 *Committee stage* (Bill examined clause-by-clause in a House of Commons committee of MPs; amendments debated and agreed)

8 *Report stage* (Amended Bill debated by the full House; all MPs may consider amendments)

9 *Third 'reading'* of Bill (final brief discussion of amended Bill)

10 *Bill is sent to the House of Lords* (where it goes through the above stages again, i.e. 6–9)

11 House of Commons considers any amendments made by the House of Lords and rejects/accepts these

12 If Bill not thrown out at any previous stage, it may now receive *Royal Assent* – the Bill becomes an *Act of Parliament*

Notes:
[a] a Private Member's Bill may be introduced to either the House of Commons or the House of Lords, but must be passed by both Houses irrespective of where it starts. Government-proposed legislation almost always begins in the House of Commons
[b] Bills are not literally read out clause-by-clause.

Numerous factors affect the way in which policy is finally developed and implemented:

- situational: local or timely factors
- cultural: the values and ideologies dominant in the political environment
- structural: the political system and its processes.

Example

Stakeholders' influence on policy direction

In July 1997 the Minister for Public Health in England announced that there would be legislation to control tobacco advertising following the Labour Party's manifesto pledge. By November 1997 the government had decided to exempt Formula One racing from this ban, arguing that prestigious sporting events might be lost to the UK. It emerged that a major sponsor of racing, Bernie Ecclestone, had given substantial funds to the Labour Party. The money was subsequently returned but it was not until May 1998 and a European Union vote to ban all tobacco promotion that the UK government agreed to phase out tobacco sponsorship of sporting events by 2005.

This example illustrates the way in which policy reflects a pluralistic society of multiple interests where groups exercise influence. Some decisions are incremental, muddling through adaptations to circumstances, rather than contributions to strategic direction.

Issue recognition

For policy to be approved and enacted, an issue has first to become relevant and identified as a problem. In general there are three ways in which issues can get onto an agenda:

- following action by community groups leading to a groundswell of public opinion
- initiated by organizations or agencies concerned with the issue
- By key political figures who then mobilise support.

In addition, key incidents may also provide the trigger for gaining support and momentum for a policy, especially if they receive widespread media coverage and spark off a public debate.

Issue recognition, or agenda setting, relies on:

- problem definition
- receptive environment
- policy proposal.

Discussion point

The UK government has identified teenage pregnancy as a major priority and developed a national strategy (Social Exclusion Unit 1999). Why was this identified as a policy problem?

Although epidemiological evidence shows a rising trend in teenage pregnancy in the UK with high abortion rates and associated risks of infant and maternal morbidity, a major driver was that teenage pregnancy disproportionately affects the poorest areas and the most vulnerable young people. The government commitment to tackling social inequalities and social exclusion meant that teenage pregnancy was part of broader policy objectives. Teenage pregnancy was therefore defined as a problem on several grounds including health, inequalities and economic. The ideological commitment to strengthening the family in order to rebuild communitarian values also meant a receptive environment where tackling the issue was seen as important. The preconditions were therefore set to ensure a policy proposal could be successfully made. In most instances there is rarely a single policy decision but a framework that shapes direction.

There is an increasing international dimension in which the European Union and World Health Organization may set international agreements. For example, the World Health Organization's first public health treaty, the Framework Convention on Tobacco Control, was agreed in 2003 (WHO 2003). It covers taxation, illicit trade, advertising and sponsorship. Globalization may offer new opportunities for cooperation in public health, but it can also inhibit healthy public policy.

Globalization has led to increased production of food and also enhanced the power of manufacturers and retailers at the expense of primary producers. Food producers are reliant on selling their products to a dwindling number of global companies, who can set their own terms and conditions. This has led to a loss of biodiversity as companies specify a limited number of crops for world markets. Whilst food scarcity is no longer an issue for the developed world, developing countries may still face food scarcity as the demand for cash crops means a loss of land available for subsistence farming. The concentration of power in the hands of a small number of global food outlets, such as McDonalds, has been blamed for contributing to an increase in unhealthy diets and the loss of home grown and home cooked products.

Globalization therefore has ambiguous effects on national goals for healthy eating. While the 5-a-day programme is facilitated by the year-long availability of fruit and vegetables, the increased reliance on manufactured and pre-cooked food with high levels of sugar, salt and saturated fats contributes to the rise of obesity and associated health problems. Yeatman (2003) argues that local food projects such as community gardens or lunch clubs are popular with local practitioners but marginal to mainstream political concerns. Local projects are acceptable and serve to divert interest away from significant issues such as the influence of global commercial food companies. Globalization has more negative effects on developing countries, for while it may foster economic growth and trade, local capacity to feed people may be lost.

The public policy environment inevitably involves struggles for power and influence in which politicians, civil servants, the media and pressure groups may try to achieve their preferred ends. One problem with public health policy is that it is not usually seen as being newsworthy. Long-term investments in health which prevent illness or disability are not as attractive to the media as topical scandals or 'feelgood' stories focused on high technology medical services and individual patients. For example, the coverage of the introduction of congestion charging in London, intended as a public health measure to reduce car use, has focused on local objections to the extra 'taxation' and stories of the effect on livelihoods. An exception to this type of coverage is the resurgence of interest in public health protection and hazard management in the wake of the 9/11 terrorist attacks in the USA in 2001 and the war in Iraq in 2003.

D iscussion point

What examples are there where increased globalization has acted against national goals for healthy eating?

Baum (2001) has shown how power is exercised in various ways and how the decision-making process can be manipulated so that certain issues are not even raised. In Australia the professional medical lobby and the private health insurance lobby are so powerful that they can ensure that the concept of an exclusively public health insurance scheme is not raised. In other cases, powerful stakeholder groups may present arguments that tap into popular sentiments and lobby support for resisting public health measures.

Discussion point	The following policies appear to be rational and effective but have not been implemented. Why not?
	<ul><li>Asylum seekers being allowed to work.</li><li>Private car owners and users pay proportionately more than those with no access to private cars for the cost of road upkeep and safety and pollution control.</li><li>Fluoridation of water.</li></ul>

In each of these cases, powerful interest groups have lobbied successfully against the introduction of policies. Appeals to individual choice and popular nationalist sentiments, and against a 'nanny state' that imposes policies, were used to counteract the arguments put forward in support of these policies.

Policy formulation

Once an issue is on the public agenda, there is an opportunity for stakeholders to influence any resulting policies. There is no single method of doing this. Baggott (2000) identifies three models of stakeholder influence on the policy process:

1. Institutional politics – policy results from the interaction of different institutions and policy networks that include pressure groups as well as government agencies. This suggests a process where consensus is arrived at through negotiation and compromise.

2. Pressure-group politics – policy results from different stakeholders and pressure groups which seek to mobilise public support through the media and direct action. Policy is not a result of consensus but more a product of the most powerful vested interests. For example, the extension of drinking hours in licensed premises has been supported by commercial licensing bodies and alcoholic drinks manufacturers, although many civic groups fear the consequences for public order and public health practitioners predict an increase in alcohol-related problems.

3. Policy knowledge and policy learning – policy results from the knowledge and experience of experts and interested parties. An example is expert committees which are set up to gather evidence to input into the policy process. This suggests a rational, scientific process driven by a clear evidence base. For example, an independent expert committee reported in 1999 to ministers, who in 2000 published the *Review of the*

Mental Health Act 1983 (DoH 2000) which sought to balance the need to protect the rights of individual patients with the need to ensure public safety. This review led to the draft Mental Health Bill 2002 which, having been through a consultation process, is currently (Spring 2004) awaiting legislation in parliament when it will become the new Mental Health Act. Scotland has a new Mental Health (Care and Treatment) Act 2003, which will come into effect in 2005.

Discussion point

How might practitioners have a say in policy formulation?

Practitioners may be involved in professional, civic or voluntary pressure groups lobbying for particular public health policies. Lobbying may involve individual action (e.g. writing to MPs), collective action (e.g. local demonstrations or petitions) or coordinated and funded media campaigns. Professional associations will have an expert view that is often sought and represented to government at the policy consultation stage.

Policies occur at many different levels. The UK government has stressed the need for 'joined up' or cross cutting policy to tackle health and social issues. The government's policy direction is underpinned by an understanding of the wider determinants of health and that the well-being of the population does not lie solely within the role of the health services. Addressing public health requires cross government, cross department focus and cross cutting policies which relate to sectors as varied as agriculture, economics, education, transport and the environment are essential. Colebatch (1998) has suggested that policy may be vertical – where those in positions of authority transmit decisions downwards for implementation – or horizontal, where those outside authority are important in mobilizing opinion and lobbying. Much of the government's public health policy is focused on interagency working and partnerships between different agencies to tackle health problems (see Ch. 7).

Policy implementation

Once a policy has been made, it is often assumed that the implementation stage is a non-problematic, administrative manner. However, many commentators have pointed out that implementation is a separate activity where policies are reinforced, changed or even sabotaged by frontline workers – the street level bureaucrats identified by Lipsky (1980). Street level bureaucrats are relatively low level employees who have considerable discretion in how they operate and who act as an interface between the public and the organization. Examples of street level bureaucrats are teachers, police officers, social workers, environmental health officers and health practitioners. Street level bureaucrats tend to be public service employees working in organizations with the following characteristics:

- demand outstrips supply
- resources are inadequate
- goals are ambiguous, vague or conflicting
- measuring employee performance to meet goals is difficult or impossible
- clients are typically non-voluntary and therefore are not a primary reference group for the organization.

In such situations, 'the decisions of street level bureaucrats, the routines they establish, and the devices they invent to cope with pressure, effectively become the public policy they carry out' (Lipsky 1980, p. xii).

Example	Many organizations are committed to anti-discriminatory practice. One practitioner comments, 'We provide individual advice and counselling on benefits and housing issues, and our services are not well used by our local Black and Asian communities. Everyone knows that's because people from these communities like to look after their own and deal with things within the family. When someone from these communities does come through the door, they're treated the same as anyone else. That to me is being non-discriminatory; not even noticing if they're White, Black, whatever. Then we had a training session, and were told we had to treat people from Black and minority ethnic groups differently, provide interpreters, give them extra time, do outreach work. To me, that is discriminatory and not being fair to our local White population. I still treat everyone as an individual and they all get the same service.'
The implementation gap	

The example above illustrates how, unless frontline practitioners are persuaded of the need to change their practice, they can effectively derail an organization's stated policies and intentions. Evaluation of the training session should have shown that additional inputs were required if staff were to be persuaded by the argument that, in order to provide an equal service for all, inputs to different communities may need to be unequal. Staff also need to be made aware of research findings that show people from black and minority ethnic groups do want access to services but are put off by barriers such as language and not knowing what is available.

At the local level, policies may be imposed on practitioners rather than developed with them so they may be subverted or even ignored to suit practitioners' ends. For example, Primary Care Trusts (PCTs) in England have received a number of policy directives and targets but without clear direction of how to achieve these.

Example	The National Service Framework (NSF) for diabetes set standards to improve services, to prevent diabetes in the population as a whole and to improve the identification of people with diabetes. A delivery strategy sets targets to be met by 2006:
National Service Framework for diabetes	

- All PCTs should be screening at least 80% of diabetes patients for diabetic retinopathy.
- All GP practices should have a register of patients with diabetes and at risk of CHD.
- All PCTs should have a diabetes network with a local patient as 'champion'.

In relation to prevention, however, decisions will be made locally. There is, for example, no guidance on screening of at-risk groups and how these should be defined. No money is earmarked to deliver the NSF and so there is likely to be some local jostling for money.

The division between policy formation and implementation – the implementation gap – is useful to both practitioners and policy makers. It allows practitioners to retain a degree of freedom and autonomy which is valued as part of the professional identity. In reality, practitioners may still refer to experience and hands-on knowledge to inform their practice rather than the latest policy directive. The implementation gap is also useful to policy makers as it allows them to blame any failures on those responsible for implementation.

Resources are crucial to the success or otherwise of policies. Most policies depend on the allocation of resources to enable their successful implementation. Setting policies without adequate resourcing means failure or other policies not being implemented as resources are diverted from them. Unless funding is ring-fenced, there is always a danger that available resources will be used to meet the current priorities of the organization. In a situation of rationed resources, the 'must haves' of key performance targets will always override the more innovative, long-term but high-risk projects.

Policy evaluation

Following implementation, policies should be evaluated to determine their impact, and this evaluation should feed back into the policy-making process. It is sometimes argued that the evaluation stage is often lacking. Policy implementation and impact may be audited, but long-term in-depth evaluation of policies is unusual. This is partly due to the complexities and difficulties of trying to evaluate policies that are intended to change practice everywhere and in a wholesale manner. There has been a plethora of health policies implemented following New Labour's election in 1997. This has led to the phenomenon of 'interventionitis' whereby practitioners are deluged by the number of new interventions, each with their own funding, criteria and targets.

Reflection point
Is there any formal evaluation (as opposed to audit) of policies affecting your work?

Reflection point
In your practice area, is the phenomenon of 'interventionitis' familiar? If it is, how do people respond to and cope with the demands this makes?

Practitioner talking	*Everywhere I go senior management tell me of progress, of targets reached and objectives met, of value for money and of real change. Everywhere I go, I also see another world – a world of daily crisis, of staff under pressure, of people working with few resources and services struggling to deliver. In this world of everyone else there is stress and low morale.*

There is often a profound implementation gap between policy and practice with a difference on the ground between senior enthusiasts who are the change agents; sceptics who tend to be the managers with a history of working in a different way and those on the front line who may feel overloaded and unable to cope with the sheer volume and pace of change. One response is to retreat into protectionism or a silo mentality whereby practitioners seek to protect their own sphere of influence and existing areas of autonomy.

VALUES AND POLICY

Policy is not primarily an empirical or pragmatic process of assessing evidence and identifying effective options, although such rational concerns may feed into the policy process. Instead, policy is clearly driven by underlying values. A value is 'an enduring belief that a specific mode of conduct or end-state of existence is personally or socially preferable' (Rokeach 1973, p. 5). In *Health Promotion: Foundations for Practice* (Naidoo & Wills 2000) we discussed the way in which certain values may influence the way in which people practise. In Chapter 1 we showed how assimilation of specific professional values is included within professional training and the adoption of a professional identity. This may relate to goals (e.g. quality of life) or certain types of behaviour (e.g. respecting clients' wishes, treating people with respect). In any society, but especially in a diverse democracy such as Britain, there will be a broad range of values that people hold with regard to these specific issues. Different groups will hold different values with respect to these topics, and often (but not always) there will be coherent groupings of value positions. Ideology is the term used to describe a coherent body of interrelated ideas and values.

The development of public health reflects different political ideologies and political systems. (These are discussed in Naidoo Wills 2000, Ch. 7.) There are alternative positions on:

- the role of the individual and that of the state
- the nature and extent of the ties that bind communities
- whether or not the economy should be managed or controlled
- the extent of legitimate state intervention in people's lives.

The spectrum of political values which underpin policy has been characterized in many different ways, and ranges from socialist to individualist, and from *laisser-faire* economics to green environmentalism to managed economies (Baggott 2000). At one end (the far right) of the spectrum are those advocating free market economics, individual liberties and minimal state regulation. At the opposite end (the far left) are those supporting a regulated economy, collective responsibilities and active state intervention. The middle ground, which New Labour in the UK has tried to colonize as its 'third way', embodies values of individual rights, duties and responsibilities as well as social justice and fairness. In the field of economics, a generally free economic market is tempered by social constraints and welfare expenditure on key services and the encouragement of joint private–public initiatives. Public sector services are to be strengthened by firm performance management coupled with a simultaneous move to devolved services, a shift from the centralized hierarchical structure or market competition of the late twentieth century.

Example

The Third Way – key values

- **Active civil society** to combat political indifference suggested by low voter turnout, e.g. teaching citizenship in schools.
- **Communitarianism** to try to rebuild societal links, e.g. New Deal for Communities.
- **Democratic family** to give stability, e.g. more generous paternity and adoption leave as well as maternity leave.
- **Mixed economy** to encourage private funding of public services, e.g. Private Finance Initiative and foundation hospitals within the NHS.

E continued

■ **Equality as inclusion** – equality of opportunity rather than equality of outcome, e.g. support for looked-after young people and children.
■ **Positive welfare** and opportunity rather than the over-dependency fostered by a commitment to protect citizens from the cradle to the grave, e.g. the establishment of the minimum wage.
■ **Cosmopolitan nation** celebrating diversity, e.g. organizations committed to equal opportunities and anti-discrimination policies.

Source: Giddens (1998)

These values give rise to specific strategies or policies:

■ public involvement – greater user participation and involvement in services
■ increased investment in public services
■ mixed economy – growing involvement of the private sector in public services
■ devolved services allowing local flexibility and freedom, with additional 'earned autonomy' for best performing services
■ quality assurance through clear standards and performance criteria
■ partnership working to erode professional barriers and enable the delivery of seamless services
■ a positive focus on disadvantaged or excluded groups
■ community focus to build capacity and encourage communities to be active providers as well as users of services
■ leadership qualities of vision, flexibility and adaptability are valued above the old style bureaucratic managerialism.

R eflection point

How many of these terms are you familiar with from your workplace? How are they interpreted and used within your workplace?

Short-term funding can be used to kick-start innovative projects but it may also lead to continued marginalization of such work, which remains on the fringes of mainstream services. Short-term funding does not facilitate long-term planning. In the UK many community projects, e.g. Healthy Living Centres, are funded by the National Lottery. In the bidding process organizations and agencies will be competing with one another when one critierion for a successful bid is the ability to work in partnership.

Contemporary debates and dilemmas

One way of viewing policy is as the arena where competing ideological values jostle for dominance (George & Wilding 1985, Malin et al 2002). There are several areas where currently different ideological values compete for dominance in the policy arena. An understanding of these helps the practitioner to identify an individual policy's drivers in terms of values, ideology and natural advocates. This will help the practitioner to reflect on their own value position and the logical interconnectedness (or not) of different policies. In practical terms the practitioner may then be better able to lobby for support for a preferred policy. Such reflection will also enable practitioners to identify those policies where they feel most motivated and committed, and able to implement policies in an effective manner.

Individual responsibility versus collectivity

- To what extent are people in charge of their own destiny?
- To what extent are people bound together through ties of kinship and community?
- What are the proper limits to individual self-determination and agency?
- How can the needs of individuals and communities be balanced?

There has been a shift in the UK from the Thatcherite Conservative ideology espousing individual free will towards New Labour's focus on collective responsibility. The Conservative ideology has been much criticized for the implication in health terms that individuals get the health status they deserve, and that individual freely chosen lifestyles are the prime determinant of health. Recognition of socially patterned inequalities in health and seeing individuals as one partner amongst many (including communities and the state) is a hallmark of New Labour's ideological standpoint.

Discussion point

One element of forthcoming Labour Party policy is to ask smokers and overweight people to sign contracts with their doctors to quit smoking and lose weight. Although there is no intention to withhold treatment as a result, it is intended to serve as a reminder to people that they must act responsibly in relation to public service use.

Are there examples from your practice of an increased emphasis on responsibility?

Equality versus inclusion

- Should our focus be on equal outcomes, or equal opportunities to participate?

A fundamental tenet of social democracy in the UK is to focus on equal opportunities. The current emphasis is to stress the need to combat social exclusion and develop an active citizenship. Equal outcomes through, for example, greater entitlement to more generous benefits has been rejected as creating welfare dependency. Instead, the focus has been on strategies designed to bring marginalized and excluded communities into the mainstream of society. There are numerous policies aimed at doing this, including economic and employment policies that make employment more economically beneficial than welfare. In the health field, initiatives such as Health Action Zones, Healthy Living Centres and Sure Start programmes are designed to target excluded groups.

Discussion point

What are the advantages and disadvantages of focusing on equal opportunities to participate rather than equal outcomes?

Proponents of inclusive policies argue that such an approach is empowering and enables people to fulfil their own potential and make choices about their lives. A criticism of such policies is that they do not necessarily reduce inequalities. The section on poverty and income in Chapter 5 discusses the problems associated with a strategy of inclusion that uses geographical targeting based on socio-economic indicators (see p. 101).

Consumerism versus empowerment

- Should the public be viewed as consumers, with the limited power that implies, or should their views shape the services we have?

Reflection point

Do you think your workplace subscribes to a consumerist or empowerment view of service users? What policies or practices support your view?

Chapter 6 discusses the current drive to involve patients and the public. One explanation for this is to see service users as primarily consumers. Services need to provide information which enables consumers to make a choice in health care – hence the plethora of comparative data showing how services perform in relation to set targets. Services need to be responsive to local views so that they are appropriately used. However, critics argue that such information does not provide an adequate basis on which to compare quality of service, merely number crunching statistics. Genuine empowerment, such as service users' decision making at executive level, is often resisted by organizations and professionals on the grounds that service users have specific concerns and lack the necessary strategic overview. Policies which embody the consumerist notion of users include the replacement of the independent Community Health Councils, which had the power of scrutiny over the NHS, with the Patients' Advocacy and Liaison Service, which is not as independent or broad in scope (the power of scrutiny has been transferred to local authorities).

Partnership versus professionalism

- Should professional identities and skills be protected?
- Or should there be moves to interprofessional working and strategic partnerships?

Reflection point

What is your experience of strategic partnerships? What factors contribute to the success of such partnerships?

Chapter 7 discusses the challenges of partnership working. Partnerships require partners to respect each other's views and skills and recognize that each brings equal value to the partnership. However, many professionals are unclear as to the role and skills of other professionals, especially if they are employed by different organizations. They may feel defensive about their own territory and remit.

The drive for partnership working may be interpreted as another attack on professionals' expertise in a situation where they already feel beleaguered by managerialism, evidence-based practice and shifting policy imperatives. However, the arguments for partnership working – to provide coherent and seamless services that meet clients' needs without duplication – are very sound. Genuine partnership working need not mean a dilution of professional expertise. What partnership working does require is the recognition and valuing of areas of knowledge and expertise of other professionals, practitioners and service users.

Need versus rationing

- How can the idea of universal needs that deserve to be met be reconciled with the reality of a limited budget and rationing of services?

One strategy is to define core services and aspects of such service provision as universal, implying universal needs that deserve to be met in a similar way throughout the country. Examples of such policies are the National Service Frameworks which outline what service users can expect of services for different conditions (such as coronary heart disease) or population groups (such as older people). However, in reality funding is always limited and hard decisions have to be taken about which services to fund and which to withhold. One casualty of rationing is infertility and reproductive services, which have been rationed and withdrawn in various areas at different times as a result of funding constraints. This dilemma is likely to become more problematic due to the ageing population, as it is generally accepted that an ageing population will have a greater level of health and social care needs. Already there have been instances of ageist policies and practices when service providers have been accused of failing to meet elderly clients' needs solely on account of their age. Chapter 6 discusses how public involvement has been extended to priority setting for health care services.

Managerialism versus professionalism

- Should services be controlled by management or professionals?
- Which form of authority is most transparent and trustworthy?

> **R**eflection point
>
> Within your workplace, do managers or professions wield the most power? Is the balance of power static or a constantly shifting battleground?

The new modernization agenda in the UK appears to prioritize managerialism over professionalism. Strategies such as performance targets and quality audits are intended to make practice transparent and accountable. While these aims are laudable, it is questionable whether the increasing use of numerical data actually provides the relevant information. Professionals complain that such monitoring leads to a 'tick box' mentality where quantity is valued over quality. This shift has been widely interpreted as an attack on professional autonomy.

Centralized versus devolved services

- Should health and social care services be nationally run?
- Or should the planning and delivery of services be locally organized?

There is a tension between providing centralised services that are the same for everyone, and providing locally sensitive services which may then vary nationwide. Equity underpins the NHS and is part of its perennial popularity – the same service for everyone, according to need not social or geographical status. Yet local services which are responsive to local circumstances are also popular and a politically sensitive issue. At least one local election has been fought and won on the issue of retaining a local hospital threatened with closure. *Shifting the Balance of Power* (DoH 2001b) is one example of devolving decision making as Primary Care Trusts take over the commissioning of local services and will eventually control 75% of the NHS budget. The existence of pressures to both centralize decision making and devolve services may make it difficult for practitioners to work in a way that supports both strategies. Practitioners may end up feeling torn between contradictory demands and as a consequence become demoralized and disillusioned.

Example	Health visitors have a long history of research-based practice to promote health. They are skilled in assessing needs and working in partnership with clients and other agencies. Recent changes in the drive for cost minimization have led to more health visitors becoming involved in management roles supervising skills-mix teams, and less involved in client contact. This has led in some instances to notable reductions in the degree of client take-up of community-based health programmes such as paediatric resuscitation training and antenatal care – an indicator of building community capacity and reducing inequalities. Thus the two policies – cost minimization and tackling inequalities – conflict with each other in practice, leading to stress and demoralization amongst the practitioners responsible for implementing both policies.

Source: Ahmad & Broussine (2003)

CONCLUSION

The policy context is one of the most important factors affecting practitioners' focus, priorities and workload. Although the policy process may appear to be remote from everyday work, this chapter has sought to demonstrate that practitioners can have an impact on policy through professional and local lobbying groups and research evidence. Policy is often presented as a rational result of weighing up the evidence, but this chapter has underlined the importance of values and ideology in the policy process. Practitioners who reflect on their own values and ideological position will be able to locate policies in terms of underpinning values, and also to identify stakeholders' views and positions. This understanding will enable practitioners to maximize their input through effective lobbying with like-minded partners.

Policies may set the overall context and direction, but there is ample scope for local and individual flexibility in the frontline implementation of policies. An understanding of the power relationships of key partners enables practitioners to reflect on their own and others' contribution to policy implementation. For the reflective practitioner, an understanding of how the policy process works and impacts on day-to-day work is fundamental for enhancing effectiveness. Policy, alongside theory, research and evidence, is a key driver for public health and health promotion practice. While there are links between all these elements, policy may also act as an independent and value-based driver for practice.

FURTHER DISCUSSION

- In what ways, both positive and negative, does policy affect your practice?
- Policy is a preferred driver for practice when compared to:
  a. economic cost-effectiveness criteria
  b. professional experience and knowledge.

  Critically discuss this statement.
- Consider an organization with which you are familiar. How, if at all, is policy resisted or transformed on the 'frontline'?

Recommended reading

- Malin N, Wilmot S, Manthorpe J (2002) Key concepts and debates in health and social policy. Maidenhead, Open University Press.

  A very useful text that identifies key social policy concepts and explores their relevance for health and professional practice. It examines ideologies of welfare using examples of recent policy shifts.

- Baggott R (2000) Public health: policy and politics. Basingstoke, Macmillan.

  An overview of public health policies which examines the history and current context for public health policies before discussing broad policy areas which impact on public health.

- Blakemore K (2003) Social policy: an introduction, 2nd edn. Maidenhead, Open University Press.

  An excellent introduction to the field of social policy, written in an accessible and user-friendly manner. Theoretical concepts and perspectives are discussed and key policy areas such as education, employment, housing and health are examined in greater detail.

- Hunter D (2003) Public health policy. Oxford, Polity Press.

  This book provides an overview of key debates about public health policy in the UK and the response of public health professionals.

REFERENCES

Ahmad Y, Broussine M (2003) The UK public sector modernization agenda – reconciliation and renewal? Public Management Review 5(1): 45–62

Baggott R (2000) Public health: policy and politics. Basingstoke, Macmillan

Baum F (2001) Health, equity, justice and globalization: some lessons from the People's Health Assembly. Journal of Epidemiology and Community Health 55: 613–616

Blakemore K (2003) Social policy: an introduction, 2nd edn. Maidenhead, Open University Press

Cabinet Office – Strategic Policy Making Team (1999) Professional policy making for the twentyfirst century. London, Cabinet Office

Cm 4310 (1999) White Paper: modernizing government, presented to parliament by the prime minister and the minister for the Cabinet Office by command of Her Majesty. London, The Stationery Office

Colebatch H K (1998) Policy. Maidenhead, Open University Press

Department of Health (DoH) (2000) Review of the Mental Health Act 1983. London, The Stationery Office

Department of Health (DoH) (2001a) Tackling health inequalities: consultation on a plan for delivery. London, DoH

Department of Health (DoH) (2001b) Shifting the balance of power: securing delivery. London, The Stationery Office

George V, Wilding P (1985) Ideology and social welfare. London, Routledge

Giddens A (1998) The third way: the renewal of social democracy. Cambridge, Polity Press.

Lipsky M (1980) Street-level bureaucracy: dilemmas of the individual in public services. New York, Russell Sage Foundation

Macintyre S, Chalmers I, Horton R, Smith R (2001) Using evidence to inform health policy: case study. British Medical Journal 322: 222–225

Malin N, Wilmot S, Manthorpe J (2002) Key concepts and debates in health and social policy. Maidenhead, Open University Press

Médécins Sans Frontières Access to Essential Medicines Campaign and the Drugs for Neglected Diseases Working Group (2001) Fatal imbalance: the crisis in research and development for drugs for neglected diseases. Geneva, Médécins sans Frontières

Milward L, Kelly M, Nutbeam D (2001) Public health intervention research: the evidence. London, Health Development Agency

Naidoo J, Wills J (2000) Health promotion: foundations for practice, 2nd edn. London, Baillière Tindall

Rokeach M (1973) Understanding human values. New York, The Free Press

Simon H (1958) The role of expectations in an adaptive or behavioristic model. In: Bowman M J (ed) Expectations, uncertainty and business behavior. New York, Social Science Council

Social Exclusion Unit (1999) Teenage pregnancy, Cm 4342. London, The Stationery Office

Sutton R (1999) The policy process: an overview, working paper 118. London, Overseas Development Institute

Titmuss R M (1974) Social policy. London, Allen & Unwin

Walt G (1994) Health policy: an introduction to process and power. London, Zed Books

Wanless D (2002) Securing our future health: taking a long-term view. Final report. London, HM Treasury

World Health Organization (WHO) (1988) Second International Conference on Health Promotion. Adelaide, South Australia

World Health Organization (WHO) (2003) Framework convention on tobacco control, A56/8. Geneva, WHO

Yeatman H R (2003) Food and nutrition policy at the local level: key factors that influence the policy development process. Critical Public Health 13(2): 125–138

2 Strategies for Public Health and Health Promotion Practice

INTRODUCTION

Part 1 has explored the drivers for public health and health promotion practice, including theoretical frameworks, research and the growing evidence base, and the policy context and underlying values that inform policies. Part 2 goes on to explore core strategies that are used in health promotion and public health. Strategy is defined as a plan of action that specifies how targets and goals are to be achieved. Health promotion and public health goals are varied and include maximizing the potential for health and well-being, the appropriate provision and use of services, and reducing mortality and ill health. Part 2 identifies four key strategies that contribute towards the achievement of these goals: tackling health inequalities, the participation and involvement of patients, users and the public, partnership working, and the provision of information, education and communication. These strategies (amongst others) have been identified in many international and national health policy documents (e.g. WHO 1986, DoH 2001a, 2001b) as the means whereby health promotion and public health goals can be translated into practice. As such, they embody core values, identified as equity, empowerment and collaboration.

Equity, defined as equal opportunity for all and social justice, was cited as a fundamental prerequisite for health by the World Health Organization (WHO 1985). Tackling health inequalities, defined as avoidable and unjust health differences, is a central UK government health strategy (DoH 2001b). Health inequalities targets have been set in a number of different areas, and tackling inequalities has been specified as a strategy contributing to the achievement of other targets and goals, e.g. the National Service Frameworks. The aim is to improve health by focusing on the most disadvantaged and deprived groups in society, rather than the simpler and easier option of improving health by addressing the most advantaged groups. Whilst many practitioners may feel sympathetic towards the underlying ethical value – equity – the required focus on the most disadvantaged groups is challenging and may sit uneasily alongside training in the provision of universal services. Chapter 5 seeks to demonstrate how practitioners can tackle inequalities in health effectively, and why tackling inequalities is a central strategy at the level of personal service delivery as well as at central government policy level.

The World Health Organization has defined health as:

> the extent to which an individual or group is able, on the one hand, to realize aspirations and satisfy needs; and, on the other hand, to change or cope with the environment. Health is, therefore, seen as a resource for everyday life, not an object of living; it is a positive concept emphasizing social and personal resources, as well as physical capacities.
>
> (WHO 1984)

Implicit within this statement is the need for information and participation in order to achieve health. Information and participation are also necessary to achieve empowerment, defined as a central goal and principle of health promotion (Tones 2001). Public participation and involvement is a key strategy for service delivery in any democracy. Robust strategies for participation and involvement ensure that services are appropriate, accessible and meet needs. Public participation and involvement also facilitates the accountability of health professionals and managers and is a mechanism to ensure services are answerable to the public who fund the services through their taxes. Participation and involvement have been recognized in many government policies and documents (e.g. DoH 2001a). Whilst practitioners may feel that participation is not an issue for community face-to-face services, Chapter 6 seeks to demonstrate the relevance and feasibility of participation strategies for everyone. Ensuring the effective participation and involvement of local communities helps to maximize the impact of service provision. Being aware of this issue, and having the skills to achieve participation, is fast becoming part of every health practitioner's repertoire.

Collaboration or partnership working is recognized as a key strategy to effectively address the multidisciplinary nature of health and the multi-agency nature of relevant service providers. In the UK the historical separation of health from other social care services has had negative effects in terms of duplication of work and service providers focusing on compartmentalized aspects of health instead of addressing health in holistic terms. The separation of responsibilities and functions can also make it hard for clients to access appropriate services. Partnership working has been identified as the solution to these problems, facilitating seamless services that meet people's needs effectively and efficiently. Working in partnerships is often assumed to be an unproblematic aspect of practice, but research and experience show it requires dedicated resources and specific skills. Working in partnerships is becoming a recognized part of the core training and education for health and social care practitioners. Chapter 7 discusses how partnership working can be facilitated and supported and identifies the resulting benefits.

The provision of information, education and communication is the fourth key strategy to be identified and discussed in Part 2. Access to appropriate information is a crucial aspect of health promotion and public health. People can only make voluntary informed choices, and thus exert power and self-efficacy, if they have access to relevant materials. The explosion of information networking and availability via the internet has demonstrated that people want information and want to be able to make informed choices. The public is bombarded with information about health matters, ranging from expert or government sponsored messages to commercial product marketing and entertainment. Such information varies widely in its accuracy, scope and persuasiveness. Health practitioners remain trusted and valued sources of information, and they have a responsibility to inform clients of relevant, up to date findings and knowledge on matters of interest. Chapter 8 discusses how practitioners can communicate effectively with clients and provide accessible and appropriate information and education.

Together, the four chapters in Part 2 discuss core strategies for health promotion and public health and explore how practitioners can most effectively use and contribute to such strategies. Policies may specify strategies and place duties on practitioners to adopt such strategies; but the degree to which this is acted upon varies widely. Part 2 aims to encourage practitioners to use strategies proactively for public health and health promotion. Each chapter discusses the strategy in the context of UK public health and health promotion policy and includes examples of good practice. We hope the chapters in Part 2 will stimulate practitioners to reflect on their potential to use the four key strategies, and to incorporate such strategies into their everyday practice.

REFERENCES

Department of Health (DoH) (2001a) The expert patient: a new approach to chronic disease management for the 21st century. London, DoH

Department of Health (DoH) (2001b) Tackling health inequalities: consultation on a plan for delivery. London, The Stationery Office

Tones K (2001) Health promotion: the empowerment imperative. In: Scriven A, Orme J (eds) Health promotion: professional perspectives. Basingstoke, Palgrave PPI ref.

World Health Organization (WHO) (1984) Health promotion: a discussion document on the concept and principles. Copenhagen, WHO Regional Office for Europe

World Health Organization (WHO) (1985) Targets for health for all. Copenhagen, WHO

World Health Organization (WHO) (1986) Ottawa charter for health promotion: an international conference on health promotion, November 17–21. Copenhagen, WHO

5 Tackling health inequalities

OVERVIEW

Inequalities in social circumstances are linked to inequalities in health via a variety of mechanisms. Whilst there is debate concerning the magnitude of effect of different factors, material disadvantages, such as low income, are generally viewed as central. Other key factors are environmental, such as poor housing and low levels of social support; psychosocial, such as low self-esteem and chronic stress; and accumulated disadvantages experienced during the life-course or concentrated into particular geographical areas (Brunner & Marmot 1999, Duggan 2002, Wilkinson 1996). The documented rise in social inequalities in the UK during the 1970s and 1980s has been mirrored by a growth in health inequalities (Acheson 1998, Shaw et al 1999). The UK government has recognized inequalities in health as a major public health issue. In 2001, two targets to reduce inequalities in infant mortality and life expectancy were set, and there has also been wide consultation around a broad range of strategies to tackle inequalities (DoH 2001).

This chapter reviews the evidence of widening social and health inequalities and then goes on to look at the mechanisms which link social and health inequalities. The current policy context is briefly reviewed, demonstrating a supportive environment for tackling inequalities. Strategies to enable practitioners to tackle health inequalities are discussed using several examples of innovative work in this area.

Key Points

- Definition and scope of inequalities
- The link between social and health inequalities
- Tackling inequalities: policies and strategies
- Tackling inequalities: the practitioner's perspective
- Evaluating what works to reduce inequalities

INTRODUCTION

For those working to promote health, a recognition and understanding of the social structural factors that underpin health experiences and health status is fundamental. Practitioners work with individuals and communities, but underpinning the experience of clients are basic social structures such as income distribution, employment prospects and housing access and affordability. These basic social determinants of health are discussed in detail in Chapter 9. One of the key characteristics of these social structural factors is their inegalitarian and inequitable distribution amongst different groups in society. For health practitioners, the link between social and health inequalities is central. Whilst it may appear at first sight to be impossible to address such structural causes of health inequality, this chapter argues that practitioners do have the potential to intervene successfully to address inequalities in health. Practitioners may feel that addressing poverty or unemployment is potentially stigmatizing and victim-blaming and therefore avoid such topics. The good practice examples in this chapter demonstrate how tackling inequalities can be undertaken in a constructive, empowering and health promoting manner. To tackle health inequalities it is necessary first to define and measure the extent of the problem.

Inequalities refers to differences in circumstances, or the state of being unequal. Its current usage in public health includes the additional element of inequity, or being unjust or unfair:

> The term inequity has a moral and ethical dimension. It refers to differences which are unnecessary and avoidable but, in addition, are also considered unfair and unjust ... Our aim is not to eliminate all health differences, for that would be impossible, but rather to reduce or eliminate those that result from factors which are avoidable and unfair ... Equity in health implies that ideally everyone should have a fair opportunity to attain their full health potential and, more pragmatically, that no-one should be disadvantaged from achieving this potential if it can be avoided.
>
> (Whitehead 1990, p. 1)

There are different types of inequalities in health, including:

- socially patterned differences in health status
- inequalities in access to, and use of, services
- geographic or regional differences
- differences in treatment outcomes.

Whilst it is unrealistic to expect everyone to have equal income or health, patterned large-scale inequalities result from social policies and action and may be reduced through positive policies aimed at reducing inequalities.

Discussion point

Look at the following list of circumstances, which are all linked to poor health status. Is it fair or just to expect poorer health as a consequence of any of them?

- living in a disadvantaged area
- being a woman
- living on a low income
- not having had any further or higher education
- living in poor quality housing
- being above pensionable age
- belonging to a minority ethnic group
- being unemployed.

Some of these factors are clearly predetermined (e.g. gender, ethnicity, age). It could be argued that some of the other factors include an element of individual choice, although this is disputed (e.g. being unemployed, not having had any further or higher education). Even where there is an element of individual choice, factors such as unemployment or education depend to a large extent on the external social environment. This is why such factors are socially patterned rather than randomly distributed. It is generally agreed that people should not suffer due to circumstances beyond their control. Suffering poor health due to factors that are beyond an individual's ability to affect them is therefore not fair or just.

THE SCALE OF INEQUALITIES

Social inequalities and poverty increased in the UK from 1979 to 1997. Although most developed countries are experiencing widening inequalities, income inequality in Britain during this time was far greater (UNDP 1996). The significant rise in poverty has been driven by low pay coupled with high unemployment rates. Unemployment, especially amongst the least educated men, has increased due to the contraction of the manufacturing industry and the shift towards the service industry. Early or lone parenthood contributes towards poverty amongst women in lower socio-economic groups. A rise in the percentage of older people who have retired from employment, and changes in farming practices and low wages in rural areas are additional factors. A shortfall in uptake of benefits amongst those entitled to receive them is a further contributory factor (McKay & Rowlingson 1999).

Most of the research which has measured the increase in social and health inequalities over the last three decades has focused on social class or socio-economic status as the key variable (Townsend et al 1988). Using social class, and the Registrar General's classification system, allows for comparisons over time and access to comprehensive data sets. However,

Box 5.1 The increase in poverty and health inequalities in the UK during the late twentieth century

- From the beginning of the 1980s to the mid 1990s average incomes rose by 40% but the number of people living in poverty doubled (using the European Union definition of less than 50% average income after housing costs).
- By the mid 1990s, 24% of the population, and a third of all children, were living in poverty.
- Between 1979 and 1995 the net income of the richest grew by 68% compared to a growth of 8% in net income for the poorest.
- Premature mortality rates overall decreased from the 1970s to the 1990s, but the decrease for the higher social classes has been much more marked than that for the lower social classes.
- Between 1972 and 1996, the difference in life expectancy between male unskilled and professional workers increased from 5.5 years to 9.5 years.
- Babies of unskilled manual workers are 2.2 times more likely to die than babies with fathers in professional occupations.
- The gap in death rates between the best tenth and worst tenth geographical areas in Britain has also increased during the 1970s, 1980s and 1990s.
- People living in the worst tenth of areas in Britain are 42% more likely to die before the age of 65 than is the average person.

Sources: Davey Smith & Gordon (2000), Drever & Bunting (1997), Shaw et al (1998)

Figure 5.1 Male life expectancy by social class, England and Wales
Source: Drever F and Bunting J (1997) In: Drever F, Whitehead M (eds) Health inequalities. Reproduced by permission of The Stationery Office

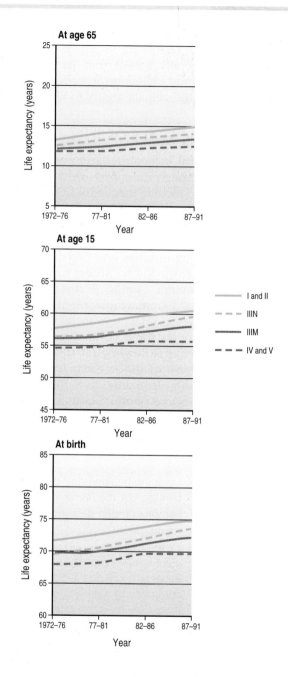

there are shortfalls with this classification system, including its applicability to women and unemployed people, its conflation of many different factors including income, education and employment, and changing employment patterns. The recently introduced new classification of social class (Office for National Statistics at www.statistics.gov.uk) has tried to address some of these problems. Other forms of inequality such as geographical area, gender, ethnicity, and the ways in which inequalities accumulate over the lifecourse are also the focus of considerable research (Graham 2000).

D iscussion point

Despite increased overall prosperity and population longevity, socially patterned health inequalities persist. How can this be explained?

The 1980 Black Report (Townsend et al 1988) offered four explanations:

- **Artefact** – inequalities result from the way data is collected and measured. This explanation is generally not accepted due to the persistence of inequalities over time and using a range of measures (Macintyre 1997).

- **Social selection** – ill health causes social inequalities via 'social drift' or the downward social mobility experienced by people with longstanding or chronic ill health. Conversely, the healthiest people, especially women, are likely to be upwardly socially mobile. Whilst the mechanism of social drift is documented, it is not seen as sufficient to explain large-scale inequalities (Bartley & Plewis 1997, Hart et al 1998).

- **Behavioural or cultural** – inequalities result from individual lifestyle choices around such issues as smoking, exercise, diet and alcohol intake. Smoking and poor diet (low consumption of fruit and vegetables coupled with high consumption of fats and sugars) are more common amongst people in the manual social classes compared to people in non-manual social classes (Drever & Bunting 1997). Whilst behavioural choices do affect health, this explanation is viewed as potentially 'victim-blaming' and neglects the social context which impacts on behavioural choices. For example, Graham's (1987) work identified smoking as a key coping mechanism used by single parents.

- **Material or structural** – material factors such as income, pollution, housing, transport, employment, education, the environment and access to services are the key factors determining inequalities. This is the explanation favoured by most sociologists and, increasingly, policy makers (Acheson 1998, Baggott 2000, Graham 2000, Shaw et al 1999).

There is a general consensus that the last two explanations are the most satisfactory in explaining health inequalities associated with social class, gender and ethnicity.

R eflection point

Smoking is the biggest single cause of the differences in death rates between rich and poor people. Which of the following views on this comes closest to your own?

- 'Poor people bring illness upon themselves. They don't care about their health, they smoke and drink too much and eat junk food. They could spend the money on healthy activities if they really wanted.'
- 'People's use of tobacco and alcohol is to a large extent determined by their social relations and social networks, which in turn affect their self-esteem and levels of stress. When social support is poor, tobacco and alcohol offer a prop of sorts.'

Research suggests that people's perceptions of risk are affected by their own situation and priorities, so that risk perception is a relative phenomenon. Epidemiological risk factors such as smoking may be constructed within people's lives as something else, for example a coping strategy (Graham 1993). Chapter 11 on changing lifestyles as a priority for practice discusses further the problems of transposing epidemiological risk factors to targeted individual education and advice.

Poverty is a key contributor to inequality (Alcock 2002). Poverty and its links with health and illness is discussed in more detail in the section on poverty and income in Chapter 9. Poverty may be defined in different ways. Objectively, poor people are defined as those living in households with incomes below 60% of the median income level of that year, taking housing costs into account. But poverty may also be defined relatively, in terms of social expectations, resources and activities. There is a strong relationship between being poor, being unemployed, having few social contacts or support, and having little say in decisions affecting one's life. The term 'social exclusion' has been defined as being unable, because of low income, to participate in many of the activities which society regards as normal or appropriate (Social Exclusion Unit 1997). Social contacts are reduced, the pursuit of individual interests is likely to be impossible, and choices are severely constrained. In a sense, poor people become socially excluded second class citizens, without the resources to enjoy what constitutes everyday life for most people.

Social exclusion is not synonymous with poverty and includes a number of characteristics that are not always included in the concept of poverty. The concept of social exclusion implies exclusion *from* something – typically 'normal society'. As we have seen in Chapter 4, policy interventions are underpinned by clear moral values. Those not working, for example, are seen as excluded but also dependent, irrespective of whether or not employment is desired (as may be the case for mothers in two parent households). Voluntary self exclusion (as in some rough sleepers) may be seen as undesirable and demanding intervention. The ways in which socially excluded groups are targeted for specific interventions are discussed in Chapter 12.

Recent research suggests that relative poverty and social exclusion are closely linked to health status (Duggan 2002). Affluent countries with unequally distributed resources have populations with poorer health status than countries with equal distribution of resources (Wilkinson 1996). Conversely, poor countries or areas with egalitarian resource distribution mechanisms and policies experience better than expected health status. This is illustrated by the example of Kerala in South India. Mortality rates in Kerala are close to those of much wealthier, industrialized countries, and very different from other states in India. Kerala has redistributive policies and many years of investing in human resources, particularly promoting women's access to education (Lynch et al 2000). Wealthy countries with redistributive policies, for example Nordic countries, Belgium and Japan, have the healthiest populations.

Health inequalities also affect people's experience of illness and disease and their quality of life as well as their life expectancy. People in the manual social classes are more likely than others to report chronic or long-standing limiting illness. Most research and statistics refer to social class, but the same explanations are used for inequalities associated with gender and ethnicity. Women and ethnic minorities in general experience poorer health than white men, although there are exceptions.

It appears that a number of factors are responsible for these patterned inequalities in health, including relative poverty, cultural stereotypes and professional and institutional inflexibility. Poverty is not the only

Discussion point

Why do you think that it is not the richest countries that have the best health, but those that have the smallest income differences between rich and poor?

Discussion point

Is poverty the explanation for the poorer health status of women and people from Black and minority ethnic groups?

explanation for observed gender and ethnic inequalities, but it plays a central role. For example, women live longer than men, yet report more ill health. Commentators (Daykin 2001, Doyal 1995) suggest no single cause but a combination of factors including continued gendered inequalities in society (e.g. the fact that women bear most of the burden of caring and domestic work and are discriminated against in the paid employment sector) and cultural stereotyping (e.g. doctors' readiness to interpret women's symptoms as evidence of mental illness). The links between ethnicity and health are complex, with some evidence of better than average health status (e.g. low mortality from cancers amongst people from the Caribbean and the Indian subcontinent) but a general pattern of poorer than average health status. There is excess mortality among migrant ethnic minority groups, higher rates of infant mortality especially among babies of Pakistan-born mothers, and a more common perception of poor health among minority ethnic groups (Daykin 2001). Material factors, including poorer living circumstances and institutional racism and discrimination, make a central contribution to these findings.

TACKLING INEQUALITIES

It is clear that inequalities in health are not just a consequence of health service delivery but have complex origins in socio-economic conditions, living and working conditions and people's lifestyles. Most public policies impact on health and can contribute to or reduce inequalities, hence the importance of 'joined up government' – a cross cutting approach that examines all policies for their impact. As we have seen, income is a major determinant of health status. Improving material conditions for the worst off is therefore an important step towards health improvement.

Traditionally, social democracy has responded to inequality with a simple solution of take from the rich and give to the poor. But most governments have pulled back from using redistributive policies that use taxation for fear of alienating better-off sections of the electorate. Instead, low income has been tackled through increased targeted benefits and the establishment of a minimum wage. The catch-phrase of American democrats is that welfare should offer a hand-up not a hand-out and is reflected in the emphasis on job creation, education for employability and flexible working. In the Netherlands for example, half the jobs created in the 1990s were part-time.

The Acheson Report (1998) into inequalities in health made 39 policy recommendations, only 3 of which related to the NHS. The report also recommended that priority should be given to improving the health of women of childbearing age, expectant mothers and young children. This reflects a focus in many developed countries struggling with welfare reform to shift redistribution forward in the life course and concentrate on the young. Giddens (1998) argues that this represents a third way between survival of the market and welfare dependency. Child care support, parental leave and subsidized pre-school education (see Ch. 9) all seek to invest in 'human capital' and build an enabling approach to inequality. A raft of interlinked policies and interventions to tackle inequalities has subsequently been launched by the UK government. Key policies are outlined in Box 5.2.

> **D**iscussion point
>
> Should governments focus on closing the gap between rich and poor or raising the floor, i.e. bringing more people out of poverty?

Box 5.2 Policies that tackle health inequalities

Early interventions to push people out of poverty
- *Sure Start* is targeted at families with under fives. Sure Start was introduced in 1998 in 60 disadvantaged areas with funding of £453 million over three years to promote early education, health and family support services to break the generational transmission of poverty.

Protection through ameliorating the effects of poverty
- *Tackling low income*   In 1999 a minimum wage was established, which in 2003 was £4.50 per hour. Over 1.5 million workers were entitled to higher pay as a result, and it appears that the majority did receive the specified wage increase. Low income workers and their families also benefited from the introduction of the Working Tax Credit and the Child Tax Credit, the introduction of a lower income tax rate and reform of the national insurance system. Benefits levels for families with children and pensioners have increased.

Tackling area based inequalities
- *Health Action Zones (HAZs)*   established in 1998, are partnerships of health organizations, including primary care, with local authorities, community and voluntary groups and local businesses, which aim to deliver innovative, measurable and sustainable improvements in the health of local people. Health care services should be improved through greater integration of treatment and care. HAZs are appointed for 5–7 years and are charged with reducing inequalities in health and tackling ill health. During 1998/99 the first wave of 10 HAZs received £4 million funding, rising to £30 million the following year, when 15 new HAZs were announced. In 1999 additional funding of £293 million over the next three years was announced.
- *Healthy Living Centres (HLCs)* were established as a UK-wide initiative in 1999. The aim of HLCs is to influence the wider determinants of health such as social exclusion, poor access to services, mental health, diet and fitness. HLCs are targeted at the most disadvantaged 20% of the population. Projects are flexible to meet local needs and local community involvement is encouraged. Examples of projects include smoking cessation, dietary advice, training and skills schemes, arts programmes and complementary therapy. HLCs are funded with lottery money and are managed by the New Opportunities Fund.
- *Single Regeneration Budget (SRB)* was introduced in 1994 in England to enhance the quality of life in areas of need by reducing the gap between deprived and other areas. SRB has since been reformed in an attempt to link resource allocation more closely to needs, promote greater involvement of communities and stakeholders, and provide a more strategic overview at regional level through the new Regional Development Agencies. SRBs focus on improving the education, skills and employment prospects of local people; reducing social exclusion; promoting sustainable regeneration through improving and protecting the environment including housing; supporting and promoting local businesses and economies; and improving community safety through reducing crime and drug abuse.

Box 5.2 *Continued*

- *New Deal for Communities (NDC)* £800 million over 10 years has been allocated to address multiple deprivation in particular neighbourhoods and bridge the gap between these neighbourhoods and others in England. NDC partnerships involve local communities in delivering change. Five key themes are: poor job prospects, high levels of crime, educational under-achievement, poor health, and problems with housing and the physical environment. Approximately £2 billion has been allocated to 39 NDC partnerships.

Promoting integration through tackling lack of work

- *New Deal – Welfare to Work* In 1998 £5.2 billion was allocated for investment on a range of New Deal initiatives to promote employment. Benefits claims and job advice agencies were merged, with the addition of intensive personalized support to find work. A requirement to take an option from a range of choices including a subsidized job, training or full-time education, or a job in the voluntary sectors or as part of the Environmental Task Force, became a condition of continued benefits for some groups.

Sources: Baggott (2000), Benzeval (2002), www.neighbourhood. gov.uk/ndcomms.asp accessed 21/11/03, www.doh.gov.uk/hlc/index.htm accessed 21/11/03

Reflection point

In your practice you may need to show that you are tackling health inequalities. What methods of monitoring would you use to show progress?

If progress is to be made towards tackling inequalities, agencies need to be able to measure local inequalities. Traditionally, data on health status and outcomes, such as standardized mortality rates (SMRs) for diseases or indicators such as the percentage of low birthweight babies, would be used. This chapter shows the complexity of health inequalities and that tackling the wider determinants of health inequalities requires action across a range of factors. Health equity audit is an important tool in reducing health inequalities strategies, and Directors of Public Health in England are required to conduct health equity audits for their areas. Equity audit is a cyclical process whereby the causes of inequities in health, access to services and treatment outcomes for a defined local population are reviewed and action taken to reduce inequities. It is important to note that equity means the fair (not equal) distribution of resources, access and opportunities according to population needs. Paradoxically, resource allocation may need to be made more unequal in order to be more equitable, i.e. to reflect a group's additional health needs. Audit involves understanding a situation, taking action to remedy a problem, and re-measuring or evaluating the situation to ensure the action has been effective. There are five key steps in a health equity audit (Flowers & Pencheon 2002):

1. Identify a broad issue – use research or local, regional or national priorities.

2. Choose a topic – it should have a significant impact on the health of disadvantaged populations.

3. Confirm and quantify inequity – this requires a measure both of service provision and of the need to which provision is related, e.g. uptake of aspirin in primary care by patients with CHD; uptake of breast screening by the eligible population; uptake of nicotine replacement therapy or buproprion on prescription amongst smokers wishing to quit.

4. Set standards or targets, define interventions and embed the outcome in mainstream NHS planning.

5. Monitor progress and evaluate interventions.

Reflection point

Consider an equity issue affecting your practice. How might you define targets and interventions and monitor progress?

Although many interventions and services are provided on a universal basis for all people within a defined population (e.g. within an age group or diagnosed with a certain condition), in practice service uptake is often poorer amongst more disadvantaged social groups. This phenomenon – the inverse care law – was first described by Tudor Hart (1971) and applies to screening and preventive services as well as for acute services. Equity audit provides a potentially powerful tool to try to tackle unequal uptake of services, and it is encouraging that equity audit has been highlighted as a required strategy in England.

Another kind of strategy involves identifying indicators that are monitored in order to assess whether or not reductions in inequalities are occurring. This could be undertaken as part of a local area needs assessment. An example of such a strategy is given below.

Example

Health equity audit

The London Health Strategy includes 10 indicators:

- unemployment rate
- percentage of pupils achieving GCSE grades A–C
- percentage of homes judged unfit to live in
- burglary rate
- air quality – number of days when air pollution exceeds set standards
- road traffic accident rate per 1000 resident population
- unemployment amongst Black and minority ethnic people
- life expectancy at birth
- infant death rate
- percentage of people with self-assessed fair, poor or bad health.

Source: www.doh.gov.uk/london/hstrat1.htm accessed 1/12/03

These indicators reflect the wide range of factors that contribute to health. For example, the burglary rate reflects community safety, whilst air quality is an indicator of environmental health. In addition, these indicators use data that is already collected and available. This is much more efficient than collecting new data.

Two 'headline' inequalities targets for England were set in 2001 (DoH 2001):

1. Starting with infant mortality rates, by 2010 to reduce by at least 10% the gap in mortality between manual groups and the population as a whole.

2. Starting with health authorities, by 2010 to reduce by at least 10% the gap between the fifth of areas with the lowest life expectancy at birth and the population as a whole.

Discussion point

Why were these chosen as the targets for reducing inequalities?

These inequalities targets were seen to be achievable yet challenging. The first target focuses on children and the next generation, an important priority group for breaking the generational transmission of poverty and disadvantage. The targets can be measured using data that is already routinely collected and available.

Four key themes for action were identified in the programme for action on inequalities (DoH 2003):

1. supporting families, mothers and children to break the inter-generational cycle of health
2. engaging communities and individuals to ensure relevance, responsiveness and sustainability
3. preventing illness and providing effective treatment and care
4. addressing the underlying determinants of health.

Some of these areas are discussed in later chapters. Several themes can be discerned from these policies and targets. First, resources are seen as needing to be channelled and targeted towards those in greatest need, e.g. families, mothers and children. Need assessment by area is also a popular option as in, for example, the establishment of Health Action Zones (HAZs). HAZs are a means of identifying and targeting disadvantaged localities, and ensuring that resources flow towards these areas.

Targeting geographical areas may seem rational and cost-effective, but it does lead to some problems. Area-based approaches to tackling health inequalities have a history of ineffectiveness (Shaw et al 1999). This is because they target help towards only a very small minority of poor people. Most poor people live outside targeted areas, and targeted areas contain a majority of non-poor households. As a policy to tackle inequalities, area-based policies are therefore severely constrained. In addition, this type of targeting means areas and localities have to compete with each other to secure funding. In order to win funding, areas have to declare themselves disadvantaged and impoverished. This is not likely to empower communities or promote their self-esteem or social capital. As an exercise, it fails to recognize that communities often achieve remarkable results in very straitened circumstances.

Tackling inequalities aims to raise the level of the less well off. This strategy ignores the fact that widening inequalities are driven not just by an increase in the poorest and most disadvantaged groups, but also by a rise in the income and wealth of the richest groups in society. The current approach is to try to break the cycle of inequalities rather than close the gap. Health promotion strategies such as those suggested to tackle coronary heart disease and cancer focus on individualized risk management and health education and are less widely taken up by disadvantaged groups. Such interventions may therefore actually increase inequalities despite improving population health overall. Chapter 11 on lifestyles discusses the approaches used to change behaviours and some of the resulting dilemmas.

The performance of agencies tackling inequalities is to be monitored against targets. Whilst the setting of national inequalities targets is important in directing strategies and funding, targets are fairly blunt instruments with which to measure change and improvement. The development and use of local targets is problematic, especially when partnership working is required. It is likely that different agencies and professional groups will have different priorities that will in turn hinder the identification of shared targets. Partnership working and community

Discussion point

What are the advantages and limitations of targeting geographical areas?

development approaches are rightly seen as the means towards achieving a reduction in inequalities. However, in order to achieve these aims, these strategies need to be resourced adequately. This is not always recognized or accounted for in funding arrangements. The challenges for practitioners of working with communities and across agencies are discussed in Chapters 6 and 7.

Reflection point

To what extent do you feel able to address health inequalities in your practice?

TACKLING INEQUALITIES: THE PRACTITIONER'S PERSPECTIVE

Many of the policies and strategies designed to reduce inequalities appear to be beyond the scope of individual practitioners, unless they are specifically employed as project workers. However, there are examples of how practitioners can routinely include tackling inequalities in their work practice. Equity audit, discussed earlier in this chapter, is one such example. Another example is given below.

Example

Nurse-led attendance allowance screening in a GP practice located in a deprived area of Glasgow

An attendance allowance screening tool was used by community nurses attached to one Glasgow general practice to opportunistically screen their elderly clients over a 3-month period for unclaimed attendance allowance. All potential under-claimants were referred to a welfare rights officer (WRO) who arranged to pay a home visit to carry out a more in-depth benefit assessment. The findings demonstrated that 86 clients had their attendance allowance status screened by community nurses; 69 clients were referred to the WRO for a home visit; and 47 clients and 4 relatives had their cases referred to the Department for Social Services for adjudication, resulting in 37 clients and 4 relatives receiving benefit awards totalling £112,892 of which over £96,000 was recurring on an annual basis. Six participants and one relative were also awarded attendance allowance and income support, thus highlighting the potential of attendance allowance assessment to act as an efficient and effective passport to other benefits.

Most of the attendance allowance benefits were awarded at the high rate, indicating a high level of frailty and unmet need. Community nurses thought that attendance allowance screening was a legitimate activity and one which added to their effectiveness. In three-quarters of cases the screening took less than five minutes to complete. WROs noted that the clinical details provided by community nurses made the GP more likely to support the application and enhanced the chances of the claim being successful. Home visits by a WRO had several advantages, including reaching people who would not be physically able or sufficiently motivated to travel for this service, and allowing other family members to be screened at the same time.

Source: With thanks to Robert Hoskins, and Hoskins & Smith (2002)

Compared to many other public health and health promotion interventions, welfare benefits screening and advice services appear to be of proven effectiveness using a variety of criteria:

- The service avoids victim blaming by focusing on benefit entitlement not unhealthy lifestyles.
- Services may be accessed by many of the most marginalized and 'hard to reach' groups.

- Quantitative positive outcomes are apparent, both in terms of numbers of users, and in terms of additional income flowing into the area.
- Qualitative outcomes are provided in the form of individual case studies where increased income leads to health benefits.

It is not easy to adapt work routines in this way, and there are cost implications. The success of the above example was due to a large extent to the availability of the WRO and effective liaison between the community nurses and the WRO. Support from management and recognition of the extra time required is essential. For overworked staff with large caseloads, any extra task may seem impossible. The historical separation of health and social care services also works against incorporating elements of welfare into health work. However the evidence now exists to show that benefits advice is a feasible and effective use of time that results in health improvements.

Practitioners can also reflect on how they deliver services to ensure that they have maximum impact on inequalities and provide accessible and empowering services. Table 5.1 below illustrates some guiding principles to help review service delivery.

Discussion point

To what extent, and how, can health and welfare services be modified to ensure they address inequalities?

Table 5.1 Helpful and unhelpful health and welfare services
Source: Laughlin S, Black D (1995) Poverty and health: tools for change. Reproduced by permission of UK Public Health Association

Helpful	Unhelpful
An integrated approach	Services that treat financial, health and social problems as unrelated
A coordinated response	Individual agencies working on separate sets of problems
Services which offer realistic advice and recognize the limitations that poverty places on people	Providing help only when families are in crisis Interventions which individualize problems
Partnerships between families and workers where families' contributions are valued	Services based on what professionals think that families want rather than what families say they want
	Failure to recognize what families do achieve in adversity
	Blaming families for their poverty
Services that are permanent	Temporary or short-term projects
Services that are relevant	Forcing families to define financial problems as emotional problems or personal inadequacy before help is given
Services that are easy to use	Only providing help when families are labelled as a problem

EVALUATING POLICIES TO REDUCE INEQUALITIES

Despite the interest in inequalities there is very little evidence of the impact of policy interventions. Little is known for example about the effects on health of redistributive fiscal policy although there is evidence of the effectiveness of income support (Mackenbach & Bakker 2002). The recommendations of the Acheson Report (1998) and its 10 steps to health equality are inevitably fairly medically focused because these are the interventions that have been evaluated and for which there is evidence of effectiveness.

Ten steps to health equality – the experts' recommendations are:

- nicotine gum and patches free on the NHS: doubles the chances of stopping smoking
- pre-school education and child care: strong evidence that it improves long-term prospects for children
- fluoridation of drinking water: cuts tooth decay
- accident prevention (e.g. fit cars with soft bumpers): accidents are principal cause of deaths in young people
- drugs education in schools: prevents pupils becoming hooked
- support around childbirth to promote breastfeeding and mental health: good evidence of long-term benefits
- improved access to NHS for ethnic minorities (e.g. by appointing linkworkers)
- adding folate to flour: prevents spina bifida in babies, and early evidence suggests it may prevent heart disease and Alzheimer's disease
- free school milk
- free smoke alarms: good evidence they save lives.
  [Source: Acheson (1998), Macintyre et al (2001)]

Policy evaluation is very difficult because of the complexities of the policy process and the pathways linking social policy interventions to individual outcomes. Experimental methodologies are usually impossible due to the broad impact of policy interventions, and the difficulty of finding comparable population groups who have not been subject to the policy in question, or one that is similar in intent. However, other rigorous methodologies, including international comparative studies and theory-based evaluation, exist and should be used when appropriate (Mackenbach & Bakker 2002).

The Dutch strategy for tackling inequalities recommends a combination of 'upstream' measures targeting the socio-economic factors that are pushing people into the river and 'downstream' measures that target the accessibility and quality of services (that might help to pull people out of the river) (Mackenbach & Stronks 2002). Upstream measures include improving the physical and psychosocial work environment, reducing smoking in lower socio-economic groups, improving nutrition (preferably through universal measures such as healthier school meals) and reducing childhood poverty. Downstream policies include health care policies that improve accessibility for lower socio-economic groups.

Whitehead et al (2000) describe a framework which is intended for researching policy impact on health inequalities (see Figure 5.2).

Figure 5.2 Framework for researching policy impact on health inequalities
Source: Whitehead M et al (2000) In: Graham H (ed) Understanding health inequalities. Reproduced by permission of Open University Press

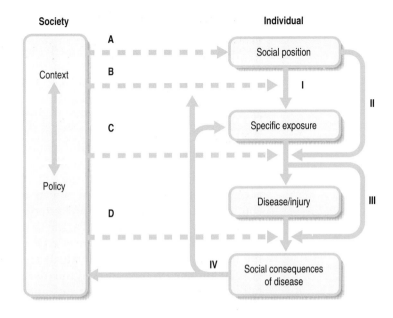

This framework seeks to evaluate the different pathways that link individuals and policies, including the impact of policies on social position (including educational policies and policies which affect social networks and social inclusion), specific exposure to risks and hazards (e.g. housing, occupational and food policies), and the impact of being ill (e.g. health care and disability policies). Whitehead et al (2000) use this framework to compare the position of lone mothers in Sweden and the UK. They conclude that whilst the magnitude of the health differential between lone and couple mothers is similar in both countries, around 50% of the health disadvantage of lone mothers in the UK is due to poverty and unemployment, exacerbated by poor access to high quality child care facilities, compared to less than 15% for lone mothers in Sweden. This suggests that benefits, employment and child care policies are all crucial in breaking the links between being a lone mother, living in poverty and experiencing poor health.

CONCLUSION

Social and health inequalities remain a significant and preventable cause of much ill health and premature death. The health inequalities agenda is now firmly established on the health agendas of many developed countries. However, the gap from policy to practitioner level can appear daunting and practitioners may feel tackling inequalities is beyond their remit and that they do not have the necessary knowledge, skills and resources to do so effectively. This chapter has sought to demonstrate that practitioner interventions to address inequalities are feasible and effective, and has argued that the extent of health problems related to inequalities makes such action a priority.

Inequalities due to socio-economic position, gender, ethnicity and geography impact on health via complex pathways involving material resources, the physical and social environment, behaviour and lifestyles, and physiological responses. Inequalities often cluster and accumulate over the course of a lifetime or may become concentrated within small geographical areas. Tackling inequalities requires policy initiatives aimed at reducing the gap between the wealthiest and the poorest sections of society. This is generally interpreted as raising the income and improving the circumstances of the poorest groups, but equally it could involve reducing the incomes of the wealthiest through redistributive taxation policies. Many countries (e.g. the UK, The Netherlands, Sweden) have adopted targeted interventions aimed at disadvantaged groups. Some commentators argue for a simpler intervention aimed at raising incomes of people living in poverty, and argue that international comparisons suggest this simpler strategy is more effective in reducing inequalities with all the benefits this brings to individuals and society in general (Whitehead et al 2000). The UK has followed the route of raising people out of poverty rather than reducing the health gap, and has achieved some success with this approach. Practitioners can support such activity by being aware of the current policy context, supporting individual clients to claim their full benefits entitlement, and working with communities to address inequalities in the local environment. Being aware of the constraints of poverty and social inequalities on lifestyles and behaviours can enable practitioners' health promotion work with individuals and families to be sensitive, appropriate, enabling and ultimately more effective.

FURTHER DISCUSSION

- With reference to your own practice, identify how (if at all) social inequalities result in health inequalities.
- What 'downstream' initiatives might help improve the accessibility and quality of services for disadvantaged clients?
- Should priority be given towards 'upstream' or 'downstream' interventions to tackle inequalities? Why?

Recommended reading

- Graham H (ed) (2000) Understanding health inequalities. Maidenhead, Open University Press.
  This book draws upon UK research to examine the relationship between social factors and health inequalities, focusing in particular on ethnicity, gender, socio-economic status, lifecourse experiences, and the home and neighbourhood environment. Links are made throughout with policies and their impact on health inequalities.
- Mackenbach J, Bakker M (eds) (2002) Reducing inequalities in health: a European perspective. London, Routledge.
  This book brings together contributions from researchers from 14 different European countries. The focus is on evaluating successful policies and interventions that aim to reduce health inequalities.

Conceptual and methodological issues relating to research in this area are also discussed.

▪ Marmot M G, Wilkinson R G (eds) (1999) The social determinants of health. Oxford, Oxford University Press.

A readable account of how a variety of social determinants affect health. Marmot and Wilkinson argue that social determinants are mediated via physiological responses and that relative inequalities are the most important in their impact on health.

▪ Shaw M, Dorling D, Gordon D, Davey Smith G (1999) The widening gap: Health inequalities and policy in Britain. Bristol, The Policy Press.

This book provides up-to-date evidence documenting the existence of a widening health gap in Britain. Different explanations for the health gap are explored, and policies to tackle health inequalities are proposed.

REFERENCES

Acheson D (1998) Independent inquiry into inequalities in health. London, The Stationery Office

Alcock P (2002) Anti-poverty strategies. In: Adams L, Amos M, Munro J (eds) Promoting health: politics and practice. London, Sage

Baggott R (2000) Public health: policy and politics. Basingstoke, Macmillan

Bartley M, Plewis I (1997) Does health-selective mobility account for socio-economic differences in health? Evidence from England and Wales 1971–1991. Journal of Health and Social Behaviour 38: 376–386

Benzeval M (2002) England. In: Mackenbach J, Bakker M (2002) Reducing inequalities in health: A European perspective. London, Routledge

Brunner E, Marmot M G (1999) Social organization, stress and health. In: Marmot M G, Wilkinson R G (eds) The social determinants of health. Oxford, Oxford University Press

Davey Smith G, Gordon D (2000) Poverty across the life course and health. In: Pantazis C, Gordon D (eds) Tackling inequalities: where we are now and what can be done? Bristol, Policy Press

Daykin N (2001) Sociology: In: Naidoo J, Wills J (eds) Health studies. Basingstoke, Palgrave

Department of Health (DoH) (2001) Tackling health inequalities: consultation on a plan for delivery. London, DoH

Department of Health (DoH) (2003) Tackling health inequalities – a programme for action. London, DoH

Doyal L (1995) What makes women sick? Gender and the political economy of health. Basingstoke, Macmillan

Drever F, Bunting J (1997) Patterns and trends in male mortality. In: Drever F, Whitehead M (eds) Health inequalities. London, The Stationery Office

Drever F, Whitehead M (eds) (1997) Health inequalities. London, The Stationery Office

Duggan M (2002) Social exclusion, discrimination and the promotion of health. In: Adams L, Amos M, Munro J (eds) Promoting health: politics and practice. London, Sage

Flowers J, Pencheon D (2002) Inphorm. Eastern Region Public Health Observatory, Issue 1, December

Giddens A (1998) The third way: the renewal of social democracy. Cambridge, Polity Press

Graham H (1987) Women's smoking and family health. Social Science and Medicine 25(1): 47–56

Graham H (1993) When life's a drag: women, smoking and disadvantage. London, HMSO

Graham H (2000) Understanding health inequalities. Maidenhead, Open University Press

Hart C L, Davey Smith G, Blane D (1998) Social mobility and 21 year mortality in a cohort of Scottish men. Social Science and Medicine 47(8): 1121–1130

Hoskins R, Smith L N (2002) Nurse led welfare benefits screening in a general practice located in a deprived area. Public Health 116: 214–220

Laughlin S, Black D (1995) Poverty and health: tools for change. Birmingham, Public Health Alliance

Lynch J, Davey Smith G, Kaplan G, House J (2000) Income inequality and mortality: importance to health of individual income, psychosocial environment or material conditions. British Medical Journal 320: 1200–1204

Macintyre S (1997) The Black report and beyond: what are the issues? Social Science and Medicine 44(6): 723–745

Macintyre S, Chalmers I, Horton R, Smith R (2001) Using evidence to inform health policy: a case study. British Medical Journal 322: 222–225

McKay S, Rowlingson K (1999) Social security in Britain. Basingstoke, Macmillan

Mackenbach J P, Bakker M (2002) Reducing inequalities in health: a European perspective London, Routledge

Mackenbach J P, Stronks K (2002) A strategy for tackling health inequalities in The Netherlands. British Medical Journal 325: 1029–1032

Shaw M, Dorling D, Gordon D, Davey Smith G (1999) The widening gap: health inequalities and policy in Britain. Bristol, The Policy Press

Social Exclusion Unit (1997) Purpose, work priorities and working methods. London, HMSO

Townsend P, Davidson N, Whitehead M (1988) Inequalities in health: the Black report and the health divide. Harmondsworth, Penguin

Tudor Hart J (1971) The inverse care law. Lancet 1: 406–412

United Nations Development Programme (UNDP) (1996) Human development report. New York, Oxford University Press

Whitehead M (1990) The concepts and principles of equity in health. Copenhagen, World Health Organization

Whitehead M, Diderichsen F, Burstrom B (2000) Researching the impact of public policy on inequalities in health. In: Graham H (ed) Understanding health inequalities. Maidenhead, Open University Press

Wilkinson R G (1996) Unhealthy societies: the afflictions of inequality. London, Routledge

6

Participation and involvement

OVERVIEW

This chapter examines the growth of participation and involvement as key strategies in public health and health promotion. The concept of public involvement is not new, and international and national bodies have advocated participation since the 1980s. However, public participation is now increasingly being seen as relevant to improvements in service delivery, monitoring and management. The NHS Plan (DoH 2000) envisages a service which is shaped around the convenience and concerns of patients. Patient and public involvement is carried out at the level of the individual, involving patients in decisions about care and treatment and at the collective level, involving patients and the public in decisions concerning the planning and delivery of services. Patient and public involvement (PPI) therefore covers a broad range of activities from providing information, to gathering feedback to involvement in decision making. This chapter discusses some of the strategies which may be used to engage the public and service users. Finally, the chapter discusses the difficulties of evaluating participation and involvement strategies and concludes with a discussion of public involvement from the perspective of a health practitioner.

INTRODUCTION

In recent years, partly at least in response to the emerging crisis in health care provision, there has been a major shift to patient and public involvement. Previously communities were seen as the passive recipients of services and patient or user knowledge or experience was not valued. This has now given way to participatory approaches intended to increase responsiveness of services and their accountability. There is a broad spectrum of attitude and purpose in relation to 'involvement'. Most definitions reflect the transfer of some aspects of service planning or delivery from providers to the individuals and the community served so that services are developed with people not for people. There is an increased awareness that being responsive to local views is likely to result in services better suited to local needs.

A commitment to a community oriented health approach informs UK government health and care programmes (see Ch. 4). The NHS Plan (DoH 2000) and section 11 of the Health and Social Care Act (DoH 2001a) ensure that patients and the public are at the centre of health care both in the patient journey through the health service and in the way in which services provided are what people want and need and monitored to ensure they meet core standards. The policy and practice guidance *Strengthening Accountability* defines involving and consulting as: 'discussing with patients and the public their ideas, your plans, their experiences, why services need to change, how to make the best use of resources and so on. It is more about changing attitudes within the NHS and the way the NHS works than laying down rules for procedures' (DoH 2003, p. 1). Examples of the ways this is shown in current policy are:

- **Patient-centred services** – e.g. integrated care pathways
- **Patients as partners in their own care** – e.g. The Expert Patient programme
- **Increased accountability of services:**
  - Patient Forums in every Primary Care Trust to bring the patients' perspective into decision making
  - Patient Advisory and Liaison Services providing on-the-spot help and advice
  - Local Authority Overview and Scrutiny Committees (OSC) to scrutinize local health services
  - Independent Complaints Advocacy Service
- **Involvement in health decision making** – the Commission for Patient and Public Involvement in Health, a national body to oversee PPI developments
- **The focus on the neighbourhood as a setting for health initiatives** – e.g. Local Authority community strategies.

'Involvement' is a principle across health and care sectors but is central to health improvement and there are specific reasons why public health and health promotion practitioners may lead on this issue. *Health Promotion: Foundations for Practice* (Naidoo & Wills 2000) highlighted how the role of communities in health improvement has been signalled in key international agreements:

- Equity and participation were central concepts of the World Health Organization Health For All 2000 strategy.
- The Ottawa Charter (WHO 1986) made community participation and strengthening communities a central principle and level of action for health promotion.
- The Jakarta conference on Health Promotion into the twenty-first Century (WHO 1997) highlighted the need to increase community capacity and empower the individual as one of five priorities for health promotion.

Patient and public involvement pose real challenges for practitioners. Although there have been moves to client-centredness in care, a professional service culture continues to be reluctant to let communities or users lead. The need to meet centrally imposed targets (see Ch. 4) means that the organizational ethos is very task focused. To increase involvement means consciously reaching out and being proactive in enabling communities to play a real role in planning services and programmes. It means discovering a community's health needs and priorities and then supporting and enabling them to improve their health. This involves uncertainty and giving up some aspects of power.

This chapter explores some of the challenges of patient and public involvement:

- How users and communities can be involved in decision making about services and generating knowledge and evidence.
- How communities can be supported to deliver health improvement.
- How the professional service culture can be changed to acknowledge the importance of users and communities as partners in health improvement.

THE CONTEXT FOR PATIENT AND PUBLIC INVOLVEMENT

A dictionary definition of 'involvement' is 'to include' or 'to be part of'. The definition of participation is simply 'taking part in'. Obviously encompassed within these definitions is the possibility of a range of activities and outcomes ranging from someone merely being present at a decision-making forum to a form of empowerment whereby people have a real say in decisions and issues that affect their lives.

Reflection point	Involving people:
Why is involving people seen as a 'good thing'?	- enables organizations to get a clearer idea of what is important to local communities - identifies unmet needs - enables resources to be targeted effectively and to prioritize future spending - ensures that services will be used and are relevant for the local context - improves quality through measuring satisfaction - encourages people to feel a greater ownership and commitment to services and projects that they have been involved in designing and may help to restore confidence in public services - contributes to greater openness and accountability.

The growth of participation can be traced through several parallel developments:

- **The growth of the power of the consumer**   There is increasing attention given to service users in all public sectors. This can be traced back to a desire to reduce the role of the state and roll back paternalistic government. The current government has prioritized quality of health services and this casts the public as consumers (NHS Executive 1998). The construction of league tables of performance and charters have introduced the concept of minimum entitlement that indicates what users have a right to expect, and is used by government to make services more accountable.

- **The growth of citizenship**   The World Health Organization identified the basic right of any citizen to participate in their health care and a 'duty' or 'obligation' to exercise that right in the Alma Ata Declaration (WHO

1978). The UK government's current commitment to a 'stakeholder democracy' has led to a much stronger commitment to 'the right to be involved'. As citizens, people have been encouraged to have a legitimate expectation to participate in decisions that affect them. Alongside rights come responsibilities. There is also therefore an expectation that citizens will use services appropriately and contribute to their own health improvement.

- **The lay voice**   In recent years there has been a questioning of professional and policy assumptions about the best way of delivering services. There is an increasing recognition that the lay perspective gives insight into patterns of behaviour and lifestyles and subjective experiences. This understanding can help to 'unpack' global concepts such as health inequalities, and enable the development of appropriate and accessible services. There is a commitment to involving patients in the management of chronic conditions and valuing individual expertise developed through experience through the 'Expert Patient' initiative (DoH 2001b).

- **Legislation**   The importance of listening to the public has been reinforced by several inquiries including the Kennedy report on the Bristol Royal Infirmary Inquiry (DoH 2001c), which recommended that the perspectives of patients and of the public must be heard, taken into account and permeate all aspects of health care.

Discussion point

What differences are implied in the different terms used to refer to public involvement – i.e. consumers, users, citizens, lay people?

These different terms, although sometimes used interchangeably, denote different levels of power. Consumers and users have limited power to affect services. Their ultimate sanction is to refuse to use services, and take their custom elsewhere. The terms originate in an economic model of relationships within capitalism, and the relevance of such terms to universal state service provision has been questioned. Most people cannot afford the alternative of private sector services, although the government has encouraged the notion of competition and 'shopping around' within the state sector for services.

The concept of citizenship implies a more active engagement and use of power to determine the kinds of services offered. Citizens hold power, even if at several removes, through the democratic process, and services need to be accountable to citizens. Lay people suggests a level of power between consumers and citizens. Lay people hold local lay knowledge, but lack expert professional knowledge. Lay people are therefore vital partners if services are to develop in appropriate and accessible ways.

Internationally, public health planning has tended to be a top-down process based on expert identification of priorities and strategies and donor agencies financing piecemeal health projects. People living in low income/developing countries often consult an array of practitioners and there are few safeguards or little monitoring of providers. Households may also make substantial contributions to health activities in cash and in kind. Many governments have tried different forms of decentralization such as district management boards and local health committees. Such structures provide a means by which local voices, particularly those of poor people and women, can be represented.

Example

Participation in health care planning

In a remote rural area of China the maternal mortality rate and infant mortality rate was much higher than the national average. A loan from the World Bank intended to improve maternal and child services stipulated that the poorest families should be allocated money from the loan to enable them to access ante- and postnatal care, hospital deliveries for emergency or high risk pregnancies and treatment for infant pneumonia and diarrhoea. But 99% of women delivered at home attended by an untrained person and some counties did not spend the money and some used it only for obstetric emergency care. A participatory planning workshop was attended by all the major stakeholders (service providers at province, district, county, township and village levels; health officials and managers; township leaders). The priorities for the loan were identified and concerns shared about its administration – that it should not be used all at once; the inability to encourage the poor to access the fund; that the limited money should be used on emergencies only; that the limited money should be used on infant disease treatment rather than maternity care. As a result of the workshop the project was able to 'correct' the misuse and under-use of the funding and ensure that the project became sustainable.

Source: Institute of Development Studies briefing papers www.ids.ac.uk

UNDERSTANDING INVOLVEMENT AND PARTICIPATION

Typologies of participation

Several writers have developed typologies of participation (Arnstein 1969, Wilcox 1994). These models make a hierarchical distinction between approaches to involvement according to the amount of power sharing involved and the degree of influence over decisions. Arnstein's model (1969) is presented as a ladder where the lower rungs are participation activities designed to give people a voice as a way of making them involved but they remain recipients of services and there is little commitment to them having real influence. The next rungs are about consultation activities that seek to identify with communities what is needed and listen to views before decisions are made. The higher rungs of the ladder identify forms of participatory activity in which the community has greater power and influence and there is a commitment to integrating their views in wider processes. The top rung is user-led activities in which agencies step back from the identification of priorities or the definition of solutions and help communities to do what they want.

Arnstein's model has been criticized as a simplistic rationalization, but it has enjoyed considerable currency as it was the first to put forward the

Discussion point

What criticisms might be made of this model of involvement?

Figure 6.1 Ladder of participation
Source: Arnstein S (1969) A ladder of citizen participation. Reproduced by permission of Journal of the American Institute of Planners

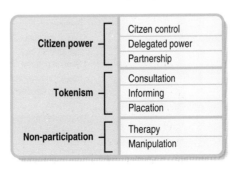

idea of establishing a structured framework of engaging a community and using consultation within the planning/participatory framework of decision making. Models of participation that are presented as hierarchies imply that projects should aspire to the highest level yet participation needs to be appropriate to its context and take account of the issues involved. A further major challenge for organizations and practitioners is to create opportunities for people to be involved. In some situations it may be sufficient to inform or consult while in others the principle of partnership and working with communities is important.

In Figure 6.2, the main dimensions of involvement are seen as at the level of the individual, involving patients in decisions about care and treatment, and at the collective level, involving patients and the public in decisions concerning the planning and delivery of services. Possible aims and objectives for local PPI may be to:

- get feedback on the quality of services
- learn more about patients' experiences of care
- identify unmet needs
- gain ideas about priorities.

The degree of involvement may therefore range from giving information through more active participation to partnerships with patients and the public. For example, Dartford, Gravesham and Swanley Primary Care Trust, as part of its strategy for patient and public involvement, held a series of 'Have your say' days with older people. The intention was to gain older people's views on their experience of health services. Key themes that emerged were the need to improve availability of information about services, the significance of having adequate income levels and how disrespectful attitudes impact on older people. The practice implications

Figure 6.2 Levels of involvement (from DoH 2003)

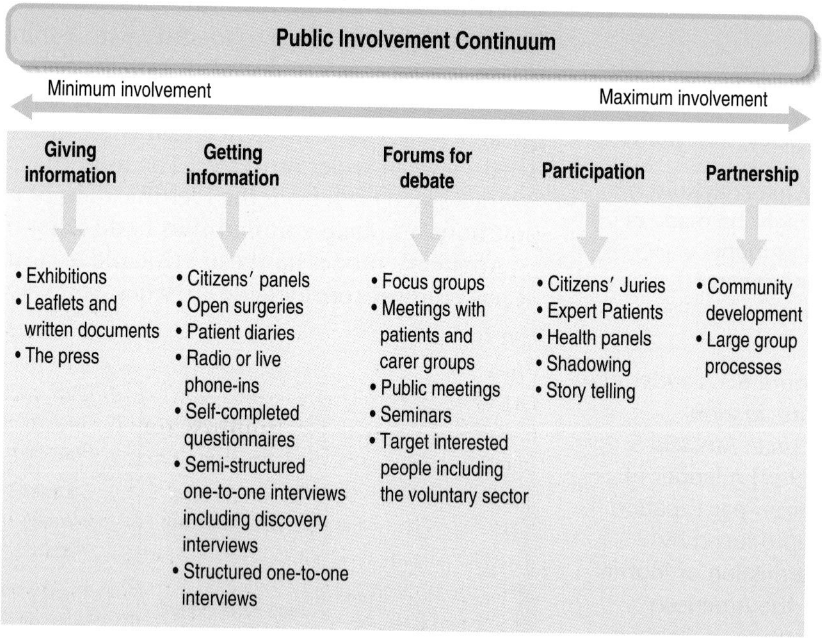

Public Involvement Continuum

Minimum involvement ←————————————————→ Maximum involvement

Giving information	Getting information	Forums for debate	Participation	Partnership
• Exhibitions • Leaflets and written documents • The press	• Citizens' panels • Open surgeries • Patient diaries • Radio or live phone-ins • Self-completed questionnaires • Semi-structured one-to-one interviews including discovery interviews • Structured one-to-one interviews	• Focus groups • Meetings with patients and carer groups • Public meetings • Seminars • Target interested people including the voluntary sector	• Citizens' Juries • Expert Patients • Health panels • Shadowing • Story telling	• Community development • Large group processes

include an information strategy across agencies and an age awareness programme (DGS PCT 2003). An alternative approach is described below in an example of a major community consultation exercise on primary care planning.

Practitioner talking

We carried out a consultation exercise with the local community about whether to set up a new health centre that would act as a local resource for advice, exercise and complementary therapies.

We held a public meeting that we advertised in the local press, community centres and libraries and in shops. About 200 people came. We then met with 23 local groups and held 6 focus groups of local people. We carried out a street survey. We also took comments in writing, on a website and in telephone calls and there were about 2000 of these. There was no problem getting a response and enormous efforts were made with the modes of communication and language.

If I were being cynical I would say that despite the number of responses, we had to be seen to be consulting. I think it was just a means of getting an existing decision across and getting public support made the case more powerful. Lots of people in the focus groups seemed to think the decision had already been made and there would not be a response to their concerns.

Commentary

Involvement in decision making is part of a new thrust to enable patient and public to engage with health services. Frequently such efforts are tokenistic and the scope for responding to views is limited. Harrison & Mort (1998) argue that involvement is frequently used as a way of legitimating corporate decisions or 'placation' on Arnsteins ladder (see p. 113) There may be a lack of openness about any decisions to be taken and the professional expectations from any consultation. Users and carers may then become cynical about the value placed on any consultation.

Diversity and representation

The current drive for 'involvement' refers to 'patients' and 'public'. These terms have been criticized. Those who use services may not identify themselves as patients or users and view their involvement as time limited and condition specific. The term 'user' signals a lack of dependency but as Ovreteit (1996) states, 'it gives the impression of someone exploiting the practitioner and does not advance the idea of partnership'. The term 'community involvement or participation' is widely used by international bodies. The concept of 'community' and the best way to define it is a long-standing debate and is briefly discussed in Chapter 10 of *Health Promotion: Foundations for Practice* (Naidoo & Wills 2000). In early work on participation, community tended to be equated with place. Geographically defined communities are convenient for agencies that want to work within boundaries, but living in the same place does not necessarily guarantee a common view. More recently, the emphasis has been on communities of interest with shared needs such as 'teenage mothers' or 'people with learning disabilities'. Marginalized communities are those whose contributions are invisible. They may experience discrimination and may not make use of traditional or mainstream services. Examples of such groups are asylum seekers, travellers and homeless people (see Ch. 12). Identifying such groups and establishing and making relationships can be challenging for practitioners.

'Stakeholders' is the term frequently used to signify those who have a personal interest in an issue. The question of who to involve in a 'community' is complicated. Early attempts to increase participation focused on a strategy of involving those who were most accessible, who tended to be local leaders. For example, attempts to reach ethnic minority groups frequently employed strategies of contacting faith leaders or using existing groups that met at religious buildings. Identifying 'activists' and those used to participating in groups – those in tenant groups or parents' associations – were also seen as ways of increasing involvement and getting a 'lay voice'. Where there is no clear constituency these representatives tend to be drawn from voluntary sector agencies. Jewkes & Murcott argue that in seeking representatives pragmatic considerations often become paramount: 'These constraints result in the community representatives being drawn from one small part of the voluntary sector, the larger funded organizations' (1998, p. 855). Organizations such as Age Concern or Mind have broad memberships but nevertheless may not enable access to harder to reach groups such as ethnic minority elders or mentally disordered offenders.

The Kennedy Report (DoH 2001c) states that the public should be represented by a wide range of individuals and groups and not by particular 'patient groups', valuing the voices of individuals and communities whose views are seldom heard. Asylum seekers, the homeless, drug users and people with a disability are examples of groups that are hard to reach, may not have a strong voice and yet have significant health needs that may not be directly addressed by services. Some groups have traditionally not had a voice. For example, in the past it has been assumed that children and young people are not able to articulate their view. A strategy for children and young people (CYPU 2001) and a National Service Framework for Children and the government's Children and Young Persons Unit (www. cypu.gov.uk, CYPU 2001) all refer to the need to involve young people in decision making. McNeish & Newman (2002, p. 200) comment that successful involvement of young people may require specific strategies:

- interesting and fun activities to hold their interest
- incentives and rewards
- ways of demonstrating respect and the value of their views
- structured activities to elicit views
- feedback about what will happen as a result of their contribution.

Discussion point

The national Teenage Pregnancy Strategy contains a commitment to involving stakeholders in the development of local responses. Who would you regard as stakeholders in relation to this issue?

Example

Involving homeless people in developing services

The 'imagine' project run by the New Economics Foundation on participative democracy encourages communities to identify what works by getting them to tell stories about the good things in their community. The method is familiar, fun and flexible enough to be used in public areas. It is then used to create a shared vision and future priorities. One group was facilitated in day centres and talked to people who were homeless about what they wanted in order to feel at home in Waterloo. One person commented 'being on the streets means that there is often nobody for homeless people to talk to as "normal" people ignore us or are frightened of us. When someone out of a crowd says "hello" and asks how you feel then that makes me feel normal again.'

Source: New Economics Foundation (2003)

TYPES OF INVOLVEMENT

Involvement in primary care is a broad concept. It may range from individual patient experience to the social and economic regeneration of communities. Opportunities exist for patient and public participation in:

- individual decisions about treatment
- user views on service provision
- health needs assessments to determine community priorities and views on an issue in order to inform service or programme development
- public consultation exercises about service provision or development
- citizen involvement in public policy panels
- strategic planning groups
- community development and neighbourhood regeneration.

Patient and user involvement

Patient involvement at an individual level involves patients in discussions and decisions about their own care and treatment or at a collective level in decisions regarding the planning, delivery and monitoring of services. The involvement may range from a one-off consultation to long-term representation on a steering group.

A fundamental shift in care has taken place that recognizes that people are partners in their own care and treatment. Many people now suffer from chronic conditions and experience physical and psychological difficulties, social and economic problems and social exclusion due to restricted work and leisure. Yet it is widely recognized that patients do not feel involved in decisions, do not feel they have anyone to talk to about anxieties and may feel unclear about tests and treatments and there may be insufficient information for family and friends (Coulter 2002). Many users and carers have not been active participants in their own care planning. Mental health and learning disability services are increasingly using advocates to increase self-assessment (DoH 2001d). Marelich et al (2002) in their work with patients with HIV/AIDS identified several ways in which patients could be involved:

Reflection point

Think of an example where you have sought the views of clients/service users. What prompted you to undertake this activity? How did you do this and what methods did you use? What did you do with the information generated?

- joint decision making
- patients taking control of treatment decisions
- patients acting as knowledge gatherers.

In many cases, however, patients are initially hesitant about participation and see their role solely as asking questions and choosing from alternatives (Sainio et al 2001). There are also real problems in involving people in discussions about service provision when the numbers with a specific condition may be low, they may not wish to associate with others and when, as is frequently the case with palliative care, there may be a difference of opinion between patients and carers.

Patient self-management programmes were first advocated in *Saving Lives: Our Healthier Nation* (DoH 1999). The government has now formalized *The Expert Patient: a new approach to chronic disease management for the 21st century* (DoH 2001b) based on the Chronic Disease Self Management Programme, a 6-week education course developed at Stanford University in the USA that covers relaxation, symptom management, fatigue, exercise, nutrition, problem solving and communication. It has been widely adopted in Australasia, the USA, Europe and China. Structured self-management programmes are said to be successful in contributing to:

- reduction in the severity of symptoms
- decrease in pain
- improved life control and activity
- improved resourcefulness and life satisfaction
- improved doctor–patient communication.

These initiatives are not about instructing or educating patients about their condition but about developing the confidence and motivation of patients to use their skills and knowledge to take control over living with a chronic illness both in the management of their own condition and helping others in education programmes. In the UK such programmes have been developed with the support of voluntary agencies in the management of arthritis, manic depression and multiple sclerosis.

Both recognize that patients have expertise in their own condition and that people with the same condition may have similar concerns and problems. Self-management is, however, intended as an integral part of the health care system, rather than as an alternative support network for those dissatisfied with their care.

The ideological tension between responsibility and involvement discussed earlier in this chapter is evident in these moves to patient involvement. There is an expectation that people want to be involved and yet this can move from empowerment to moral coercion – that with the rights to treatment and care come responsibilities. As Small & Rhodes put it: 'Problems arise where opportunity turns into obligation and user involvement comes to be seen as a condition of receipt of services and more widely of responsible citizenship' (2000).

The 'Expert Patient' document recognizes that practitioners may have concerns and asserts that the Expert Patient programme is not an 'anti-professional initiative but one based on partnership. The expertise of professionals is no less essential in treating chronic disease when patients are involved in self-management' (DoH 2001b, p. 6). What does change with

---

Discussion point

What factors are likely to promote patient participation in decision making?

Discussion point

How do patient management groups differ from the self-help groups that have mushroomed since the 1970s?

Reflection point

What challenges would be posed to your practice by greater patient involvement?

the Expert Patient programme is that the relationship between patient and professional is enhanced through a recognition that the patient holds expert knowledge too, of how the chronic disease impacts on their life and how it may best be managed. The relationship thus becomes one between equal partners who each have a valuable expertise and perspective.

Patients as service users may also be involved in an advisory or management capacity as part of quality standards monitoring or strategic planning. The Community Health Councils that served as a local forum to comment, monitor and observe local health services have now been replaced by Patient Advisory and Liaison Committees whose role is as a point of contact and information for patient concerns, but with the monitoring function taken over by local authorities. Ensuring that such processes are productive and not tokenistic conduits for involvement is a major challenge.

Practitioner talking

I was part of a multi agency group carrying out a review of mental health services. We hired an independent researcher to lead focus groups of users and carers, health professionals and the general public. The members of the public and users were paid and this ensured good attendance. But those who didn't use the services found they had little to contribute and those that did had plenty to say about their experience but very little about how the services could be better organized or delivered. Some of the health professionals didn't listen when the users were talking and dismissed what they said as 'just their opinion'. The carers were worried about saying anything that could be seen as critical. The health professionals did not attend regularly and were not a cohesive group with different responsibilities and roles. The process was valuable but I think overall people were disappointed.

Commentary

The level of involvement expected here was not great and the exercise was a consultation with little opportunity to develop plans from the views expressed. Health professionals may see any views expressed as a challenge to their expertise and users do not feel they are taken seriously or fear their care might be affected. It is important that users do not feel they are merely commenting on issues but can be consultants. Some users have begun to develop research skills in order to find out about issues in a 'scientific way'. In other situations Anderson et al (2002) describe how the 'outsider voices' may be strong enough to have input because they are seen as representative of a wider community. The legitimacy of views can be called into question when the organizational culture is professionally dominant.

In order to avoid accusations of tokenism, organizations need to be clear about why they are seeking participation, what they want it to achieve and what level of involvement is appropriate. There needs to be transparency about which decisions are open to change so expectations aren't raised or organizations presented with a long list of actions that they are unable to deliver on. Preparatory work before any consultation is therefore vital to ensure a commitment to the process and so that everybody is clear about what is achievable and why the process is being undertaken. Clear mechanisms for feeding back information and decisions are also needed. As Brooks & Gillam found in their case studies of patient and public involvement in primary care, 'the single biggest criticism made of public involvement work by professionals and lay people alike is that it fails to bring about change. It simply doesn't make any difference' (2002, p. 55).

Participation should be a mainstream part of health and social care not a marginal activity or one left to a few 'experts' such as advocates or 'champions'. It is not easy to manage effectively. Avon and Wiltshire Mental Health Partnership NHS Trust (2002) set out standards for drug and alcohol services to ensure user involvement in the decision-making process. Suggested strategies include:

- asking more than one user to attend
- using language that is free from jargon
- meeting all expenses for travel, time, child care and being aware of the effect of payment on benefits (e.g. payment in vouchers)
- explaining the structure of meetings to the attendees beforehand
- providing training, e.g. assertiveness skills, chairing meetings, confidentiality
- offering appropriate settings that are comfortable and accessible
- ensuring that there is feedback about the ways in which user views have influenced decisions.

R eflection point

What further guidelines for user involvement would you add to the list above?

Participatory needs assessment

Comprehensive health and social needs assessment is the starting point for the development of any intervention strategy, service development or health improvement programme. Most national priority areas demand local strategies based on local knowledge of local needs. In Chapter 17 of *Health Promotion: Foundations for Practice* (Naidoo & Wills 2000) we discussed the question of what needs are and different ways of assessing needs. A health needs assessment is a systematic review of the health issues of a population leading to agreed priorities that will improve health and reduce inequalities.

Needs assessment uses quantitative and qualitative methods to investigate and understand:

- demographic and social characteristics of the population (its structure, socio-economic environment, lifestyles, history, culture and religion, its social institutions and interaction patterns)
- what medical conditions have the most impact: extent and scale of the issue (incidence and prevalence) and the burden and impact on those affected, their families and society
- current services and their utilization, unmet needs or excessive levels of service provision
- people's perception of what services and interventions should be developed and how they should be delivered
- views of professionals, managers and policy makers about the type and prevalence of problems and the best means to deliver services
- views of policy makers on resource feasibility.

'Community Oriented Primary Care' (COPC) is the term used in many countries to describe the process whereby a population's health needs are identified and addressed with the community as partners in the process. As Hooper & Longworth (2002) point out, health needs assessments need to be underpinned by the involvement of 'those who know, care and can make things happen'.

All too often in health needs assessments, health professionals take the lead and define 'health needs and services' from their perspective, which usually means what the epidemiological data suggest as the main priorities and what they are able to provide. New methods and techniques prioritize the involvement of communities and members of the public in the process. Rapid appraisal and participatory needs assessment are techniques which increase the participation of the community in defining needs and solutions.

<table>
<tr><td>

E xample

Rapid Appraisal as a method of needs assessment

</td><td>

Rapid Appraisal is a professionally led research approach that aims to provide policy makers with an understanding of communities. Rapid Appraisal gathers information about the health situation of a particular community in a short period of time and without large expense and is based on a community's own priorities (see Ong 1996). Rapid Appraisal typically involves interviewing a range of key local informants, collecting existing records and making observations in the neighbourhood. This information is then collected into an information 'pyramid' that describes the neighbourhood's issues and priorities. The validity of the approach depends on triangulation – data from one source is cross-checked against data from at least two other sources or methods of collection.

</td></tr>
</table>

Participatory needs assessment (PNA) emphasizes participatory processes which enable community members to set the agenda, analyse their situation and identify their own plans for action. This approach provides a useful starting point for engagement with a community and provides policy makers with quick and accurate assessments of the implications and impact of policies and services. PNA utilizes various methods including problem solving, community walks, force field analysis and ranking exercises that are highly visual. The use of several different methods increases the likelihood of engaging different groups within the community, including people who might be excluded by formal paper exercises. The collected data forms the basis for dialogue and can be discussed and modified.

D iscussion point

What criticisms could be made of these methods of community needs assessment?

As only limited data is collected it could be argued that the resulting needs assessment is superficial and partial. Qualitative data which is collected can be hard to analyse and 'pool'. The rapidity of the process means that relevant key informants may be missed and it may be difficult to move beyond individual agendas. The process can exclude people from particular cultural backgrounds or social groups.

The advantage of such methods is that they are participatory processes that enhance people's understanding of their problems and enables them to have a voice in defining local priorities. It is also a way to encourage policy makers to have contact with the communities they serve and build confidence in communities. The example below shows how needs assessment is not just a listening process but one where people can translate their solutions into actions.

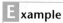xample

Figure 6.3
Roundshaw
Participatory Health
Needs Assessment
Source: Cornwall A.
Reproduced with per-
mission

The focus of this participatory needs assessment on a housing estate in South London was residents' views on well-being on the estate and their suggestions for improving the quality of life. Recommendations from the residents ranged from the provision of general and dog litterbins to establishing community run facilities such as a centre for the unemployed, greater support from health professionals with well woman clinics, community dentist and a female GP. Community members explored their priorities and then categorized them according to those they could undertake for themselves, those that could be undertaken in partnership with agencies working on the estate, and those that external agencies should undertake for, or on behalf of, the community. Representatives from a range of agencies expressed their preferences for action based on evidence of effectiveness and community-perceived needs.

Source: Cornwall (1997)

By Us/With Us	For Us	'Professionals' Priorities
• GP monitoring group	• Wardens to visit elderly once a month and to know where the elderly are on the estate	• Community-run unemployed centre
• Aromatherapy sessions		• General help for alcohol/drug related problems
• Dogs' mess/dog-free zones	• Make the estate cleaner: find ways to deal with the dog problem (i.e. dog-free zones, dog areas)	• A community advocate
• Domestic violence support *on* the estate		• A cook and eat club
• Alcohol/drug support	• GPs: need a new one in the health centre, improve old ones	• Wardens to visit all older people monthly
• Leisure facilities for older people		• GP monitoring group linked to the Community Health Council
• Youth facilities	• Need a dentist on the estate	
• A community advocate	• Advice/information on what's available and where to go for help: medical, social services, other kinds of help	• Domestic violence support
• Build an adventure playground		• Furniture project – involving younger people
• A support group for people with mental health problems		
• A cook and eat club	• A higher police profile: a police base on the estate	• Health information and health provision

'The process highlighted the extent to which the residents on Roundshaw were and are aware of the challenges that face them and were able to offer many workable solutions to address the needs they perceived as most pressing' (Rowley and Bhuhi 1999, p. 29).

Priority setting

One way in which individuals or groups may be involved in service planning is through deciding the priorities of different services or the allocation of resources. The mechanism used by many Local Authorities is the Citizens' Panel, which typically comprises 1000–2000 local residents who are presented with information and asked to help in decision making. An early exercise in community priority setting was that started in 1982 by Oregon Health Council to decide health service priorities and which services should be part of the local health plan. This eventually developed into an independent civic organization that has focused on access to health care, allocation of resources and which services should be included as part of Medicaid (Ham 1998, Hogg 1999).

In Canada, day-long dialogue sessions with representative groups of ordinary 'unorganized' citizens have been used to draft the health care policy. This process involves complex value judgements about responsibilities and choices and begins to redefine the role of a citizen from a passive consumer to an active participant in the governance of the health care system (Maxwell et al 2003).

Priority setting in citizens' panels typically takes place within a policy vacuum and on the basis of little information. This often leads to a majority view predominating depending on which professional discourses have entered the public domain. Decision making favours services that have impacted on participants' own families. Conversely, marginal or specifically targeted services and the needs of the most excluded get selected out.

Discussion point

What factors are likely to influence the decisions made by citizens' groups?

Community development

Community development involves active engagement with a defined group of people over an extended period of time in order to identify and tackle some of the social, economic, environmental and political issues that determine their health and quality of life. As well as leading to desirable outcomes, the process itself is important because its aim is to encourage participation and involvement and this is in itself beneficial to health.

Even when there is a commitment to community development and participation, its practice poses many challenges for practitioners. Community development includes a range of strategies and methods but fundamentally it involves the nurturing and release of talents, skills and capabilities. This requires time and trust in order to develop relationships, networks and effective ways of working. Goals may be initially unclear, become clarified and change over time. The process of community development therefore sits uneasily with the pressure on many practitioners to meet predetermined targets and objectives. Much of this work is resourced by short-term funded projects which do not recognize the time required to work successfully in this way. Experienced practitioners report that typically the time needed to establish relationships is underestimated but vital. 'This is the project worker's dilemma. If s/he involves people it may limit what can be done but if s/he doesn't what will be achieved anyway? Change isn't just an objective it must be part of the process. *How* you do it, really is what you get' (Beresford & Croft 1993, p. 119).

There may be longstanding feelings of disaffection, suspicion or powerlessness or a lack of structures to enable people to become involved. Freire (1972) argued that liberation requires people to develop a critical awareness of the world in which they live (conscientization) and to define problems as well as being involved in decision making to resolve problems. Communities cannot become active if people are not willing or able to give time or energy, where there are high levels of distrust or where

Discussion point

Why might it be difficult to engage communities?

people do not know each other and there are no networks that link people together.

The Standing Conference on Community Development published a definition of community development that clarifies it as a process:

> Community development is a way of working that encourages individual and collective action around the common needs and concerns identified by the community itself... It is about changing power structures to remove the barriers that prevent people from participating in the issues that affect their lives.
>
> (Standing Conference on Community Development www.sccd.org.uk accessed 10/5/03)

Barr & Hashagen (2000b) describe community development as an approach that uses various activities to help communities to exercise greater control and personal effectiveness:

- **Profiling and analysis** Getting to know the community including identifying its assets and strengths.
- **Capacity building** Building confidence in people as individuals and collectively so that they may become more active and interested in local issues and creating opportunities to develop new skills and gain new knowledge.
- **Organizing** Making contacts and bringing people together.
- **Networking** Provide support for people to come together and build networks, helping people to identify their priorities.
- **Resourcing** Gaining access to funds and resources.
- **Negotiating** Helping the community negotiate with service providers.

Discussion point

What community abilities might need to be developed?

The concept of community capacity has become widely used in recent years to describe the ability of a community to identify, mobilize and address social and public health problems and may be used synonymously with community development.

Capacity building may include resource building; personal development; skills training including literacy and numeracy and accredited schemes such as NVQs; and organizational development activities. Frequently there are few resources for this work and practitioners need to think creatively about the opportunities available.

Involving people in shaping and influencing decision making about health increases interaction between people which will have positive health outcomes. A high level of social capital is related to lower crime rates, better health and higher educational qualifications. Social capital is a relatively new concept that has aroused considerable debate about how it should be defined and measured. It originated with the work of Robert Putnam in Italy and the USA (Putnam 1993, 2000). Putnam found that in the USA the very poor living in urban areas who have a few relatively intense family or neighbourhood ties are trapped in their poverty whereas those with a wider network of weaker contacts do better. Social capital is the term used to describe networks and shared norms that facilitate coordination and cooperation for mutual benefit and create civic engagement. Developing communities then means developing the organizational structures, leadership and channels of communication that may help a community to:

- raise money
- comment or complain
- help others through volunteering or activism
- become involved in planning and decision-making processes.

Example

Housing and Regeneration Community Association (HARCA)

Seven housing estates in East London voted to be managed by HARCA but resident involvement was low and the estates housed diverse communities with diverse needs. The aim of the community development project was to assist the communities to become engaged in urban renewal initiatives. The community development worker spent considerable time scoping – getting to know the community, building contacts and identifying formal and informal networks and structures, finding out, identifying and prioritizing main concerns. The next stage was to clarify goals and priorities and identify what might need to change through a series of problem-solving questions:

- What are the main areas of dissatisfaction?
- What do people want to change?
- What needs to happen to bring about the changes?
- What can the people do themselves, who will do it, when and how?

The development stage of the project entailed:

- working with tenant boards and supporting them to be more active and effective
- setting up priority committees through community centres
- working with individuals, providing training and opportunities for development
- developing projects.

The outcomes for the residents:

- many residents have moved from volunteering to paid work
- specific projects for the community including play scheme, food coop, community newspaper, second hand shop, annual community festival
- greater levels of involvement
- breaking down isolation and a 'shut in culture' and increasing contacts and communication
- greater trust and confidence in public sector agencies.

Source: www.poplarharca.co.uk

EVIDENCE OF EFFECTIVENESS

In this chapter we have explored the current drivers towards patient and public involvement and some of the health outcomes expected from greater participation by individuals and communities:

- increased access to information
- greater ability to identify and articulate health needs
- increased self esteem and confidence in individuals
- more responsive services

- better relationships and greater understanding between stakeholders
- stronger community networks, relationships and support.

Evaluating each of these outcomes poses difficulties because they refer mainly to qualitative changes in people's perceptions rather than quantitative factors which can be counted. For medical practitioners especially, such evaluation may seem too vague to be credible. However, it is important that such outcomes are not ignored or devalued simply because they are hard to evaluate.

The methodological challenges of evaluating community development initiatives are common to many health promotion interventions (see Naidoo & Wills 2000, Ch. 19, and Ch. 3 in this volume).

Community development typically involves different partners, each with their own agenda, criteria for success and preferred method of evaluation. Deciding what to measure, when, and what threshold to accept as evidence of success, are current dilemmas for many community development projects. There is often a tension between funders of projects, who require relatively 'hard' quantitative data, and project workers or participants, who are often more drawn to 'soft' qualitative data. This may be crudely stated as a preference for outcomes (e.g. How many people became involved? In what ways did their behaviour change?) versus impact (e.g. What did people gain as a result of participating? How do people feel the project has affected their health and that of the community?), although the reality is more complex than this. There are frameworks for evaluating community development approaches to improving health and well-being. For example, the Achieving Better Community Development (ABCD) framework (Barr & Hashagen 2000a) and the Learning Evaluation and Planning Model (LEAP) (Barr 2002) both provide a structure within which community development work to promote health may be measured and evaluated.

The ABCD framework is built on the following principles:

- Planning and evaluation – needs to be built into projects and will be context specific.

- Empowerment – ways of defining and measuring participation and empowerment need to be included.

- Learning organizations – community organizations need to be flexible, adaptable and able to monitor their environment and react to change.

- Participative evaluation – the community itself is a key partner in any evaluation, and clear goals and criteria for success need to be identified collaboratively.

The LEAP model is characterized by the following features:

- Needs, problems and issues are defined by communities.

- Participative learning based on dialogue and equality rather than top-down expert led notions of learning.

- Partnership based.

Discussion point

Why might it be difficult to evaluate community development initiatives?

LEAP for Health (Hashagen 2003) suggests three broad outcomes areas which can be divided into several dimensions. The key outcomes are:

1. *Healthy people* who have:
   - awareness and knowledge
   - confidence, choice and control
   - independence and self-reliance
   - connections to community.

2. *Strong communities* characterized by:
   - community skills
   - equalities
   - community organization
   - community involvement.

3. *Quality of life* – likely to be context-specific but include indicators of the following:
   - community economy
   - community services
   - community health and safety
   - community culture
   - local democracy.

Discussion point

How could you use the LEAP model to evaluate a community gardening project which provides community allotments for young people, people with learning disabilities, and people with mental health problems?

An evaluation of such a project might include an assessment by project users and other key partners such as carers, parents and project workers of changes in users' confidence, social skills and independence since starting the gardening club. The development of community skills and organization linked to the gardening and sale of produce in the local farmers' market could be documented. The enhancement of quality of life through access to fresh vegetables and an income from sales of produce could be included, as could the respite offered by the project to carers. The increased physical activity of participants could also be noted. In this way, the multiple benefits of such a project on a community's health and well-being could be documented. By contrast, the traditional quantitative evaluation would probably only have counted the number of people involved, and missed the evidence of multiple and synergistic positive outcomes linked to the project.

INCREASING INVOLVEMENT: THE PRACTITIONER PERSPECTIVE

Reflection point

What opportunities are there for you to work in this way? What would be the main barriers?

Many of the barriers to involvement are linked to the culture of health care professionals and their employing agencies. This culture fosters a belief in professional expertise and often reinforces the dependent status of patients. The shift required to move from this position to one where members of the public are valued as equal experts is significant. In many instances public involvement is regarded as a 'time-consuming indulgence' – desirable and helpful but not necessary. Public and patient involvement is not yet mainstreamed into all areas of service delivery. Many PCTs have responded by appointing champions – people who will ensure this happens and remind people of what needs to be done and the mechanisms that need to be in place and ensure that there is feedback.

Reflection point

What arguments could you put forward to colleagues to support greater public or user involvement in your work?

For the individual practitioner working in primary care, for example, there are considerable disincentives to work in this way. It is time consuming and challenging to professional authority. It is likely that a practitioner would have to work alone and is unlikely to be supported by other members of the team. An individual practitioner would probably not be able to respond positively to many issues raised.

Practitioner talking

Staff attitudes to Patient and Public Involvement

Ironically staff at the coalface who interact every day with patients and public see the concept of involvement as an additional task. Managers and commissioners of services also have a dilemma in prioritizing the views of local service users when bound by their own professional judgement, targets, planning constraints and finite resources. To make public involve-ment their business, staff have to see it as part of the organizational culture and they need to have some decision-making power to improve services for patients. Opportunities need to be taken to involve the public within working and development groups, team meetings and larger conferences and events. Rich patient stories about patient experience, outcomes of care, environment and the organization of care are everyday bread and butter for community staff. They may need to tweak their listening skills but at the individual level, patient involvement can be easily facilitated. A more difficult area is how staff involve patients in their own care and treatment. It may feel a bit messy and out of control for the clinician to give the patient more responsibility but patient involvement and increased self-management will shift the balance of power. Staff should see this opportunity as another string to their bow not the straw that...well you know the rest...

Commentary

Greater public involvement can be supported on many grounds – professional, ethical and practical. From a health practitioner perspective, greater public involvement will ensure that services provided are accessible and appropriate, and are therefore used more effectively by patients. The new public health and health promotion are characterized by a concern to start with people's self-defined health needs and issues, which means taking a broad social perspective on health. Integral to this is the need to foster public involvement, both as a means of establishing public priorities and as a means of increasing public health and well-being through the participatory process. From an ethical perspective, greater involvement fosters autonomy and helps reduce inequalities associated with socio-economic factors as well as bringing additional benefits to service users. From a practical point of view, greater involvement will mean that resources are used efficiently and not wasted or duplicated, because services will be more closely tailored to needs. Public involvement may pose challenges, but this is part and parcel of the quest to broaden and develop practitioner expert-ise. As public involvement appears to be a permanent fixture on the public health agenda, developing expertise in this area will enhance professional and career development.

CONCLUSION

This chapter has located the current shift towards greater public involvement in health and public services within various policies. The rationale for public involvement includes enhanced efficiency, effectiveness and quality. Public involvement is a diverse phenomenon that refers to different models of 'the public', including patient, consumer, citizen and lay person. The implications of these different ideal types in terms of the kind of relationship and activities envisaged in public involvement have been discussed. Four particular strategies for public involvement – patient and user involvement, participatory needs assessment, priority setting and community development – have been explored in more detail. Particular challenges facing practitioners who wish to support greater public involvement have been identified and discussed throughout the chapter. A key challenge, which has been discussed in more depth, is the need to evaluate public involvement activities in ways which are appropriate and meaningful.

Public involvement is a relatively new concept within the health services, and health professionals are unlikely to have received training to support efforts in this field. As well as being an unfamiliar field for many practitioners, public involvement may also be viewed as a threat to professional expertise and autonomy, and a waste of time and resources. However, this chapter argues that public health and health promotion are inseparable from public involvement and participation. This is because the content of efforts to improve public health must relate to public perceptions and priorities and also because the process of participation is a key factor in health and well-being. Reliance solely on the medical model of health and professional expertise ignores many fundamental socio-economic determinants of health and fosters an unhealthy dependency and passivity amongst patients. An understanding of the benefits of public involvement and skills in supporting public involvement are vital aspects of the role of the public health and health promotion practitioner today.

FURTHER DISCUSSION

- Do you think public involvement knowledge and skills should be part of every health practitioner's training? Why?
- What strategies and techniques can be used to increase the involvement of the poorest and most marginalized groups in your community?
- What opportunities are there to encourage participation in your organization? Where are these on Arnstein's ladder of participation?

Recommended reading

- Anderson W, Florin D, Gillam S, Mountford L (2002) Every voice counts. Primary care organization and public involvement, London, King's Fund.
- Brooks F, Gillam S (2001) New beginnings: why patient and public involvement in primary care. London, King's Fund

Two guides that explore the current policy drive to patient and public involvement and examine how this is being implemented in several case study Primary Care Trusts.

- Orme J, Powell J, Taylor P, Harrison T, Grey M (eds) (2003) Public health for the 21st century: new perspectives on policy, participation and practice. Maidenhead, Open University Press/McGraw-Hill Education.

A useful text that explores participation and partnership as part of contemporary public health practice.

- Rifkin S, Lewando-Hundt G, Draper A (2000) Participatory approaches in health promotion and health planning – a literature review. London, HEA.

A comprehensive review that examines the various definitions of 'community' and 'participation' and discusses the methods and tools used in participatory approaches.

- Smithies J, Webster G (1998) Community involvement in health: from passive recipients to active participants. Aldershot, Ashgate.

An accessible guide to the origins and development of community development approaches.

REFERENCES

Anderson W, Florin D, Gillam S, Mountford L (2002) Every voice counts. Primary care organization and public involvement. London, King's Fund

Arnstein S (1969) A ladder of citizen participation. Journal of the American Institute of Planners 35(4): 216–224

Avon and Wiltshire Mental Health Partnership NHS Trust (2002) Service user involvement. Avon and Wiltshire Mental Health Partnership NHS Trust

Barr A (2002) Learning evaluation and planning. London, Community Development Foundation

Barr A, Hashagen S (2000a) ABCD handbook: a framework for evaluating community development. London, CDF Publications

Barr A, Hashagen S (2000b) Achieving better community development. London Community Development Foundation

Beresford P, Croft S (1993) Citizen involvement: a practical guide for change. Basingstoke, Macmillan

Brooks F, Gillam S (2001) New beginnings: why patient and public involvement in primary care. London, King's Fund

Children and Young People's Unit (CYPU) (2001) Learning to listen: core principles for involving children and young people. Nottingham, Department for Education and Skills

Cornwall A (1997) Roundshaw participatory health needs assessment www.ids.ac.uk/ids/particip/research/health.html accessed 10/5/03

Coulter A (2002) After Bristol: putting patients at the centre. British Medical Journal 324: 648–651

Dartford, Gravesham and Swanley Primary Care Trust (DGS PCT) (2003) Towards a strategy for public involvement. Dartford, Gravesham and Swanley Primary Care Trust

Department of Health (DoH) (1999) Saving lives: our healthier nation. London, The Stationery Office

Department of Health (DoH) (2000) The NHS plan: a plan for investment, a plan for reform. London, DoH www.nhs.uk/nationalplan

Department of Health (DoH) (2001a) The Health and Social Care Act (Section 11 Public involvement and consultation). London, The Stationery Office

Department of Health (DoH) (2001b) The expert patient: a new approach to chronic disease management for the 21st century. London, DoH

Department of Health (2001c) Learning from Bristol: the report of the public inquiry into children's heart surgery at the Bristol Royal Infimary (Kennedy Report) 1984–1995. London, DoH www.bristol-inquiry.org.uk

Department of Health (DoH) (2003) Strengthening accountability: involving patients and the public policy guidance. London, DoH

Freire P (1972) Pedagogy of the oppressed. Harmondsworth, Penguin

Ham C (1998) Retracing the Oregon trail: the experience of rationing and the Oregon Health Plan. British Medical Journal 316: 1965–1969

Harrison S, Mort M (1998) Which champions, which people? Public and user involvement in health care as a technology of legitimation. Social Policy and Administration 32(1): 60–70

Hashagen S (2003) Frameworks for measuring community health and well-being. In: Orme J, Powell J, Taylor P, Harrison T, Grey M (eds) Public health for the 21st century: new perspectives on policy, participation and practice. Maidenhead, Open University Press/McGraw-Hill Education

Hogg C (1999) Patients, power and politics: from patients to citizens. London, Sage

Hooper J, Longworth P (2002) Health needs assessment workbook. London, Health Development Agency

Jewkes R, Murcott A (1998) Community representatives: representing the 'community'. Social Science and Medicine 46(7): 843–858

McNeish D, Newman T (2002) Involving children and young people in decision making. In: McNeish D, Newman T, Roberts H (eds) What works for children? Maidenhead, Open University Press

Marelich W, Roberts K, Murphy D, Callari T (2002) HIV/AIDS patient involvement in antiretroviral treatment decisions. AIDS Care 14(1): 17–26

Maxwell J, Rosell S, Forest P G (2003) Giving citizens a voice in health care policy in Canada. British Medical Journal 326: 1031–1033

Mitcheson J, Cowley S (2003) Empowerment or control? An analysis of the extent to which client participation is enabled during health visitor/client interactions using a health needs assessment tool. International Journal of Nursing Studies 40(4): 413–426

Naidoo J, Wills J (2000) Health promotion: Foundations for practice. London, Baillière Tindall

New Economics Foundation (2003) Participation briefing on the Imagine Project. London, NEF

NHS Executive (1998) First class service: quality in the new NHS. London, DoH

Ong B N (1996) Rapid appraisal and health policy. London, Chapman Hall

Ovreteit J (1996) How patient power and client participation affects relations between professions. In: Ovreteit J, Mathias P, Thompson R (eds) Interprofessional working for health and social care. Basingstoke, Macmillan

Putnam R (1993) Making democracy work: civic traditions in modern Italy. Princeton, NJ, Princeton University Press

Putnam R (2000) Bowling alone: the collapse and revival of American community. New York, Simon & Schuster

Rowley J, Bhuhi J (1999) Participatory Needs Assessment: a practical approach in partnerships between local residents and professionals. Public Health Medicine 1: 27–30

Sainio C, Eriksson E, Lauri S (2001) Patient participation in decision making about care: the cancer patients' point of view. Cancer Nursing 24(3): 172–179

Small N, Rhodes P (2000) Too ill to talk? User involvement and palliative care. London, Routledge

Tudor Hart J (1971) The inverse care law. Lancet 1: 405

Wilcox D (1994) A guide to effective participation. Brighton, Pavilion

World Health Organization (WHO) (1978) Alma Ata 1978 Primary Health Care. Copenhagen, WHO

World Health Organization (WHO) (1985) Health for all in Europe by the year 2000. Copenhagen, WHO

World Health Organization (WHO) (1986) Ottawa charter for health promotion: an international conference on health promotion. Geneva, WHO

World Health Organization (WHO) (1997) New players for a new era: leading health promotion into the 21st century. 4th International Conference on Health Promotion, Jakarta, Indonesia. Conference Report. Geneva, WHO

7 Partnership working

Key Points

- Defining partnership working:
  - types of partnerships
  - features of successful partnerships
- The impetus for collaboration
- Understanding partnership working:
  - organizational theory
  - groupwork theory.

OVERVIEW

Partnership working is now a central feature of all public services and the modernization agenda. It is based on the understanding that individual and community well-being is determined as much by social, environmental and economic systems as health-care provision. It follows then that the promotion and maintenance of health does not belong to one professional group or sector. The World Health Organization (WHO) states that intersectoral collaboration across different public sectors is central to achieving the goal of Health For All and to the development of a healthy public policy. National health strategies also support the concept of partnerships as the key way to deliver health improvement, better integrated services and reduce health inequalities. This chapter looks at the context in which this current emphasis on collaboration has arisen and explores the tensions underpinning current practice. It outlines how an understanding of organizational theory and groupwork theory can help to identify key themes in successful partnership working.

INTRODUCTION

Partnerships appear to be a rational response to service delivery and professional working. They expand the budget available to tackle an issue, they may help to achieve better coordination and through the pooling of ideas and resources may achieve 'added value'. The benefits of partnership working are:

- a greater mix of skill and knowledge
- the sharing of common concerns and information
- the ability to influence decision making
- avoiding the duplication of, or gaps in, a service response so making better use of existing resources
- a more comprehensive and holistic approach to problems
- synergy – the effect of collaboration being greater than that achieved alone.

The term 'partnership' has become rather a catch-all phrase for a range of different concepts of joint working. The Department of Health initially used the term 'healthy alliance' to define the way agencies can work together to promote health, emphasizing cooperation and partnership: 'A healthy alliance is in effect a partnership of individuals and

Reflection point

How many partnerships are you aware of in your area? What is their purpose? Who do they involve?

organizations formed to enable people to increase their influence over the factors that affect their health and well-being' (DoH 1993, p. 22).

WHO used the term 'Intersectoral Collaboration' to emphasize that collaboration should take place across public sectors and involve a wide range of agencies. The Alma Ata declaration (WHO 1978) stated that health could only be attained by action in spheres additional to the health sector, in particular: agriculture, animal husbandry, food industry, education, housing, public works and communications. By the late 1990s a new partnership culture had emerged. The White Paper *Working Together for a Healthier Scotland* (Scottish Office 1998), as its name suggests, places partnership working as the cornerstone of health improvement strategy. Similarly, *Well Being in Wales* (Welsh Assembly 2002) requires local health boards and local authorities to work in partnership to develop health and well-being. In England all NHS partners are expected to work with Local Authorities to produce health improvement plans (HiMPs) showing how public services would be integrated. A commitment to partnership as a means of planning underpins Local Strategic Partnerships (LSPs). Other initiatives such as Sure Start and the National Strategy for Neighbourhood Renewal also bring together different organizations. 'Successful partnership working is built on organizations moving together to address common goals: on developing in their staff the skills necessary to work in an entirely new way – across boundaries, in multidisciplinary teams, and in a culture in which learning and good practice are shared' (DoH 1999, p. 123).

Partnership working has come to represent a new means of governance – instead of hierarchies or competition, the dominant mode of organization is networks. Networks are based on trust. Yet to expect this to happen automatically is unrealistic. Indeed, many practitioners' experience of collaborative working is of intense competition and rivalry and a reluctance to share information or 'give up' areas of work. Many professional training and education programmes stress the unique perspective and skills of the profession, which may lead to 'protectionism' when professionals feel threatened by rapid organizational change. In such uncertain situations, instead of recognizing the potential for partnership working, professionals may retreat within their own professional role and identity.

There are also the differing perspectives that organizations have on what exactly constitutes promoting health. There is no identifiable theory of collaboration which can help to illuminate this.

> Collaboration is a paradoxical concept in the field of social welfare. There can be little doubt that the notion is in vogue. The desirability of some form of collaborative activity has become a *sine qua non* of effective practice within the welfare professions, both at practitioner and policy making levels. However we know remarkably little about how collaborative activity works, why it may initially be developed, how it may be measured or even how it may be defined.
>
> (Hudson 1987, p. 175)

There are only a small number of studies which focus on collaborative activity and these are principally in the fields of child protection where

---

R **eflection point**

Has your professional training included partnership skills? What would these be?

inter-agency cooperation is a high priority (Birchall & Hallett 1992, DoH 1991) and the working of primary health care teams (Ovreteit 1993). There are a few empirical studies in the UK of intersectoral collaboration in the health promotion field which attempt to develop a theory of collaboration (Davies et al 1993, Delaney 1994a, Springett 1995) but otherwise most of the conclusions about the features of successful collaboration draw mainly on the experience of practitioners (see, for example, Balloch & Taylor 2001). These accounts tend to be enthusiastic about the prospects but pessimistic about the actual outcomes of partnerships. This chapter draws on organizational studies and groupwork theory to explore why collaboration is a difficult principle to put into practice.

DEFINING COLLABORATION AND PARTNERSHIP

'Partnership' is a slippery concept that is difficult to define precisely (Audit Commission 1998). The World Health Organization uses the term 'collaboration' and the Department of Health in the 1980s used the term 'healthy alliance' and now uses the term 'partnerships'. Networks or coalitions may also be used to describe health and welfare practitioners working together. Table 8.1 shows the distinctions made by Leathard (1994) between

- concept-based terms
- process-based terms
- agency-based terms.

The underlying assumption of partnerships is that agencies work together. In Table 8.1 there are many process-based terms to describe working together. Many of these terms are used synonymously, although there are differences. Ovreteit (1993) when discussing how people from different professions and agencies work together gives emphasis to three key words:

- Coordinate – to bring into order as parts of a whole
- Collaborate – to labour together, to act jointly
- Cooperate – to unite for a common effort and shared goals.

The experience of partnerships is that partners have different expectations and degrees of real and perceived power. Plampling et al (2000) distinguish coordinating partnerships where the partners agree the nature of the problem and its solution from corporate partnerships in which partners pursue their own goals most effectively by working with others. In a review for the King's Fund, Pratt & Plampling (1998) comment on the processes of joint working, noting that shared goals do not usually predominate in partnerships. Where these do exist (such as tackling inequalities) then partners cooperate. They may even engage in 'co-evolution'. Where, however, there is a single goal (such as cancer prevention) then partners may at best collaborate to achieve a plan, but at worst they may compete.

Table 7.1 Alternative terms used variously for inter-professional work denoting learning together and working together
Source: Leathard A (1994) Going Inter-professional: Working Together for Health and Welfare. Reproduced by permission of Routledge

Concept-based	Process-based	Agency-based
Interdisciplinary	Joint planning	Inter-agency
Multidisciplinary	Joint training	Intersectoral
Multiprofessional	Shared learning	Trans-sectoral
Transprofessional	Teamwork	Cross-agency
Transdisciplinary	Partnership	Consortium
Holistic	Merger	Commission
Generic	Groupwork	Healthy alliances
	Collaboration	Forum
	Integration	Alliance
	Cooperation	Centre
	Liaison	Federation
	Synergy	Confederation
	Bonding	Inter-institutional
	Common core	Locality groups
	Interlinked	
	Interrelated	
	Joint project	
	Collaborative care planning	
	Locality planning	
	Unification	
	Coordination	
	Multilateral	
	Joint learning	
	Joint management	
	Joint budgets	
	Working interface	
	Participation	
	Collaborative working	
	Involvement	
	Joint working	
	Jointness	

'The general pattern of collaboration would seem to be one of the health service eliciting support of other sectors for the implementation of NHS initiated policies' (Farrant 1986).

Do you agree with the above statement? Can you identify any changes in collaborative working since 1986?

Concept-based terms include those most commonly used in the health sector of 'interdisciplinary' or 'multidisciplinary' working. These terms both refer to a team of individuals with different professional or training backgrounds (e.g. nursing, education, social work) who make different contributions to the team. Interdisciplinary means within the same professional group, e.g. community nurses and acute sector nurses, whereas multidisciplinary is normally taken to refer to a wider group which includes members from different professions.

Partnerships can:

- link individuals, informal networks or agencies and organizations
- be loose networks or formal arrangements
- be single issue or broad based
- have a fixed timescale or an on-going remit
- be neighbourhood, community, nationally or internationally based
- be concerned with a client group, a health issue or broader issues such as environmental responsibility
- be strategic, facilitative or implementing.

The partners are determined largely by the nature of the task and how broadly the coordinating agency interprets 'health'. A review of HiMPs in 1999 (Hamer 1999) found considerable variety ranging from complete NHS dominance to the involvement of different local authority tiers and departments, voluntary sectors, the police, the probation service, a university and the private sector. Increasingly partnerships are part of mainstream working and attempt to address major issues where the problems are hard to define and the causal chains hard to unravel (Henwood & Hudson 2000).

From the NHS, there might be community nurses, GPs, health promotion, nutrition and dietetic services, occupational health, physiotherapy, smoking cessation services, community pharmacists. From the Local Authority there might be representatives from leisure services, regeneration and planning, social care services, transport, road and highways. From the voluntary sector there would be organizations with a remit for CHD prevention or which address risk factors for CHD and organizations with links with target groups such as Black and ethnic minority groups or older people. There may be representatives for the private sector including food retailers, large local employers, private sector leisure providers, restaurateurs and caterers.

Partnership means different things in different contexts. It can cover a variety of arrangements, ranging from parallel working with some informal contact through to integrated working on many different levels. Table 7.2 illustrates this.

Table 7.2 Degrees of partnership

Isolation	No relationship, agencies work in isolation. No partnership exists.
Encounter	Some informal ad hoc contact between agencies, e.g. the day-to-day liaison that takes place between health and social care professionals about clients and service delivery.
Communication	Formal joint work undertaken but not seen as central, e.g. working groups on issues of shared concern or collaborative projects.
Collaboration	Joint working seen as central to organizations' purpose, e.g. the formal arrangements that exist for the providing or commissioning of local services. The coordination of policy and priorities across key agencies such as Sure Start programmes.
Integration	Organizations may be willing to integrate. An alternative to partnership.

Source: Adapted from Peckham (2003)

THE DEVELOPMENT OF PARTNERSHIPS AND HEALTH POLICY

An acceptance of the impact on people's health of all sorts of policies and programmes outside of the health service sector requires the development of mechanisms so that policy makers are aware of the consequences for health of their actions. The WHO Health For All strategy stressed the need for intersectoral collaboration for just this reason (WHO 1985). The revisited Health for All strategy, 'Health 21: 21 targets for the 21st century' contains a specific target (number 20) on mobilizing partners for health: 'By the year 2005, implementation of policies for health for all should engage individuals, groups and organizations throughout the public and private sectors and civil society, in alliances and partnerships for health' (WHO 1998, p. 200).

Peckham (2003) identifies three broad strategies which have been used to develop partnerships:

- Cooperation based on agreement. The healthy alliances policy initiative originating in 1992, for example, encouraged the formation of focused partnerships at local level such as 'Stepping Stones' a project in Lancashire in which social services, health services and voluntary groups helped people with mental health problems return to education. In most cases, the alliances were operational and incremental – one project leading to more general collaboration.
- Incentives to encourage partnerships through funding and more flexible resource allocation. In the mid 1990s for example, the need for urban regeneration provided the impetus and cash incentives for numerous projects under the umbrella of 'City Challenge' or 'Drug Prevention Initiatives'.
- Authoritarian approaches requiring organizations to work in partnerships such as the duties on local health boards in Wales and Primary

Care Trusts in England to work with Local Authorities. Since 1997 'partnership has become a legal, almost moral imperative in the health and social care world' (Plampling et al 2000, p. 1723)

Table 7.3 shows how the concept of partnership working has slowly been endorsed in the UK. Inter-agency working in areas of need was evident in the 1960s in Educational Priority Areas and through the early community development programmes. By the 1980s, however, the introduction of a market system of welfare led to a fragmentation of services.

Discussion point

What makes a partnership strategic?

Table 7.3 The impetus to partnership: selected policy initiatives

1980	WHO Health For All European Strategy
1984	WHO Healthy Cities settings approach
1986	Development of primary health care teams
1989	Public inquiries into child abuse cases (Beckford 1985; Carlisle 1987; Cleveland 1987) highlight lack of coordination between relevant agencies. Department of Health publishes guidelines on child protection
	NHS and Community Care Act: To provide seamless care for those needing care in the community – elderly, disabled and mentally ill
1992	Health of the Nation: English national health strategy
1993	Agenda 21 UK strategy for sustainable development requires Local Authorities to show how they will protect the environment for the twenty-first century
1998	Modernizing Social Services: promoting independence, improving protection, raising standards
1998	Health Improvement Programme: A three-year framework to improve health and social care with NHS, local authority, voluntary organizations and community partners
1998	Health Action Zones: To develop local strategies for improving the health of people and tackle health inequalities
1999	National Service Frameworks: Set out performance standards for services and recommend pooled budgets, integrated provision
	Childrens' Fund: Education, health and social care partnerships to support the well-being of school age children and their parents
2001	Local Strategic Partnerships (England): A single body to prepare and implement a community strategy to tackle deprivation (crime, jobs, education, housing, health)

Example

Local Strategic
Partnerships

Local Strategic Partnerships (LSPs) bring together the main public service providers in an area along with local communities and the voluntary, public and private sectors. Their purpose is to coordinate improvements in public services to achieve sustainable economic, social and physical regeneration and to narrow the gap between the quality of life in deprived areas and the rest of the country.

Manchester LSP has seven thematic partnerships:

- Economic and Local Employment
- Children and Young People
- Sustainable Neighbourhoods
- Crime and Disorder Partnership
- Health Inequalities
- Transport
- Culture Contact.

UNDERSTANDING PARTNERSHIP WORKING

Although little is known about collaboration for health, there is a substantive body of theory on inter-organizational coordination in general which suggests that organizations have conflicting interests and degrees of power. Another body of literature on occupational cultures suggests that professions are basically autonomous and resistant to crossing boundaries. The assumption then that organizations can, and want, to work together is somewhat unrealistic. The concept of exchange is therefore seen as the key to understanding collaboration. Regardless of the overt purpose of an organization (e.g. to provide services or meet client needs), most organizations are also concerned to preserve their interests – to ensure adequate resources, their autonomy, status and authority. Working with other agencies results in some loss of independence and control and necessitates the investment of scarce resources into building partnerships, the outcomes of which are by no means clear. Consequently, organizations only enter into collaborative working if they can see the needs of their organization are being met and will benefit in some way.

The Department of Health (1999) identified the following benefits from joint working:

- the ability to plan jointly for the commission and delivery of services across a health community
- sharing skills and resources, economies of scale
- the opportunity to develop programmes of work which directly support the delivery of plans for improving health and health care within the community.

Yet there is an increasing acceptance that partnership working is neither easy nor a panacea for tackling big issues. As a Health Education Board for

Scotland report comments (HEBS 2000, p. 7) 'many writers stress the inevitability of conflict and the need to accept it and work with it'.

SUCCESSFUL PARTNERSHIP WORKING

Plampling et al (2000) identified a series of steps that are important when establishing a partnership:

1. Find a shared goal.
2. Build trust gradually.
3. Find a common currency/fair exchange.
4. Clarify vision and objectives.
5. Include a wide range of stakeholders.
6. Have good communication, visibility and transparency of working.
7. Develop human resources.

Find a shared goal

For participants to believe that the partnership is beneficial, there needs to be a clear, shared vision of what it is intended to achieve (Delaney 1994a, DoH 1993, Nutbeam 1994, Powell 1992). When partnerships to promote health try to identify their goals, a lack of agreement comes to the fore with competing rationales. Delaney thus calls the basis for developing a shared vision in many partnerships 'rather flimsy' (Delaney 1994a, p. 220). Taking the time to identify shared values and a common starting point through workshops and open discussions is deemed to be the first task of a partnership.

Build trust gradually

It cannot be assumed that a partnership will fall into place because there are structures and processes supporting it. Building trust is an important ingredient in successful partnerships. Trust includes recognizing the purpose and value of partners' work, and knowing that others value one's own contribution, skills and knowledge. Powell (1992) found that to be effective, partners need to discover how each other's organizations are structured; how decisions are taken and by whom; their financial and planning processes and the ways in which information is communicated. This vital stage may be overlooked when partnerships see their priority as getting things done.

The fragmentation and compartmentalizing of practitioners and services which is typical of the role culture of the NHS can make collaboration difficult. Recent guidance on partnership working (DETR 2001) recommends that individuals clarify what they bring to a partnership as representatives of their community, as a service provider and as a partner. Those working in the NHS may be particularly bound by their roles and hierarchical structures. Participants may lack the status to make decisions or commit money or be unclear about the roles of other departments within the organization. Representatives who are committed to the partnership and who share the same values as the other members may not be

---

Discussion point

To which culture does your organization belong? How does the leadership and decision making in this kind of culture affect partnerships with other organizations?

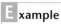xample

Organizational
cultures

A recognition of different organizational cultures is an important element in the understanding of the partners in an alliance. Handy (1976) has identified organizations as like tribes and families, with their own ways of doing things. He uses the symbolism of four gods to describe the varying types of management that can be discerned in organizations:

▪ The club culture symbolized by Zeus. This organization is characteristic of small family type companies. Control is exercised from the centre with little bureaucracy.

▪ The role culture symbolized by Apollo. This a typical bureaucracy with different departments for different functions such as finance, purchasing, marketing, etc. These are coordinated by a hierarchy of managers.

▪ The task culture symbolized by Athena. This is a matrix organization with a team culture. Expertise rather than position is important and management is flat and low key.

▪ The existential culture symbolized by Dionysus. This organization is a cluster of individuals, each of whom is fairly autonomous.

representative of their organization. Glover describes a workplace project in which 'building on an individual's enthusiasm without getting the agreement of the organization they represented created a problem. Consequently, when there were changes of personnel, commitment to the project was lost and support had to be renegotiated with the individual's successor' (Glover 2001, p. 213). Where partnerships have a strategic role, partners need to have enough influence within their own organization to secure a commitment to the policy.

Find a common currency/fair exchange

One of the key factors in effective collaboration is achieving an inter-agency equilibrium where power is balanced among the participating agencies. A sense of equality among partners is important in generating commitment. This can be problematic when partners vary widely in terms of size, status and funding. The source of power for an organization varies. Local authorities are controlled by elected politicians; voluntary organizations are accountable to management committees and their client group, health authorities have a duty to develop mechanisms for consultation but have no direct local accountability. The different basis of Local Authority and Health Authority membership can create different priorities. Local Authority officers who have to work from election to election can find longer-term strategic planning difficult (Delaney 1994b). Health services' accountability is governed by the Patient's Charter and various statutory responsibilities but have only recently embraced the principle of participation and the need for consultation and involvement.

D **iscussion point**

What factors might constitute 'power' for an organization in a partnership?

Power might include information, access to important networks or groups the organization is intended to serve and, crucially, sources of funding. Power also manifests itself in partnerships through the way participating organizations negotiate the remit of the partnership and whether they are 'invited' to join a partnership by a lead agency. This can lead to the work and contribution of partners not being equally valued.

E **xample**

Regeneration partnership

Regeneration partnerships exist in many disadvantaged areas. They need to work across boundaries beyond the usual focus of NHS and Local Authority coordinating services. The 'Health Ladder' scheme in East London was funded by the Single Regeneration Budget and is an example of NHS and social care working together to tackle economic development, employment strategy and the regeneration of the local area. Local Authorities are charged with creating employment and reducing the social exclusion of vulnerable groups. The NHS is often the largest employer in a locality yet in many urban areas finds it difficult to recruit enough staff. Under the 'Health Ladder' scheme, refugees are helped to qualify for work in the NHS and young people are provided with work experience in the health service and mentoring by NHS staff. The evaluation of the programme is built around three principles:

- sharing lessons (because this is the first scheme designed to improve an area through health care it is vital to understand how successful it is)
- giving communities a say and identifying what communities consider the markers of success
- making the scheme responsive by feeding back into the scheme results of on-going evaluation.

Source: www.lsbu.ac.uk/regenva

The exchange theory of organizational relations suggests that for partnerships to develop there needs to be some brokerage and matchmaking, recognizing what each brings to the task and negotiating on points of conflict. Financial clout is at the heart of power relations. Organizations may be wary of joint working if they are concerned about their partner's commitment but may equally embrace it if they believe it will increase access to other pots of money.

Clarify vision and objectives

Partnerships often emerge as strategies to bid for specific funding streams. This can lead to conflict. In a resource starved environment, different imperatives become clear. The pots of money that are available for new initiatives such as Sure Start or Neighbourhood Renewal can lead to competition rather than developmental commissioning. Differential budget growth, a reluctance to share resources and different budget cycles may all be barriers to successful public sector partnerships. Partnerships where time has been taken to allow a common shared vision and objectives to be defined are much stronger, more stable, and stand a better chance of survival. It may be difficult to take time out at the outset of partnerships to establish a shared vision, but experience suggests this is time well spent.

Practitioner talking

This isn't a very successful partnership as we seem rather peripheral. There isn't a stable and linked structure for the Sure Start programme so we don't link in with people as well as we should. Where we do, it's because I go round chasing and go out to meet people. But I am not sure we know who are the key partners. Certainly I don't think I know much about what is happening. There's supposed to be a system of communication and feeding back but it doesn't filter through to the ground and there isn't a good uptake of people at the meetings. We just don't have time and it doesn't get prioritized.

This partnership includes a major agency from the voluntary sector. What they seem to be doing is trying to promote themselves. They want an active role like having their facilities used even when it isn't necessarily the most effective or cheapest option. It's like they are competing for resources and leadership. I know it's important within such a tight geographic boundary to include all the organizations but everybody needs to be considered and acknowledged equally.

Commentary

A shared set of values is deemed the most important prerequisite for a partnership (DETR 2001). In this Sure Start partnership there appear to be different priorities. Large-scale programmes such as this have major funding attached that provides an incentive to organizations to work together. This seems to have supported innovative projects but not had much impact on departmental ways of working. Existing power relationships remain and practitioners (and service users) are at the margins of the partnership process. The partnership 'table' takes people away from 'the frontline' and their constituency. Those left delivering the service can become resentful as they get stretched and may feel they have been neglected for more attractive work. As well as the cultural challenge, there are structural and managerial challenges requiring ways of sharing and disseminating information.

Include a wide range of stakeholders

Some partnerships tend to focus on statutory agencies only. Although there may be professional barriers, there are also commonalities – a professional work role, a service sector employer and bureaucratic work cultures – which make it relatively easy to work together. To embrace voluntary agencies and service users as equal stakeholders represents a much greater challenge. Voluntary sector organizations sometimes find it difficult to be active partners. They are unable to commit funds to joint working and their organizational culture is different from the statutory and private sectors. Although they are not bound by the roles of the statutory sector, they may be perceived as amateurish and as not accountable and unable to deliver. Voluntary groups may feel compelled to be part of partnerships because of access to extra funding but also feel that their lobbying role is thereby compromised. What voluntary organizations do bring is the understanding of the perceptions, attitudes and values of service users which will ultimately determine how acceptable and effective service provision is. Understanding this different, but equal basis for stakeholders is one important aspect of successful partnerships.

R eflection point

To what extent are members of the general public (or their representatives) seen as equal partners within your organization?

Have good communication, visibility and transparency of working

Good communication, including the transparency of decision making, is a central factor underpinning effective partnerships. Communication includes face-to-face contact such as in meetings as well as written documentation, and increasingly, email networks. Every avenue of communication needs to be scrutinized to ensure that it is inclusive, accessible and understandable to all partners.

Develop human resources

Most studies on inter-agency working have concentrated on the structures of organizations and the context in which it takes place. Nevertheless most partnerships attribute their success or failure to 'personalities' and individual members. Whilst the role of personalities can be overplayed, most studies suggest that 'networking' is at the heart of collaboration and that nurturing relationships is crucial. Group theory can help us to understand how networking takes place, how groups can fail to achieve their task, and how conflict can arise.

D iscussion point

What reasons might there be for conflict in joint working?

As we saw in the previous section, organizations have partisan interests and want to hold on to their resources and autonomy. In addition, there are professional constraints on collaboration. Lack of role clarity is often cited as an explanation for conflict when members are not clear about their contribution or that of others. Sentiments such as these are commonplace:

- I don't know what I'm doing here or why I've been invited. I've got nothing to do with health.'
- 'The PCT (or any of the other participants) are just doing this to get more money for themselves.'
- 'This is just a talking shop. It's got nothing to do with our priorities.'

Simnett states:

R eflection point

Think of a partnership where you have been a partner. Were there any partners who questioned their participation? What did each of the partners bring to the alliance?

> Once members of a team understand how they can best contribute to a team, in terms of their roles and know they are valued for their unique contributions, then they no longer need to compete against each other. In this way, teams or groups can begin to achieve more – what has been called synergy, something that is more than the sum total of that produced by individuals.

(1995, p. 156)

Davies et al (1993) identify a key role in alliances for the mediator, who can resolve conflicts through bargaining and exchange. They also identify a role for 'the reticulist' – someone who plays a bridging role, spanning organizational boundaries, and who can harness energies and skills. It is often necessary for a formally appointed coordinator to take on this bridging role.

Tuckman's model of group development (Tuckman 1965) has been influential in showing how groups have common characteristics in their development. Tuckman describes groups as moving through five identifiable stages:

Reflection point

Belbin's research into the working of teams (Belbin 1981) has been extremely influential in understanding the particular problems which may arise in groups and how the contribution of individuals can be enhanced. Belbin identified eight roles which together create a balanced, high-performing group:

- leader (the coordinator)
- task leader (the shaper)
- ideas person (the plant)
- analyst (the monitor/evaluator)
- practical organizer (company worker)
- fix it (the resource investigator)
- mediator (the team worker)
- details person (the finisher).

Can you identify the role you normally play in groups?

1. **Forming** – in which a group first meets and works out the roles of members and tries to agree a task and some way of working.

2. **Storming** – in which the group becomes polarized and may form subgroups. There may be reactions to power distribution and some resistance to the task.

3. **Norming** – in which the group begins to establish some shared goals and to find a way of working. Members take on roles to support the group in its task or to help the group work well together.

4. **Performing** – in which the group begins to work well. There is more trust and acceptance of the contribution of each member. Interpersonal issues get resolved. Members approach the task with energy.

5. **Mourning** – the group disbands, sometimes reluctantly and there may be attempts to continue the life of the group.

Reflection point

Think of a partnership where you have been a partner. Can you identify stages in the 'life' of the partnership? What helped to move the group through the stages or did it get stuck?

In the initial stages of partnerships, there may be competition (the storming phase) as the balance of power within the group is worked out. For a group to move on, however, a safe enough environment has to be created.

Participants have to relinquish some control in joint working. For professions in health and social care which have been seeking to define their professional competence and difference such as nurses and health promotion specialists, crossing professional boundaries and finding ways to work together can be challenging. Beattie (1994) cites the following as common barriers to intersectoral working:

1. professional ambition and competition
2. territoriality and protectionism
3. information used as a major source of power and shared only reluctantly
4. different terminology and jargon.

In partnerships, participants often focus on the task for which they have come together. Difficulties arise over the nature of the task and the role of the participating agencies in the partnership. What often gets ignored in partnership working is the 'maintenance' of the partnership – those ways of being which help people to work together. Markwell (1998), for example, identifies the importance of making sure that participants are acquainted. The motivation of someone drafted in or someone who has little influence or knowledge of the echelons of their own agency may be limited. So effort in communicating about the work and keeping participants on board is vital. Having a task focus with equal opportunities for contribution and responsibility through, for example, the setting of the criteria for the alliance and chairing meetings, can help to defuse power conflicts. Conventional ways of working, such as committees, steering groups and formal minute taking can hamper the development of ideas and inhibit the contribution of community representatives who may be unused to such ways of working. Many studies of collaborative working suggest that informal arrangements can be more productive and cooperative (Delaney 1994b, Springett 1995).

Beattie argues that groups also need to develop the ability to give feedback on how the group is working and that there is a strong case for drawing on 'the theory and practice of psychodynamics of relationships within institutions to explore the significance of emotional processes and interpersonal defence mechanisms' (Beattie 1994, p. 119). Members need to spend time talking over differences and reviewing relationships within the partnership. The Health Education Board for Scotland (HEBS 2000) also identified 'transparency', 'mutual trust and confidence', 'open and honest communication' as key indicators of successful partnerships.

This section has looked at organizational and interpersonal issues drawing on established theories from management and organizational studies and social psychology and psychodynamic work. These ideas help us to make sense of those factors, identified from empirical studies, which are the ingredients for successful collaboration. The insights gained from practice can also help us to 'test' these theories to see if they do offer explanations of what goes on in collaborative and alliance work.

CONCLUSION

The theoretical frameworks and variety of experience which characterize collaboration for health reveal a number of common themes concerning the difficulties and opportunities for successful collaboration. There are obvious costs and benefits involved. Partnership working is about compromise and entails some change in normal patterns of working. It may require additional and specific skills such as effective group working and management skills. Partnership means relinquishing control and the inclination to put one's own interests first and it entails crossing professional boundaries. It is very expensive in terms of time and resources and so it must have top-level commitment. On the other hand, at the level of a specific project or campaign, partnership working may lead to synergistic working with the achievement of more significant and long-term outcomes than would be achieved by agencies working in isolation. It may have a 'trickle down' effect whereby partner agencies become more committed to public health and health promotion and gain new insights into problem definitions and possible solutions. Where partnerships include voluntary organizations and members of the public, there may be additional benefits of empowerment and increased social capital. Partnership working offers the potential of more 'transparent' ways of working, with greater accountability to a variety of interest groups. Most fundamental of all, however, is that it can bring about a cultural change that recognizes health as a multidimensional concept not merely confined to health services.

FURTHER DISCUSSION

- Is partnership a consequence of joint working?
- Is the commitment to partnership working by government more rhetoric than reality?
- Do professional education and training courses equip people to work effectively in partnerships?

Recommended reading

- Balloch S, Taylor M (2001) Partnership working: policy and practice. Bristol, Policy Press.

  A collection of case studies of partnerships in health, social care and regeneration. It examines the theoretical and practical reasons why partnerships do or do not work.
- Glendinning C, Powell M, Rummery K (2002) Partnerships, new labour and the governance of welfare. Bristol, Policy Press

  An edited collection examining the political drivers to partnership working as a means of 'joined up' government.
- Health Development Agency (2003) The working partnership. London, HDA

  A manual that examines the evidence from community involvement, business excellence and partnership dynamics for common features of successful partnership working. It includes assessment tools so that partnerships can identify their achievements and areas for improvement and capacity building.
- Watson J, Speller V, Markwell S, Platt S (2000) The Verona Benchmark – applying evidence to improve the quality of partnership. Promotion and Education, VII(2): 16–23.

  A benchmarking and assessment tool to enable participants to share good practice. The Verona Benchmark focuses on leadership, organization, strategy, learning, resources and programmes.
- Health Education Board for Scotland (2001) Partnerships for health: a review, HEBS working paper No. 3. Edinburgh, HEBS.

  A paper that provides a useful overview of the published literature and a critical examination of the issues involved in successful partnership working.
- Peckham S (2003) Who are the partners in public health? In: Orme J, Powell J, Taylor P, Harrison T, Grey M (eds) Public health for the 21st century: new perspectives on policy, participation and practice. Maidenhead, Open University/McGraw Hill Education.

  This chapter examines different meanings and frameworks for partnerships, and focuses on the necessity of partnerships for public health and the barriers and opportunities for partnership working at local level.

REFERENCES

Audit Commission (1998) A fruitful partnership: effective partnership working. London, Audit Commission

Balloch S, Taylor M (eds) (2001) Partnership working: policy and practice. Bristol, Policy Press

Beattie A (1994) Healthy alliances or dangerous liaisons? The challenge of working together in health promotion. In: Leathard A (ed) Going interprofessional: working together for health and welfare. London, Routledge

Belbin R M (1981) Management teams: why they succeed or fail. Oxford, Butterworth Heinemann

Birchall E, Hallett C (1992) Coordination of child protection. London, HMSO

Davies J, Dooris M, Russell J, Pettersson G (1993) Healthy alliances: a study of inter-agency collaboration in health promotion. London, London Research Centre report for South West Thames Regional Health Authority

Delaney F (1994a) Muddling through the middle ground: theoretical concerns in intersectoral collaboration and health promotion. Health Promotion International 9(3): 217–225

Delaney F (1994b) Making connections: research into intersectoral collaboration. Health Education Journal 53: 474–485

Department of Health (DoH) (1991) Working together: a guide to arrangements for inter-agency cooperation for the protection of children from abuse. London, HMSO

Department of Health (DoH) (1993) Working together for better health. London, HMSO

Department of Health (DoH) (1999) Partnership in action. London, DoH

Department of Transport and the Regions (DETR) (2001) Local Strategic Partnerships: government guidance. London, DETR

Farrant W (1986) Health for all by the year 2000? Radical Community Medicine. Winter 1986/7: 19–26

Glover M (2001) Alliances for health at work: a case study. In: Scriven A, Orme J (eds) Health promotion: professional perspectives, 2nd edn. Maidenhead, Open University Press

Hamer L (1999) Health improvement programmes 1999–2000: a national review. London, Health Development Agency

Handy C (1976) Understanding organizations. London, Penguin

Health Education Board for Scotland (HEBS) (2000) Partnerships for health: a review, HEBS working paper No. 3. Edinburgh, HEBS

Henwood M, Hudson B (2000) Partnership and the NHS plan: cooperation or coercion. The implications for social care. Leeds, Nuffield Institute for Health

Hudson B (1987) Collaboration in social welfare. Policy and Politics 15: 175–182

Leathard A (ed) (1994) Going interprofessional: working together for health and welfare. London, Routledge

Markwell S (1998) Exploration of conflict theory as it relates to healthy alliances. In: Scriven A (ed) Alliances in health promotion: theory and practice. Basingstoke, Macmillan

Nutbeam D (1994) Intersectoral action for health: making it work. Health Promotion International 9(3): 143–144

Ovreteit J (1993) Coordinating community care: multidisciplinary teams and care management. Maidenhead, Open University Press

Peckham S (2003) Who are the partners in public health? In: Orme J, Powell J, Taylor P, Harrison T, Grey M (eds) Public health for the 21st century: new perspectives on policy, participation and practice. Maidenhead, Open University/McGraw Hill

Plampling D, Gordon P, Pratt J (2000) Practical partnerships for health and local authorities. British Medical Journal 320: 1723–1725

Powell M (1992) Healthy alliances: report to the Health Gain Standing Conference. London, Office of Public Management

Pratt J, Plampling D (1998) Partnership: fit for purpose. London, King's Fund

Scottish Office (1998) Working together for a healthier Scotland. Edinburgh, Scottish Office

Simnett I (1995) Managing health promotion: developing healthy organizations and communities. Chichester, Wiley

Springett J (1995) Intersectoral collaboration: theory and practice. Liverpool, Institute for Health, John Moores University

Tuckman B W (1965) Developmental sequence in small groups. Psychological Bulletin 63: 384–399

Welsh Assembly (2002) Well being in Wales. Cardiff, Welsh Assembly Government

World Health Organization (WHO) (1978) Alma Ata 1978 Primary Health Care. Copenhagen, WHO

World Health Organization (WHO) (1985) Health for all in Europe by the year 2000. Copenhagen, WHO

World Health Organization (WHO) (1986) Ottawa charter for health promotion: an international conference on health promotion. Geneva, WHO

World Health Organization (WHO) (1988) Adelaide recommendations on healthy public policy. Adelaide, WHO

World Health Organization (WHO) (1998) Health 21. 21 targets for the 21st century. Copenhagen, WHO Europe.

8

Information, education, communication

OVERVIEW

An integral part of the World Health Organization definition of health promotion is empowerment – people's ability to increase control over their health. Information, and the skills to use this information to effect change, are central to empowerment. This chapter explores the ways in which individuals and communities can be empowered through education. Information, education, communication (IEC) is an approach commonly understood and adopted across the world but variously termed. It includes elements of health education, communication for behaviour change and social marketing, but can be defined as an approach which attempts to enhance health or prevent disease through learning – whether through the provision of information, education programmes or through mass media campaigns. Education for empowerment includes a number of different stages, e.g. creating awareness, increasing knowledge, changing attitudes and motivating people to change or continue their behaviour or to adopt an innovation. This chapter explores some of the challenges for practitioners in ensuring that the planning and development of IEC strategies are equitable, ethical, client-centred and participatory.

INTRODUCTION

The Ottawa Charter (WHO 1986) emphasizes the centrality of participation and collaboration through all stages of health promotion interventions. The concept of 'enablement' in the Charter is 'premised on the idea that in order to realize their freedom and assume greater responsibility for their health, individuals may require help in the form of know-how, resources and power to assume greater control' (Yeo 1993, p. 233). This 'know-how' or health literacy may include knowledge, personal skills and education concerning the determinants of health as well as risk factors and behaviours and the use of health care systems and is part of achieving effective participation.

The term 'health education' has been used in the past to describe learning opportunities about:

- health risks and behaviours
- use of health services
- the wider environment in which health choices are made.

D iscussion point

How can individuals take control over their health?

Tones (1999) has argued that the key to health improvement is education. He argues that it is through the process of communicating, informing and educating individuals and communities that people gain control over their health.

The term 'empowerment' is used to describe a process through which individuals and groups 'are able to express their needs, present their concerns, devise strategies for involvement in decision making, and to achieve political, social and cultural action to meet those needs' (Nutbeam 1998, p. 354). For people to be empowered then they need to not only feel strongly enough about their situation to want to change it but also feel capable of changing it by having the information, support and skills to do so. Tones outlines how the rhetoric may be operationalized 'as part of client contract behaviour modification, people might learn how to avoid environmental circumstances which trigger consumption of tobacco or alcohol, acquire skills in resisting social pressures and they might learn how to resist temptation by applying social regulatory skills' (1999, p. 71). Whilst health communication is an important element of empowering individuals and communities, it can in this way be seen as a way of achieving support for compliance with predetermined objectives (Nutbeam 1998, p. 355). Education for empowerment means client-led learning, where people define for themselves their own needs and objectives, and what methods are best suited to their needs. However, much education in the health field is 'expert-led', where agendas and methods are predetermined by experts or practitioners.

D iscussion point

At what point does information-giving become persuasion?

Information, education, communication (IEC) is an accepted set of strategies for learning that enable people to make decisions for health. These strategies may range from:

- mass media communication such as the health messages of campaigns and other forms of one-way communication such as leaflets and posters
- health messages incorporated into existing communication media
- interpersonal communication such as individual/group discussions, community meetings or counselling sessions
- patient/client information
- skills development.

A major plank of the modernization of the NHS is to improve access to information on health and health services (DoH 1998). Part of the rationale for this is that a better-informed population is better able to look after themselves. The development of new media such as internet and digital television offers enormous opportunities to widen access by the public to information about health and health services. At the same time sections of the population are 'information poor' and unable to access new technologies.

UNDERSTANDING COMMUNICATION

For most practitioners, communication to a client/audience is about conveying a message about reducing risks, compliance or the effective use of services, and to do this effectively means understanding the audience, the channels and the mode of communication and its effects. There are many process models of communication, all of which adopt a mechanistic and linear orientation. The American Yale–Hovland model of communication which was designed to develop ways of influencing public attitudes and was later elaborated by McGuire (1978) is shown in Figure 8.1. It suggests that the process of mass communication entails five variables: source, message, channel, receiver and destination. This type of model of communication underpins most IEC strategies. The effectiveness of the communication depends on:

- the extent to which the source has credibility and trustworthiness
- the way the message is constructed and distributed
- the receiver's receptiveness and readiness to accept the message.

Figure 8.1 A model of communication

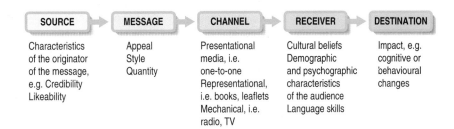

Theories on behaviour change suggest that the adoption of healthy behaviours is a process in which individuals progress through various stages until the new behaviour is routinized. Behaviour models, such as the Health Belief model (Becker 1974) or the Theory of Reasoned Action (Ajzen & Fishbein 1980) or Ajzen's later Theory of Planned Behaviour (Ajzen 1988) which were discussed in *Health Promotion: Foundations for Practice* (Naidoo & Wills 2000) are based on a set of assumptions about the change process. These models show that the simple provision of information without some modification of attitudes and beliefs, has little effect on behaviour. Nevertheless, IEC strategies do draw on the factors highlighted in these models as influencing behaviour.

Emphasis may be placed on making the audience aware of the issue's relevance to them by, for example, stressing individual susceptibility through specific risk factors. The severity of the disease may also be stressed but specific changes to behaviour or lifestyle will be suggested to emphasize the individual's feelings of self-efficacy. Particular benefits from making a change would be highlighted and barriers to change addressed.

Reaching people through the mass media has been a major activity in health promotion. The belief that the mass media could provide a panacea for health professionals in which they could convey a health message to large numbers of people who would then be persuaded to change their behaviour has been tempered by numerous research studies (see Tones & Tilford 2001 for a useful summary). Most of these studies suggest that the mass media can be successful in raising awareness of health issues.

Discussion point

How and what might a health adviser at a clinic communicate to a young client about chlamydia?

A mass communication programme dealing with sensitive issues socially validates open discussion of these issues, thus making them part of the everyday agenda. However, to be effective, mass media must be supported by interpersonal and group communication. Communication channels should ensure availability of feedback mechanisms. People need to be actively involved – articulating their concerns, setting goals, discussing how changes can be made – and this can only be done in two-way communication which is tailored to the needs of a specific individual or group.

The theory of Diffusion of Innovations (Rogers & Shoemaker 1971) illuminates the process whereby an idea or practice comes to be adopted or rejected by a community. Reassuringly for health promoters, Rogers & Shoemaker (1971) point out that the rate of adoption of new ideas is slow. It will be influenced by the nature of the community – traditional communities will have fewer opinion leaders or what are termed 'innovators' and 'early adopters'. IEC strategies thus need to know and incorporate community traditions (e.g. the International Planned Parenthood Federation (IPPF) refer to the importance of respecting health traditions concerning the disposal of placenta and preferred birth position (IPPF 1999)).

The whole process of a public health communication approach thus needs to be carefully researched and planned to understand what the health problem really is, who it affects, how people understand and respond to the problem, what actions need to be taken, what obstacles people are likely to encounter, and how the client/target audience can be influenced to change. This means having:

■ clearly articulated objectives, keeping the client at the centre of what is being designed
■ conducting appropriate research to understand the needs and values of the target audience
■ undertaking audience segmentation, carefully crafting and testing messages
■ knowing and using appropriate channel choices, and planning for monitoring and feedback.

D iscussion point

An IEC strategy recommends 'following the community at its own rhythm'. What do you think is meant by this phrase? Think of an example from your practice where you want a group/community to adopt a particular action – what would it mean to be 'following its rhythm'?

E xample

Behaviour and communication change in reducing HIV in Uganda

In Uganda HIV prevalence declined nationally from 21% to 9.8% between 1991 and 1998. The major factor in this decline is the decrease in non-regular partners by 65% during 1989 to 1995. Other countries in east and southern Africa have committed greater resources and established more comprehensive programmes of action including condom provision, treatment of STIs, testing and counselling and media programmes but have not seen the same decline in infection as that in Uganda.

Uganda has adopted the ABC message to reducing HIV: *Ab*stain (from sex), *B*e Faithful (together), or use *C*ondoms. Basic knowledge about AIDS was similar to other countries but rather than use a population-based media programme or a message that focused on condom use which would run counter to the values and structures of Uganda, there was a widespread community-based communication process using personal and social networks, faith organizations, prominent cultural, political, military and community figures

E *continued*

and non-governmental organizations (NGOs). Key features in Uganda included:

■ a clear message that focused on reducing sexual partners or 'zero grazing', 'loving faithfully' and caring for those with AIDS
■ the disease was made notifiable and case surveillance ensured that there was a direct response to AIDS locally and that it was talked about
■ strong care and NGO organizations that offered support and talked openly about AIDS, for example at funerals.

Source: Low-Beer & Stoneburner (2003)

R eflection point

Think of a client with whom you have worked to achieve a change. What factors do you need to take into account when devising a suitable communication approach?

TARGET AUDIENCE

Understanding the perceptions, motivations, behaviour and needs of people enables the message to be matched to the client/audience. For populations, IEC programmes use audience segmentation (i.e. the grouping of audiences by demographic, social and psychographic variables). The assumption behind market segmentation is that the population is made up of groups of individuals who share particular values, attitudes or consumption patterns. Targeting specific 'segments' of a population enables messages to be more closely tailored to fit that group's existing predispositions. We shall see in Part 3 that targeting is usually on the basis of professional perceptions of risk and thus relates to epidemiological and demographic classifications. Table 8.1 shows the range of social, behavioural and psychological variables that might be used to differentiate a target population.

Table 8.1 Market segmentation Source: Lefebvre R C (2002) In: Bunton R, Macdonald G (eds) Health promotion: disciplines and diversity, 2nd edn. Reproduced by permission of Routledge

Sociodemographic	Behavioural	Psychological
Location (community, neighbourhood)	Use of product/service	Self-esteem
Household size	Benefits sought	Readiness for change
Age	Level of activity	Introspection
Sex	Use of leisure	Sensation seeker
Ethnicity	Level of sexual activity	Hedonism
Nationality	Health professional utilization	Achievement orientation
Religion		Need for independence
Marital status		Societally conscious
Education		Belongers
Occupation		Need for approval
Income		Need for power
Social class		

Discussion point

The 11–18 age group is a large segment of the population. Psychographic profiles will state that there are divisions or groups within this age group. How might this affect the development of a message to wear bicycle helmets?

Population strategies may also segment on the basis of attitudes to health issues and disposition to change. Egger et al (1993) explore the similarity between Prochaska et al's (1992) concept of an individual's readiness to change with marketing's concept of 'buyer readiness' which states that at any point there are those in the population who are aware of the product, those who are informed about the product, those who are interested in buying the product, those who are motivated to buy and those who have formed an intention to buy. This awareness of the stages in behaviour change means that a target audience can be segmented according to the degree of positive attitudes to the behaviour or action and different messages tailored accordingly. Thus in a health promotion intervention designed to increase activity levels, the positively disposed moderately active person may get a reinforcing message to ensure they maintain the behaviour, the positively disposed sedentary person might get an incentive message and the sedentary person who does not want to be more active and sees no value in it may get a confrontational message such as stressing the health risks of inactivity.

Example

Targeting smoking campaigns

The Health Education Authority targeted its mass media campaigns on the basis of socio-demographic factors such as age or family-focused messages on the benefits of quitting for children. Research has also analysed smokers' position on a quitting continuum – younger smokers being less motivated than middle-aged smokers. Older smokers may have more reasons for quitting but are also likely to have experience of previous quit attempts and need support and encouragement to try again. Targeting a campaign according to readiness to quit proved difficult. The objectives of the 'John Cleese' campaign in 1992–3 were therefore developed for all smokers as:

- to encourage smokers to believe that giving up was both possible and worth doing
- to increase the feeling among smokers that their lives would be improved if they quit
- to support ex-smokers in the determination not to lapse.

Source: Health Development Agency (2000)

IEC strategies increasingly are 'bottom up' in that they are informed by the precise interests and needs of particular groups. For example, patient and carer views are important to the development of health information and focus groups, surveys, interviews and panels are all methods of collecting information about the type of information people want. Health information for the public should reflect the client group's perceived needs and they should be consulted about what they want, need and already know. In this respect, the community is vital; it is not simply a message channel or a passive recipient of services or information. Figure 8.2 shows the process of involving consumers in the production of health information.

The message

Any health promotion communication may be used to try to influence the acceptability of an idea or it may be providing information. The idea

Figure 8.2 Involving consumers in the production of information Source: Centre for Health Information Quality (1999) Topic bulletin No. 4, with permission

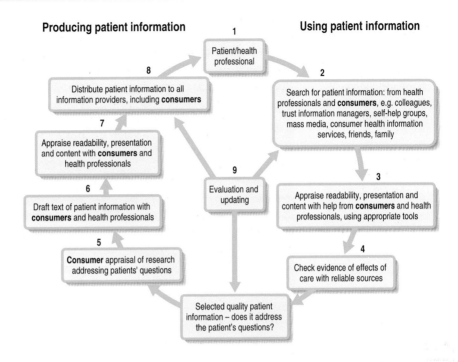

Producing patient information

Using patient information

1 Patient/health professional

8 Distribute patient information to all information providers, including **consumers**

2 Search for patient information: from health professionals and **consumers**, e.g. colleagues, trust information managers, self-help groups, mass media, consumer health information services, friends, family

7 Appraise readability, presentation and content with **consumers** and health professionals

9 Evaluation and updating

3 Appraise readability, presentation and content with help from **consumers** and health professionals, using appropriate tools

6 Draft text of patient information with **consumers** and health professionals

5 **Consumer** appraisal of research addressing patients' questions

4 Check evidence of effects of care with reliable sources

Selected quality patient information – does it address the patient's questions?

may be quite general such as 'good health' or it may be a specific behaviour such as using a condom or breastfeeding. A message and image has to be developed which will appeal to the client/target audience. The assumption of social marketers is that given the right message in the right way at the right time, people will accept and act upon it. Most texts on health promotion offer similar advice on how to 'get the message across' (e.g. Egger et al 1993, Ewles & Simnett 2003).

Make it relevant

Research will identify the beliefs and attitudes of the target audience and their information needs. Health communications then need to be in the language of the target audience and use appropriate vocabulary. For example, an attempt to get young men to access primary care services to reduce mental health problems used posters in public lavatories with the slogan 'Pissed Off?' 'Honesty is the Best Policy' is a project supported by young people to develop drug information resources. In Figure 8.3 text messaging is used to suggest to young people the importance of communicating about their health decision making.

The communication needs to emphasize the similarity between the consumer and the source of the message, so that the targeted group sees the issue as affecting 'someone like me'. AIDS campaigns in most countries of the world have used personal testimonies from a wide range of HIV-positive people to show that HIV is not confined to particular population groups, that it is not possible to guess the HIV status of others and to challenge the stigma associated with a positive status. Similarly, current tobacco campaigns include a number of life histories (www.givingupsmoking.co.uk) under the tag line 'True Stories'.

Discussion point

What message and image would be appropriate to persuade people over 65 to get a flu jab in the winter?

Figure 8.3 Communic8 campaign (reproduced by permission of Wyvern Community School and University of the West of England, Bristol)

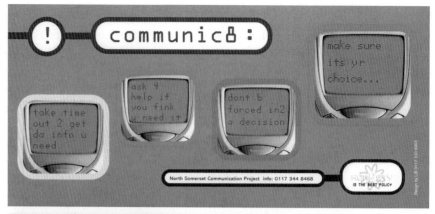

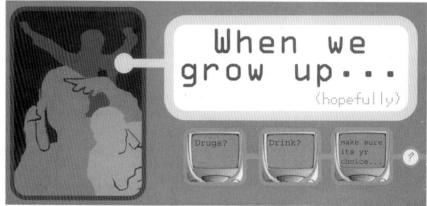

Make it credible

The acceptability of a message is influenced by the credibility of its source (Hovland & Weiss 1951). On the one hand, people are influenced by the similarity of the image with themselves. On the other hand, when recommendations are made for change, expert knowledge is seen as most credible. The AIDS campaign decided to use doctors and public health specialists as 'talking heads' in a series of advertisements in 1990 partly on this basis, but also in order to adopt a deliberately unsensational approach.

People are also more likely to adopt the attitudes of those they admire and with whom they wish to identify. Research is used to identify opinion leaders and 'significant intermediaries' for the target group. Thus many campaigns use celebrities as role models. The person chosen has to be acceptable to the target audience. The youth market, in particular, is segmented according to music and clothes tastes and celebrities may appeal to a very narrow segment. The influence of role models may also be transitory – people may identify with the person and the message but not necessarily internalize it so that if the role model fades then the attitudes may change too. The person must be credible – figureheads may end up doing the thing they are supposed to be against or vice versa.

Discussion point

What are the drawbacks of using a figurehead to lead a campaign?

Make it motivational

A client/target audience needs to have reasons to adopt positive attitudes to an issue. This is where initial formative research or discussion with a client will have highlighted likely values such as family responsibilities or personal well-being. In commercial marketing, a product is linked to a desired value or attribute, e.g. cars and sexual attractiveness, chocolates and escapism. When health is the product, the motivating values are often youth, or energy.

Marketers state that buying a product or adopting a health message involves an exchange. The consumer pays a price, either in financial terms or in terms of time or physical or psychological effort. The price must therefore be fixed at a level which makes the benefit of the product outweigh its costs. The art of marketing according to Lefebvre lies in 'communicating effectively the benefits of behaviour change and making the price worth it' (2002, p. 167). In some instances, this may mean offering incentives to change such as a basket of fruit or leisure club voucher for quitting smoking. In health information campaigns it is more ethical and effective to make explicit the costs of adopting a change in behaviour. A two-sided message may be recommended which acknowledges the benefits of a health behaviour (e.g. drinking is sociable and an aid to relaxation) but also its adverse consequences (e.g. drinking too much can lead to hangovers, driving when over the limit, unwanted sexual activity) (Hovland et al 1949). However health promoters often assume that such messages will be confusing and so simple imperatives characterize many IEC strategies, e.g. the 'Just Say No' of drug prevention campaigns.

For practitioners, there is often a tension between persuading people to adopt a recommended behaviour or giving them fuller information and enabling them to choose. In *Health Promotion: Foundations for Practice* (Naidoo & Wills 2000) we discussed the ethical dilemmas of creating and respecting people's autonomy and the tension between individual choice and the social good. Practitioners have to manage this tension when working with individual clients about whether there is ever *a* healthy choice. Communicating about the probability of risk, the nature of the risk and knowing how people make choices is an important part of a health practitioner's skills.

Most media, other than print, make the communication of complex information difficult. To convey the contentiousness of much health information (e.g. the contribution of alcohol as a protective factor in coronary heart disease) demands time (and therefore considerable expense) and a commitment to increasing awareness as much as changes in behaviour. Taking the example of oral health, the message to cut down on sugar is deceptively clear. But does it refer to the added sugar in drinks or cereals or the hidden sugar in most processed food? It is not possible to convey complex information about the sources of sugar or its relative risks to oral health or weight gain in an advertising campaign and so consumers are presented with insufficient information to make an informed choice about their health behaviour. Persuading people of the benefits of oral health is also difficult.

Discussion point

What other motivating values are commonly linked with health messages?

Discussion point

What message(s) would you give to a parent of a young child due to have its MMR immunization?

Which of the following images would you adopt for an oral health campaign:

- a young woman with sparkling white teeth
- a child crying in a dentist's surgery after having a tooth filled
- a toothbrush and pink, glossy gums with the message 'Massage your gums'?

Dental decay has declined with the introduction of fluoride-based toothpaste and additions to the water supply in many areas; thus the main emphasis of oral health promotion is to encourage healthy gums. The first of these images emphasizes the appearance of teeth. The second image creates anxiety and deliberately emphasizes risk. The third image encourages healthy gums but seeks to convey this message using sexual imagery. The first and third images both use people's anxiety to appear physically attractive to sell the message.

Figure 8.4 Examples of dental health campaigns (reproduced by permission of NHS Greater Glasgow)

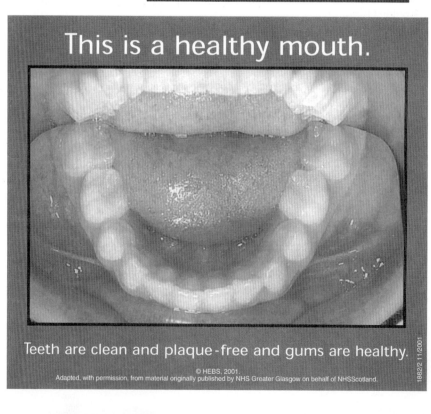

Points to Note

No tooth decay present

Colour Pale pink

Shape Gum margins taper to a fine point between teeth

Texture Gums are firm, flat and stippled (like orange peel)

NHS
SCOTLAND

This is a healthy mouth.

Teeth are clean and plaque-free and gums are healthy.

© HEBS, 2001.
Adapted, with permission, from material originally published by NHS Greater Glasgow on behalf of NHSScotland.

1882/2 11/2001

Make it seem possible

Significant changes in lifestyle may seem daunting. The individual's feelings of control and self-efficacy can be enhanced if specific actions are suggested such as calling a helpline, signing a contract with a friend to take action or specific tips on how to make a change. Health communications frequently make choices seem easy. Most HIV/AIDS campaigns, for example, have presented a simple message – use a condom. The latest campaigns such as those by Gay Men Fighting Aids acknowledge the difficulties of sexual decision making and maintaining safer sex (www.gmfa.org.uk).

Arouse emotional involvement

Commercial advertising attracts attention in a variety of ways but dramatic images often feature prominently. When people are asked what message or image should be used for health communications they often respond that something frightening or a stern warning is needed to jolt people into action and make then 'sit up and take notice'. Health promotion campaigns have frequently used appeals to anxiety or fear. The 1986 AIDS campaign used images of tombstones carved with the word AIDS. The 1995 Drink-Driving campaign used contrasting images of young people enjoying a happy summer pub lunch with a horrific car crash. A 1994 Scottish stop smoking campaign used images of a young child visiting a grandparent in an oxygen tent.

The use of fear in campaigns has had a varied history but strong imagery has by and large been eschewed recently in the light of research that shows that people do not necessarily respond rationally to avoid the threat which has made them frightened and high levels of fear or repeated exposure to it can often lead to denial and disassociation from the message. On the other hand, fear may be a powerful motivator in the short term (Montazeri 1998).

Reflection point

The mother of a young woman who died from a heroin overdose in 2002 has asked that a photograph of her daughter taken at her death should be widely distributed to act as a deterrent for young people. What is your reaction to the use of this imagery in health information?

CHANNELS OF COMMUNICATION

Having identified the target audience and developed an appropriate message or information, the main channels or mode of communication need to be identified. Different channels do different jobs and the choice of channel is determined by this and by cost, literacy levels, extent of penetration of a medium and its availability in the target population. Written information is, for example, usually the cheapest and requires least specialist expertise to produce.

It may not be suitable for communities with low levels of literacy or who do not speak English. Translation is not an add-on part of an initiative – literal translations may not exist and word-for-word substitution may distort meaning.

Discussion point

When would it be appropriate and when would it not be to use written patient information?

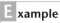

E xample

Communication channels

Nepal is an example of a country where there is lack of access to information about contraception options and particular cultural perceptions in which husbands disapprove of family planning. Culturally defined gender roles emphasize the importance of sons to the family and limit women's participation in decisions related to their fertility.

Radio is used as a way of increasing contraceptive information because it has the most potential for reaching rural families and health workers. Only 5% of women read a newspaper or magazine at least once a week, and 12% watch television at least once a week, but 36% listen to the radio daily. Furthermore, the reach of radio is consistent across all age groups of women and is the most likely to reach isolated, poorer, less educated women.

Cut Your Coat According to Your Cloth was broadcast nationally on Radio Nepal from December 1995 to December 1996. This Entertainment Education (Enter-Educate) radio drama serial aimed at improving public perceptions of health service providers and repositioning contraception away from its historical focus on sterilization toward a broader notion of 'the well-planned family'. It also modelled men and women actively seeking better health conditions for themselves and their village with the help of a community health worker who represented a new generation of client-oriented service providers. It was broadcast once a week (57 episodes) in the Nepali language.

R eflection point

What do you understand by the term marketing?

D iscussion point

What benefit does the health promoter get from the exchange?

D iscussion point

How would you market the idea of hand washing in a hospital?

SOCIAL MARKETING

The term social marketing was first used in 1971 by Kotler & Zaltman who described it as: 'the design, implementation and control of programs calculated to influence the acceptability of social ideas and involving considerations of product, planning, pricing, communication, distribution and marketing research' (1971, p. 5). They argued that just as there is a marketplace for products, there is a marketplace for ideas and the same techniques which are used to sell products can be used to sell an idea or cause or to persuade, influence or motivate people to change their behaviour or use a service. The process is based on the concept of a mutually beneficial exchange. In commercial terms, the consumer gets a product they want at a price they can afford and the producer gets a profit. In the marketing of health, the consumer gets the promise of improved health and quality of life at a possible cost of giving up a pleasure (e.g. chocolate, cigarettes) or making some physical or psychological effort (e.g. going to a gym).

According to Hastings & Haywood commercial marketing is 'essentially about getting the right product, at the right price, in the right place at the right time presented in such a way as to successfully satisfy the needs of the consumer' (1991).

The marketing mix is thus said to be made up of:

- the product and its key characteristics
- the price and how important it is for the audience
- the place (where the message would be promoted)
- the promotion (how the message is to be presented).

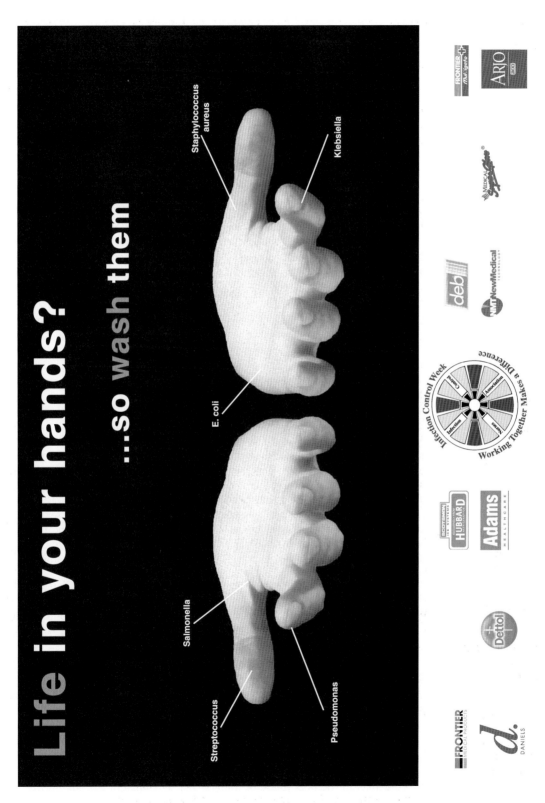

Figure 8.5 'Life in your hands?' campaign (reproduced by permission of Infection Control Nurses Association)

Health promoters believe that social marketing can help them to use advertising techniques to package 'health' to various target groups. Values which are seen as desirable – youth, attractiveness, being slim, self-discipline, belonging – would thus be used to 'sell' health.

Discussion point

Consider the following messages which are used in health promotion campaigns. Do you regard these messages as 'healthy' or 'unhealthy'?

- Eat well to keep in trim
- Drink sensibly to be sexy
- Exercise to keep the body toned
- Avoid ageing skin by protecting yourself in the sun

Branding plays a major part in selling commercial products. People buy things not just to satisfy a functional need but also to be seen to identify with a group. A very successful example of the development of a tangible product that indicates support of a cause is the Red Ribbon first used by a small charity in New York in 1991 as a symbol to unite the various groups working to get the AIDS epidemic acknowledged. The Red Ribbon is recognized by 50% of the population as 'something to do with AIDS' (Freeman 1995). Its success has led to the wearing of a coloured ribbon being adopted by other groups, e.g. those working for awareness of breast cancer use a pink ribbon.

Discussion point

A national campaign is being organized to raise awareness of incontinence. What could be its message?

Example

Branding a way of life

loveLife is a campaign in South Africa, largely funded by a US charitable foundation, targeted at the 12–17 age group with the overall aim of reducing the rate of HIV infection in 15–20-year-olds by 50% in five years. loveLife uses media awareness, education, outreach and youth-friendly reproductive health services. The aim has been to position the loveLife brand as part of youth culture. The key to loveLife's approach is to get young South Africans to talk about sex, sexuality and gender relations. The loveLife media campaign has concentrated on brand awareness and promotion, through an initial teaser campaign designed to create intrigue, to a clearer focus on sex and HIV. The three objectives for the campaign in the first year were to:

- Initiate a national conversation about the loveLife brand and excite the popular imagination about loveLife.
- Guide this dialogue towards sex and specifically adolescent sexuality with an emphasis on inter-generational communication about sexuality.
- Make explicit the link between sexual behaviour and HIV.

The start to the whole of the campaign was a series of billboard teasers titled 'Foreplay'. In Phase 2 of the campaign, the payoff line 'Talk about it' was introduced and the youth sex talk show loveLife 'JikaJika' launched, as well as the toll-free telephone helpline. In Phase 3, the second television series 'S'camto' was launched and billboard messages designed to shock complemented the series. The publication *The Impending Catastrophe* was widely distributed in the print media aiming to inform the broader South African public of the ramifications of the epidemic. In the final phase of the first year's campaign, the link between

E *continued* behaviour and HIV was made more explicit by using the theme 'The future ain't what it used to be'. The print media was more targeted in this phase, challenging parents to talk to their children about sex. The evaluation of loveLife is still taking place and it has achieved a high level of awareness of a campaign message but is not yet adopted as a 'brand'.

Source: www.lovelife.org.za

Developing a message to promote continence is particularly difficult. It is a taboo issue which is rarely discussed in public. In addition, the term itself may not be understood. The negative effects of incontinence may be stressed such as loss of self-esteem, effects on social and sex life or the costs of sanitary protection, but this is not likely to break the taboo or encourage sufferers to seek help. Therefore the message that incontinence is both common and curable is more likely to be effective.

The dilemma for health promotion is that if it uses advertising techniques, it is most likely to be effective if it employs the images and values with which people are familiar. Those images are ones produced by a consumer culture which attempts to sell products by associating them with desirable attributes – sex, power, wealth, success, escape, fantasy, glamour, energy, fitness and youth. For health promoters, adopting marketing principles means endorsing these very stereotypes which many health promoters claim are unhealthy. Such stereotypes reinforce sexism and ageism and damage many people's self-esteem. The alternative for health promoters is to emphasize *moral* values such as responsibility, safety, conformity and social acceptance. It is precisely this difference between the worlds of commerce and health which makes the marketing of health difficult and, in the view of many, inappropriate.

Marketing is predicated on the basis that individuals have the 'freedom' to choose and to buy what they want and that there will be a reward or benefit from the exchange, what is termed a 'voluntary and mutually beneficial exchange'. The consumer gets the goods they want at an acceptable price and the manufacturer gets a profit. Yet the process is not straightforward in health promotion. The product of better public health and quality of life are distant and unlikely returns. The consumer thus sees the marketing of health not as a mutually beneficial exchange but as overt persuasion. Lupton (1995) argues it is this fundamental difference in the 'product' rather than any disparity in available resources between health promotion and commercial companies which makes for success in commercial marketing and makes health marketing unsuccessful.

D iscussion point

Can health be sold like a washing powder?

- A health message is more difficult to define than the attractions of a product and there may be different views on its benefits.
- The target audience for the health 'product' are those least interested in it.
- The benefits from adopting a health message are long term as opposed to the instant gratification from using or acquiring a product.
- Health messages often involve giving up something which people value.
- The decision to adopt a health message is more complex than the relatively simple decision to purchase a product.

It is through attempts to identify the benefits from an exchange that social marketers are led to construct health in ways borrowed from commercial marketing. Health must be seen as both desirable and a product, a tangible thing which it is possible to acquire.

Marketers argue they are meeting consumers' needs by identifying what people want from a product or service. Critics argue that marketing is about the artificial creation and stimulation of wants and needs which can be met by commodities. In terms of health promotion, if a certain health behaviour is desirable, then people need to be made aware of it and why it is of value and why it would be good for them. Although people value their health as something to have, there is no actual demand for it. In fact, quite the opposite. In marketing health, health promoters are often trying to get people to give up what they perceive as desirable such as sweet things or cigarettes. The provision of health information is not meeting an unmet demand as a commercial manufacturer would argue about their product.

It could be argued that the process of surveying needs as part of social marketing is a participative strategy ensuring better targeting and meeting unmet needs. This is in contrast to the authoritarian paternalism of most health persuasion which Beattie describes as 'employing the authority of public health expertise to re-direct the behaviour of individuals in top-down prescriptive ways' (1991, p. 168). On the other hand, critics of a marketing approach to health promotion argue that it is actually a process of constructing needs according to a market model. Health promotion is constructing the individual as a health consumer who wants and needs health (Grace 1991). This process reflects a rise in consumerism in health and social care (Bunton et al 1995). People are deemed to be consumers with choices about what they use and what they do. They are thus responsible for their own health, preventing ill health by 'purchasing' relevant health information and services when necessary.

Advocates of social marketing in health promotion argue that the consumer is an active participant. People's views are sought to identify needs and then a message is developed *for* them. The lessons from these sophisticated research techniques do not, however, hide the fact that, as Lupton puts it: 'social marketers seek knowledge of consumers better to influence or motivate them, not to ensure that the objectives of social marketing are considered by consumers as appropriate' (1995, p. 112).

Reflection point	Think of an example where you have received health advice that has made you feel uncomfortable or resistant – was this because it made you feel guilty or uncomfortable?
	Did you feel it promoted choices for you or did it present only partial information, not exploring its contentiousness or inconclusiveness and thereby become prescriptive?

CONCLUSION

In this chapter we have seen the paradoxical relationship of health promotion with the mass media. On the one hand, health promotion is highly critical of the mass media and its influence. Considerable efforts are devoted to campaigning against tobacco advertising on the grounds that it encourages new smokers. Many of the risk factors for disease – sedentary lifestyle, unhealthy eating, unprotected sex – are shaped by a consumer culture which promotes unhealthy products such as junk food and confectionery and presents risky behaviours such as excessive alcohol intake or fast and reckless driving as acceptable. Health promoters criticize how the public perception of health issues is generally related to illness rather than positive health due to the reporting of hospital-based medicine and technological wizardry (Naidoo and Wills 2000).

On the other hand, health promotion endeavours to use marketing techniques (which it sees as effective) to promote health. In so doing, it is in danger of reinforcing some of those negative attributes so readily seen in the marketing of commodities. The argument presented in this chapter is that although a social marketing approach to health promotion may be an effective way of targeting information and changing attitudes and behaviour, it still tends to be professionally and epidemiologically driven. In particular, there may be a conflict between marketing's concept of the individual as a consumer and health promotion's concept of individuals as participating and autonomous citizens. Health promoters swayed by the idea that marketing techniques may be more equitable and empowering for target groups need also to weigh up the ethics of attempts to persuade people that health is something they need and want.

The practice of understanding the client group through careful and systematic research rather than professional assumptions is important. Equally important is to recognize the diversity of health beliefs and to move beyond simple socio-demographic categories for targeting. Information and messages can be tailored to particular audiences and do not need to follow the common sense assumption that 'short and simple' is best. On the other hand, marketing's use of the concepts of both 'individual' and 'health' constructs health as a personal choice, ignoring the role of poverty as the principal determinant of ill health.

FURTHER DISCUSSION

- Are marketing and health promotion fundamentally compatible or incompatible?
- How does marketing construct health as a personal choice?
- Four key principles of health promotion are:
  - equity
  - collaboration
  - participation
  - empowerment.

How do these relate to the concept of marketing?

Recommended reading

- ▣ Egger G, Donovan R, Spark R (1993) Health and the media: principles and practice for health promotion. Sydney, McGraw Hill.

  A comprehensive and accessible guide to using different media for health promotion. Combines practical advice, examples (mostly from Australia) and some underpinning theory.
- ▣ Coulter A, Entwistle V, Gilbert D (1998) Informing patients: an assessment of the quality of patient information materials. London, King's Fund.
- ▣ Duman M (2003) Producing patient information: how to research, develop and produce effective information sources. London, King's Fund.

  Two guides to patient information and the importance of identifying needs, developing and piloting materials, methods of dissemination and how to obtain consumer feedback.
- ▣ Tones K, Tilford S (2001) Health promotion: effectiveness, efficiency and equity, 3rd edn. London, Nelson Thornes.
- ▣ Tones K, Green J (2004) Health promotion: planning and strategies. London, Sage

  Both texts summarize the main studies on the effectiveness of health promotion using the media and include a section on education and communication for health.

REFERENCES

Ajzen I (1988) Attitudes, personality and behaviour. Maidenhead, Open University Press

Ajzen I, Fishbein M (1980) Understanding attitudes and predicting behaviour. Englewood Cliffs, NJ, Prentice Hall

Beattie A (1991) Knowledge and control: a test case for social policy and social theory. In: Gabe J, Beattie A, Gott M, Jones L, Sidell M (eds) (1993) Health and wellbeing: a reader. Basingstoke, Macmillan/Open University

Becker M H (1974) The health belief model and personal health behaviour. Health Education Monographs 2: 324–508

Bunton R, Nettleton S, Burrows R (1995) Sociology of health promotion. London, Routledge

Centre for Health Information Quality (1999) Topic bulletin No. 4. Winchester, CHIQ

Department of Health (DoH) (1998) Information for health: an information strategy for the modern NHS 1998–2005. London, The Stationery Office

Department of Health (DoH) (2000) The NHS plan: a plan for investment, a plan for reform. London, The Stationery Office

Department of Health (DoH) (2003) Information for health. An information strategy for the modern NHS 1998–2005. London, DoH

Egger G, Donovan R, Spark R (1993) Health and the media: principles and practice for health promotion. Sydney, McGraw Hill

Ewles L, Simnett I (2003) Promoting health: a practical guide, 5th edn. London, Baillière Tindall

Freeman D (1995) World AIDS Day evaluation report. London, Health Education Authority

Grace V M (1991) The marketing of empowerment and the construction of the health consumer: a critique of health promotion. International Journal of Health Services 21(2): 329–343

Hastings G, Haywood A (1991) Social marketing and communication in health promotion. Health Promotion International 6(2): 135–145

Health Development Agency (2000) A breath of fresh air: tackling smoking through the media. London, HDA

Hovland C I, Weiss W (1951) The influence of source credibility on communication effectiveness. Public Opinion Quarterly 15: 635–650.

Hovland C I, Lumsdaine A A, Sheffield F D (1949) Experiments on mass communication. Princeton, NJ, Princeton University Press

International Planned Parenthood Federation (1999) Reproductive health in refugee situations: an inter-agency field manual. Geneva, WHO

Kotler P, Zaltman G (1971) An approach to planned social change. Journal of Marketing 35: 3–12

Lefebvre R C (2002) Social marketing and health promotion. In: Bunton R, Macdonald G (eds) Health promotion: disciplines and diversity, 2nd edn. London, Routledge

Low-Beer D, Stoneburner RL (2003) Behaviour and communication change in reducing HIV: is Uganda unique? African Journal of AIDS Research 2(1): 9–21

Lupton D (1995) The imperative of health. London, Sage.

McGuire W J (1978) Evaluating advertising: a bibliography of the communication process. Advertising Research Foundation

Montazeri A (1998) Fear-inducing and positive image strategies in health education campaigns. International Journal of Health Promotion and Education 36(3): 72–75

Naidoo J, Wills J (2000) Health promotion: foundations for practice, 2nd edn. London, Baillière Tindall

Nutbeam D (1998) Health promotion glossary. Health Promotion International 13(4): 349–364

Prochaska J, DiClemente C, Norcross J C (1992) In search of how people change. American Psychologist 47: 1102–1114

Rogers E M, Shoemaker F F (1971) Communication of innovations. New York, Free Press

Tones K (1999) Health education and the promotion of health. In: Kendall S (ed) Health and empowerment. London, Arnold

Tones K, Tilford S (2001) Health promotion: effectiveness, efficiency and equity, 3rd edn. London, Nelson Thornes

World Health Organization (WHO) (1986) Ottawa charter for health promotion. Geneva, WHO

Yeo M (1993) Toward an ethic of empowerment for health promotion. Health Promotion International 8(3)

Priorities for Public Health and Health Promotion

We have investigated the key drivers for public health and health promotion in Part 1 of this book and core strategies in Part 2. In Part 3 we take an overview of the current priorities for public health and health promotion. The focus here is on the UK, but many of these priorities are the same for other developed and developing countries. Health is created through the interplay of many factors including:

- economic status
- the environment
- genetic disposition
- how people behave
- people's ability to satisfy basic needs
- the quality of people's social relations
- access to prevention, treatment and care services.

This gives rise to a broad, and at times bewildering, array of priorities, encompassing addressing the underlying socio-economic determinants of health, preventing illness through early detection and intervention, improving access to effective treatment and care, reducing the risk factors for ill health and death (smoking, nutrition, physical activity and accidental injury), and meeting the needs of specific population groups who are seen as vulnerable or over-represented in ill health statistics.

The history of public health demonstrates a particular concern with the physical aspects of the environment that may influence health directly such as water purity and housing quality. Other factors may influence health indirectly and interact with each other – poverty, for example, is associated with poor housing, diet and education. Figure S3.1 illustrates some of the links between socio-economic circumstances and health outcomes including the ways in which social attitudes and contexts facilitate or hinder individual health behaviours and the resources that promote health.

Figure S3.1 Socio-economic circumstances and health outcomes Source: Acheson (1998)

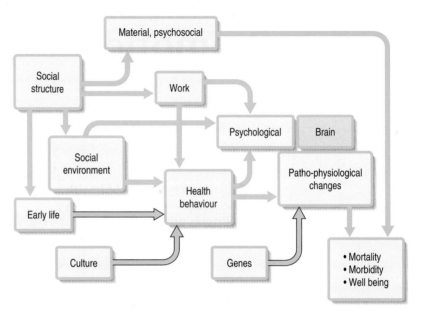

Public health and health promotion recognizes that a tension exists between agency and structure – whether people are autonomous free agents who choose the behavioural choices that promote or threaten their health, or a deterministic view that sees social and environmental factors as shaping health outcomes. These elements are often seen as discrete and independent variables to be addressed separately. Dahlgren & Whitehead's diagram (see p. 177), however, shows the health of the population as affected by interlocking factors: broad, societal or 'upstream' forces such as poverty and unemployment, 'midstream' factors that have a direct influence on people's lives and reflect broader social issues such as living and working conditions and the individual lifestyle, or 'downstream' factors that are also affected by the broader conditions in which individuals and families live their lives.

Different theoretical approaches explore the relationship between the social environment and health. Positivist sociologists focus on the impact and constraints of social determinants on individual choices, behaviours and health status. For example, poverty and a polluted environment will disadvantage people, lead to 'poor' health choices, and impact negatively on their health. Postmodernists place a greater stress on the cultural meanings and significance of factors affecting health – for example, risk behaviours may be positively valued by some groups, leading to adverse health consequences. Life course perspectives analyse the ways in which biological risk interacts with economic, social and psychological factors in the development of chronic diseases throughout life. A person's social experience is influenced by their genetic endowment, biology and physiology – for example, low birthweight is linked to physical and social disadvantages in later life.

The role of individual lifestyles in determining health status is undisputed, although there are different theories as to what factors affect lifestyles, and how lifestyles impact on health. Whilst the focus is usually on negative effects, the salutogenic approach seeks to explain the factors responsible for creating and maintaining good health. In particular, Antonovsky (1987) focused on how a 'Sense of Coherence' within individuals can explain the relationship between life stress and health status. The challenge for public health is being able to identify, promote and protect the salutogenic factors that promote health even amongst disadvantaged people.

The medical origins of public health are apparent in the focus on communicable diseases and chronic conditions that impact on quality of life and longevity. This is reflected in policies such as the National Service Frameworks (NSFs) for England and Wales. NSFs set standards for the provision of high quality services relating to major diseases and client groups. NSFs also aim to reduce unacceptable variations in care and treatment. NSFs have been introduced on a rolling basis and to date are planned for the following disease conditions: cancer, coronary heart disease, diabetes, mental health, renal disease and long-term neurological conditions. In addition there are NSFs for older people and children. The control of communicable diseases is another priority in public health, and one that is receiving increased attention as a result of the worldwide increase in HIV and outbreaks such as SARS.

Public health refers to the health of the whole population, but within that category certain groups of people may be prioritized. The rationale for focusing on specific groups is usually that their health potential is not being met. This often emerges from research that demonstrates a specific population group has a high level of health needs that are often unmet due to problems with service access and availability (e.g. asylum seekers and migrants). Targeting can, however, stigmatize groups. HIV, for example, is concentrated in social groups who are already marginalized such as commercial sex workers, injecting drug users and men who have sex with men. It can also lead to oversimplification in categorizing the targeted group. Black and minority ethnic groups for example, are frequently treated as a homogenous category for interventions.

Interventions to improve health are necessarily complex and interlinked. For many years, the emphasis was on lifestyles and behaviour change through education and awareness raising programmes. The focus of many interventions was on defined diseases targeted at changing the behaviours of high risk individuals. In recent years there has been a shift to introducing systemic and structural changes to create environments for better health. Public health and health promotion strategies thus range from the macro structural level via the meso community level to the micro individual level. There are numerous policy initiatives that seek to address the social determinants of health from housing to transport. The challenge for many public health and health promotion professionals is how to be involved in the political processes and policy making that bring about social change to structural problems. Adopting the lens of a social model of health through which to tackle priorities is also challenging. At the meso community level local interventions and projects seek to address priority areas using local knowledge, resources and skills. For many health and welfare workers, individual clients remain their focus. Working with individual clients does not exclude a consideration of how social determinants impact on their health, or how their individual behavioural choices result from community and peer pressures. Whilst it may not be the immediate focus of practitioner–client contacts, a recognition of the impact of broad structural factors on individuals can only increase the effectiveness of work with individual clients.

In practice, public health strategies often use a mix of interventions spanning all three levels. For example, food and diet is a public health and health promotion priority area, and poor diet is responsible for a great deal of associated ill health and disease. Food and diet may be construed as an individual lifestyle choice, and many interventions take this approach, focusing on education or weight monitoring to try to effect changes in diet. Many people work with individual clients or patients to raise awareness of health issues and provide information and counselling to change knowledge, attitudes and behaviour. However, research has also pointed out that diet is related to socio-economic determinants of health, and therefore a useful focus may be on communities rather than individuals. Community interventions rely on strategies such as partnership working and building and releasing community capacity and capability. Many of the necessary skills and solutions exist within communities but may require facilitation and networking in order to materialize. For example, interventions such as food cooperatives, allotment and food growing projects and breakfast clubs in schools all rely on the skills and resources that exist within communities. Community interventions seek to model healthier food options and make them accessible and appropriate for local populations. Finally, many of the factors affecting diet are structural, such as the loss of local shops due to supermarkets' aggressive marketing and pricing policies, inadequate food labelling, and poor dietary choices in workplaces and schools. These factors require lobbying at local or national levels to tackle relevant structures. Features of successful and effective interventions at each level are identified, and evidence showing that tackling this kind of priority area is effective is collated and presented.

Part 3 therefore explores four public health and health promotion priorities: the social determinants of health, the major causes of ill health and mortality, lifestyles and behaviours, and population groups. Each of these is the focus of a chapter where the rationale for prioritizing this category is explored and justified. Each chapter then goes on to identify how this factor has been addressed and examples are given of work at different levels – macro (structures), meso (communities) and micro (individuals). We hope Part 3 of this book will prove inspirational in identifying the huge range of skills, interventions and activities that can impact positively on the public health and health promotion. Many of these activities are not primarily concerned with health although they may be pivotal in promoting good health. For example, tackling poverty is a key government policy area because it is seen as crucial to creating a more egalitarian, inclusive and democratic society. However, it is also true that reducing poverty is one of the most effective, if not the most effective, means of promoting the health of the poorer sections of society, and hence of society at large. We therefore hope that everyone, whether or not they work in the health services, will be able to identify in Part 3 relevant issues, skills and interventions which they can use and adapt within their own workplace to improve the health of the people they work with.

REFERENCES

Acheson D (1998) Independent inquiry into inequalities in health. London, The Stationery Office

Antonovsky A (1987) The salutogenic perspective: towards a new view of health and illness.

Advances. The Journal of Mind-Body Health 4: 47–55

Dahlgren G, Whitehead M (1991) Policies and strategies to promote social equity in health. Stockholm, Institute for Future Studies

9 Social determinants of health

OVERVIEW

Health determinants are those factors that influence health. Several models of health have attempted to show the interconnectedness of social, economic, environmental, behavioural and biological factors. Dahlgren & Whitehead's (1991) model for example (see Figure 9.1 below) defines the determinants of health as individual lifestyle factors, social and community influences, living and working conditions and general socio-economic and environmental conditions.

The Toronto Health Department (City of Toronto Community Health Information Section 1991) refers to the social determinants of health as 'risk conditions' and includes poverty, low social status and social exclusion as well as dangerous working conditions and polluted environments. *Saving Lives: Our Healthier Nation* (1999) also distinguishes the determinants of health as socio-economic conditions, physical conditions and social, community and working conditions. This chapter discusses the social determinants of health – those structural factors that impact on health and are beyond any individual's ability to change. Social determinants of health is a broad term encompassing both socio-economic factors, such as income, and environmental factors, such as housing. Both these categories are fundamentally shaped and determined by collective societal choices embodied in social policies and regulatory and legislative frameworks. Such policies exist at different levels – global, national, regional and local.

Figure 9.1 The main determinants of health (from Dahlgren G & Whitehead M (1991) Policies and strategies to promote social equity in health. Reproduced by permission of Institute of Future Studies)

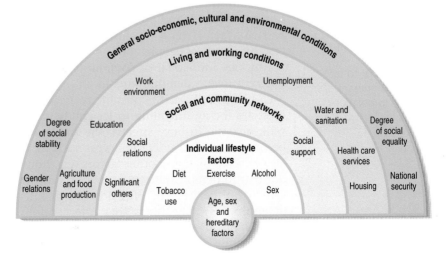

These determinants are amenable to change, especially at the collective, community or social policy level. At the macro level the social, economic and physical environment can be changed in significant ways, affording more health promoting choices and opportunities to people. At the meso level, communities can be supported to address collectively the impact of social determinants on their health. At an individual level, practitioners can work with clients to enable them to overcome the constraints and limitations on their lives and health imposed by social determinants. This chapter first discusses the concept of health determinants and the evidence showing their impact on health. It then goes on to consider action and interventions at different levels to implement change in health determinants. Evidence demonstrating the effect of interventions tackling socio-economic conditions, environmental conditions and social and community life on health status and examples of effective interventions are given to illustrate the range of health-promoting and health-developing activities.

INTRODUCTION

Risk conditions are social structures such as poverty or poor quality housing that are associated with poor health. Figure 9.2 shows how the effect of risk conditions (e.g. social marginalization) is directly linked to risk factors (e.g. lack of social support) and is also mediated by risky behaviours (e.g. drug use). Risk conditions and risky behaviours give rise to physiological and psychosocial risk factors that are in turn recognized precursors to many causes of ill health and premature and preventable death. Figure 9.2 also shows how certain groups of people are more likely to experience both risk conditions and risky behaviour, leading to poorer health status. For example, unemployed people are more likely than the general population to be living in poverty and to be socially marginalized. This in turn leads unemployed people to be more likely to participate in risky behaviours such as smoking and the use of legal and illegal drugs, and thus to be at increased risk of developing a variety of diseases causing ill health and premature death. Risk conditions, risky behaviours and risk factors tend to cluster together and disproportionately affect certain groups of people.

Any one individual or community tends to experience the impact of different health determinants in an integrated way, as 'quality of life' or 'well-being'. Whilst it is possible to isolate the effect of heavy traffic on lifestyles (being unwilling to let children play outside, unwillingness to walk or cycle in busy streets), the sum total of all the effects of traffic become subsumed under concepts such as stress or isolation, which are also affected by many other factors (e.g. housing, income). It is therefore difficult to demonstrate that any one health determinant is the primary cause of ill health. The plus side of this interconnectedness of different determinants of health is that interventions in any one field tend to have ripple effects in other fields. Social and community interventions demonstrate that it is possible to increase health and well-being through

Figure 9.2 The relationship between risk and health (adapted from City of Toronto 1991)

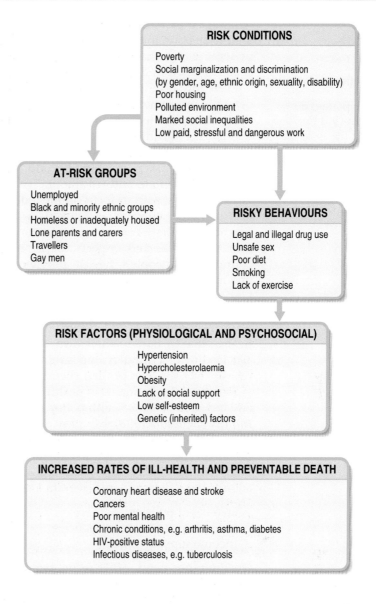

RISK CONDITIONS

Poverty
Social marginalization and discrimination
(by gender, age, ethnic origin, sexuality, disability)
Poor housing
Polluted environment
Marked social inequalities
Low paid, stressful and dangerous work

AT-RISK GROUPS

Unemployed
Black and minority ethnic groups
Homeless or inadequately housed
Lone parents and carers
Travellers
Gay men

RISKY BEHAVIOURS

Legal and illegal drug use
Unsafe sex
Poor diet
Smoking
Lack of exercise

RISK FACTORS (PHYSIOLOGICAL AND PSYCHOSOCIAL)

Hypertension
Hypercholesterolaemia
Obesity
Lack of social support
Low self-esteem
Genetic (inherited) factors

INCREASED RATES OF ILL-HEALTH AND PREVENTABLE DEATH

Coronary heart disease and stroke
Cancers
Poor mental health
Chronic conditions, e.g. arthritis, asthma, diabetes
HIV-positive status
Infectious diseases, e.g. tuberculosis

building and supporting factors that improve health, such as community safety, social capital and local income.

Addressing the social determinants to enable them to become health promoting is a daunting task that requires many discrete skills. First there is a need to establish the health links, proving that determinants can affect health both positively and negatively. This has already been accomplished by a variety of research studies endorsed by official reports such as the WHO European Regional Office publication *The Social Determinants of Health: The Solid Facts* (www.who.dk/document/e59555.pdf) and inquiries such as the Black Report of 1980 (Townsend et al 1988) and the Acheson Inquiry (Acheson 1998). Although the evidence exists, it still needs reinforcing in many different forums because traditionally public sectors have worked in isolation. Establishing that, for example, regeneration and renewal are part and parcel of health development work leads to the next logical step of joint planning, funding and working. This stage still presents many challenges and dilemmas for practitioners, which have been discussed in detail in Chapter 7.

Even for those public health practitioners who recognize the social determinants of health, other barriers remain. Acknowledging the scale of the problem can lead to a feeling of helplessness. Health care professionals may feel ill-equipped to address such problems, and relevant activities, for example supporting communal interventions such as food cooperatives, are often seen as falling beyond their remit. Such a situation can lead to low morale and frustration. The professional training of many health workers, with its focus on the individual client, has been identified as a barrier to effective anti-poverty work (Blackburn 1993). For many practitioners there is a strong professional ethos of one-to-one intervention that values and respects the individuality of each client. Factors common to people's health problems, such as social isolation or unemployment tend to be overlooked or are seen as posing additional burdens on health instead of being seen as the fundamental cause of much ill health and premature death. Blackburn (1993) found that practitioners consistently underestimate the extent and impact of poverty on health, due in part to their own distance from poverty. This distance can lead to practitioners imposing advice or information that has little relevance to the lives of their clients.

Structural determinants of health have been recognized by government and included in some health policy and strategy documents. The Acheson Inquiry (Acheson 1998) was a key document that fostered recognition of the need to address health inequalities and their underlying social determinants. The Acheson Inquiry included 38 recommendations covering many health determinants, and led to a plethora of policy making to address these determinants (see Ch. 5):

- area-based policies
- individual employment policies
- income support policies.

On the other hand, other recommendations such as water fluoridation have been neglected. Whilst there is much support for tackling inequalities and health determinants in a joined-up way, certain strategies need to be implemented in order to achieve results (Exworthy et al 2003):

- mainstreaming funding and interventions so that tackling inequalities becomes part of the health or other service's core business
- closer monitoring of the impact of interventions designed to tackle health determinants
- evaluation and research designed to assess the impact and outcomes of strategies.

Legislation and regulation are two of the most effective means to change infrastructures. They demonstrate a common view of what constitutes health risks and what actions should be taken to minimize harm. Legislation often sets minimum standards that have to be met, e.g. for air quality, wages, safety in the workplace and housing. This approach

> **R**eflection point
>
> How important do you think it is to address the social determinants of health in your work practice? Do you feel you have the skills and resources to do so effectively?

requires agreed standards based on some form of evidence plus a monitoring and enforcement body to ensure compliance. There also needs to be an adequate infrastructure of trained and resourced inspectors to enforce standards. Different professions each have a distinctive role to play. For example, environmental health officers (EHOs) are responsible for monitoring and enforcing standards for many health determinants including air pollution, food safety, housing and workplaces, whilst the police force is responsible for public protection and crime detection, and public health specialists are responsible for managing and controlling outbreaks of infectious diseases. Trading standards officers have also been identified as contributing to public health through their role in monitoring faulty goods and workmanship and enforcing the laws regarding the sale of tobacco, alcohol and solvents.

There may be tensions in the practitioner–client relationship if the practitioner has an enforcement or regulatory role. Having a regulatory role gives added authority to the practitioner, but this may have a downside. Some practitioners may feel clients will be less open and trusting if they feel they are being checked up on. Conversely, practitioners may feel clients will be more receptive and willing to take advice on board if they know there is an element of enforcement of standards involved.

One of the benefits of legislation is that it is an 'upstream' intervention that directly addresses the social determinants of health. For example, if poor quality housing is upgraded using minimum standards, then eventually no one will be living in substandard housing. This is of course an over-simplification. In practice, standards are constantly being revised, and there is always a shortfall between standards and what happens in real life. Some practitioners feel in addition that tackling determinants of health is a diversion from their primary role and expertise, which is working with individual clients. Many practitioners shy away from activities at a policy level regarding this as political action. As noted in Chapter 4, practitioners are engaged in political activity when they are implementing policy. They also have a clear role in influencing the policy agenda (for example, the input of learning disabilities nurses into government policy in the White Paper *Valuing People* (DoH 2001)) and in monitoring the effects of policy.

Strengthening disadvantaged communities through targeted interventions and regeneration and renewal is another popular approach to addressing the social determinants of health. This aims to strengthen the community fabric, building and releasing social capital and thus enhancing skills and self-esteem. *Health Promotion: Foundations for Practice* (Naidoo & Wills 2000) outlines the role and challenges of community development in promoting health including the non-statutory nature of the activity and the ambiguities surrounding professional education and training in a field which aims to break down professional/lay barriers and promote participation and equality.

The third distinct approach is targeted at individuals and aims to provide opportunities for people to tackle or overcome constraining influences on their health. For example, providing opportunities for adult education and training will help people find and retain paid employment,

Reflection point

Is there an enforcement or regulatory aspect to your role? Do you regard it as health-promoting?

thus enhancing employment and income, two key health determinants. Developing and recognizing skills that people may already have (e.g. child caring) through accreditation may reduce dependency and enhance self-esteem and self-efficacy. Providing services for individuals also has the benefit of providing direct inputs to those most at need. The direct face-to-face interaction implied by such an approach readily conforms to the model of individual client–practitioner relationship underpinning most professional education in the health care services. A major limitation of this approach is that it follows a 'downstream' rather than an 'upstream' approach. Supporting people to overcome the constraints of their circumstances will help those individuals, but if nothing is done at source to tackle the causes of their disadvantage, other individuals will take their place, living in poor housing, on low incomes, without secure employment. This cycle will only be disrupted by removing the causes of disadvantage at their source.

In practice, all three approaches are used by practitioners, and the strongest effects are found when the three different approaches build on and complement each other. Most practitioners will feel more at ease with one approach, and this provides another reason for partnership working (see Ch. 7) where different practitioners work together, each developing their own area of expertise but working alongside others. So, for example, in any one locality, environmental health officers may be working to enforce quality standards in housing and minimum exposure to pollutants in the air; youth and community workers may be facilitating and supporting community projects such as walking and exercise programmes or peer education arts projects to reduce problematic drug use; and health visitors may be providing postnatal support programmes for new mothers to reduce social isolation.

Reflection point

How does where you live affect your health?

Area of residence affects many factors that are known to independently impact on health. The type of housing and socio-economic profile of the area and its residents will affect local income levels, housing quality and exposure to overcrowding or damp, cold housing. The nature of local neighbourhoods will affect employment opportunities and levels of crime. Local transport facilities will affect the ability to travel beyond the local area for work and services, and will also have an impact on pollution levels. These factors collectively will have a big direct and indirect impact on the health of local residents.

This chapter considers the following socio-economic and environmental health determinants:

- income and poverty
- employment and unemployment
- crime
- housing
- regeneration and neighbourhood renewal
- transport.

For each health determinant, the research showing its impact on health is first reviewed, followed by examples of different kinds of strategies and interventions designed to tackle the determinant. In particular, interventions that can be undertaken by health and welfare practitioners are highlighted. Evidence about the effectiveness of different strategies is reviewed and discussed.

INCOME AND POVERTY

Box 9.1 The gap between the poorest and the richest people in the UK

- The definition of poverty used by the UK government in Opportunity for All (DWP 2002) is where household income falls below 60% of the median income level in that year.
- Society became more polarized during the last quarter of the twentieth century as the gap between the poorest and the richest widened, driven not just by increasing poverty but also by the increased wealth of the richest.
- The number of people living in poverty in Britain escalated in the last 30 years of the twentieth century from 1 in 10 to 1 in 4 of the population, rising to 1 in 3 of all children.
- The poorest 10% of single adult households were, on average, £208 per year worse off in 1995/96 than in 1979.
- During the same period, the richest 10% became £6,968 per year richer in real terms.
- People living in poverty have become more concentrated in particular areas of the country, leading to significant geographical inequalities in wealth and health.
- The most recent research shows that there has been a reduction in the number of people living in poverty.

Sources: Shaw et al (1999), Sutherland et al (2003)

Income is a key determinant of health because it is the mediating factor that determines access to a host of variables related to health. The relationship between poverty and ill health can be seen in:

- reduced access to material resources such as income and good quality housing, neighbourhood and work environments
- constrained behavioural choices such as increased rates of smoking as a coping mechanism or reduced access to healthy food due to price and local availability
- psychosocial factors such as reduced social networks and feelings of low self-worth and self-esteem.

There is now an accepted evidence base that clearly demonstrates that poverty leads to poor health outcomes and excess mortality (Acheson 1998, Benzeval et al 2000, Gordon & Pantazis 1997, Shaw et al 1999). Newer research supports the view that it is low income rather than income inequality that is the key factor determining chronic ill health and mental ill health (Sturm & Gresenz 2002) as well as perceived health (Shibuya et al 2002).

Reflection point

How would you
define poverty? Is
poverty different to
inequality? How?

Income, and hence poverty, is both absolute and relative. Absolute poverty refers to an income that is insufficient to pay for the basics of a healthy life – adequate nutrition, heating and housing (although defining basic minimum needs is not easy and is affected by cultural norms). Relative poverty is 'when (individuals) lack the resources to obtain the types of diet, participate in the activities and have the living conditions and amenities which are customary, or at least widely encouraged or approved, in the societies to which they belong' (Townsend 1979, p. 31). The key issue is whether a poverty line should be set in relation to a basic survival budget, or at a level of income that would enable people to participate in society and meet social and cultural needs. The definition of poverty used by the UK government (DWP 2002) is a household income below 60% of the median income level in that year. Other methods of establishing poverty levels may be the proportion of income needed to cover a basic food basket (used in the USA) or whether people can afford what are perceived to be necessities for life. 'Necessities for life' is a relative concept although there is considerable consensus about basic requirements. For example, a survey conducted by the Joseph Rowntree Foundation (Gordon et al 2001) found beds and bedding for everyone and adequate heating were commonly accepted as necessities for life.

Poverty is both a structural issue, affecting large sections of the population in a patterned and predictable way, and an individual issue, affecting and constraining every aspect of individual people's lives. Practitioners need to be aware of the constraints poverty places on people's lives, and take this on board in their interactions with clients living in poverty.

Reflection point

In what ways do you
tackle poverty in
your work?

Tackling poverty requires a multi-layered response that addresses the causes and effects of poverty. The government is committed to eliminating childhood poverty by 2020 and there is widespread support for policies to reduce poverty in the UK. Tackling the causes of poverty involves social policies focusing on:

- benefit levels
- access to employment
- access to child care
- tackling low wages.

The biggest and most significant anti-poverty policy is the social security system. Each year over £100 billion in social security benefits is distributed to over half the population (Alcock 2002). Universal benefits are paid in the UK on the basis of age or family circumstances, e.g. pensions and child allowances, but a significant element is also welfare benefits, such as income support or unemployment benefit, which aim to relieve poverty. In addition to social security benefits, policies such as the introduction of a minimum wage, changes to the tax system, e.g. working tax credit and child tax credit, and changes to the national insurance system, are designed to ensure that being in employment leads to a higher income than being on benefits, and to help working people escape the trap of low income. Practitioners can help to ensure that clients are receiving their full benefit entitlement. Some practitioners may view such work as beyond their remit and area of expertise, but such schemes are practical and effective (see for example p. 102 in Ch. 5).

Example

Social policy interventions to tackle poverty

Between 1996/7 and 2000/1 poverty in the UK has fallen by approximately one million, including about half a million fewer children living in poverty although this trend will become harder to sustain. Greater employment, or 'work for those who can' has made the most significant contribution but there is a limit to how much further these measures can contribute. Changes to the tax and benefits system have particularly benefited those with children and low earners but has disadvantaged others such as those receiving incapacity benefit. Changes in indirect taxation (such as increases in tobacco tax and TV licence) negatively affect those on low income, for whom such taxes represent a significant proportion of total income.

Source: Sutherland et al (2003)

At a local level, initiatives such as credit unions or local exchange trading schemes (LETS), which allow local trade by using credits instead of money, are an important means of facilitating and supporting local economies. LETS are also intended to maximize employment opportunities by building up skills. Schemes that maximize or increase income, or provide services and stimulate trade via credits, provide the most direct example of tackling the links between poverty and health.

Other strategies to tackle poverty may aim to strengthen individuals. For example, brief behavioural counselling to increase the consumption of fruit and vegetables amongst low income adults was found to be more effective than nutrition education counselling. Brief behavioural counselling led to a 42% increase in the proportion of participants eating five or more portions a day (Steptoe et al 2003). Other interventions may focus on 'living on a budget', such as community kitchens. These schemes can be effective in getting people together to think about common problems and encourage social support networks. The challenge for practitioners is to avoid exacerbating problems by blaming people, explicitly or implicitly, for any unhealthy behaviours.

There is ample evidence of the link between low income and poor health, but historically there has been a separation between health and social care professionals, with income support work being undertaken by social care professionals. However, there are examples of interventions tackling poverty and low income where health practitioners play a key role. With training, support and resources, addressing low income and its effects on health can become a realistic and effective task for health practitioners. At a basic level, awareness and acknowledgement of the effects of low income on clients can enable practitioners' core work, for example health promotion advice and education, to become more sensitive, appropriate and effective.

EMPLOYMENT AND UNEMPLOYMENT

There is a strong link between employment and health. For some people, the work environment can present hazards and health risks. Health and safety legislation covers employers' statutory responsibilities to protect the health of their employees, but occupational ill health remains a significant problem. Social inequalities are reflected in the workplace, with workers from low socio-economic positions, Black and migrant workers disproportionately employed in the most hazardous and unhealthy jobs.

Box 9.2 The links between work and health

In the UK conservative estimates of the contribution of work-related conditions to health each year are:

- 2000 premature deaths are caused by occupational disease
- 8000 deaths are caused in part by work conditions
- 80 000 new cases of work-related disease are registered
- 500 000 people continue to suffer from work-related ill health
- ill health accounts for 18 million lost working days
- occupational accidents and ill health are estimated to cost £7 billion.

Worldwide each year:

- 250 million occupational injuries are reported
- 160 million cases of occupational disease are reported.

Source: Watterson (2003)

Discussion point

Think of your own employment and workplace. What factors there contribute to your health and well-being, and what factors contribute to stress and ill health?

Stress at work plays an important role in contributing to the large differences in health, sickness absence and premature death related to social status. Marmot et al (1999) researched civil servants at varying grades within the civil service to determine the effect of work-related status and control on health. He found that having little control over work demands and processes, and being relatively low down in the work hierarchy, is linked, via a variety of physiological changes, to an increased risk of ill health. Attempts to foreground health within the workplace and make the workplace a healthy setting have been patchy and uncoordinated although there are some success stories. Occupational health services are voluntary and remain relatively underdeveloped in the UK, with many workers lacking access to these services. Occupational health policies are not prioritized, for example, they are absent in many Health Action Zones and Health Improvement Plans. More could be done to prevent occupational ill health and protect the health of people in the workplace. For the majority of people, however, the association between paid employment and health is overwhelmingly positive. Paid employment provides people with an income, feelings of self-esteem, purpose and self-efficacy, and a social network. Employment provides goods or services that contribute to the national economy.

Unemployment is a greater health risk than employment, and is strongly related to ill health and mortality. A good case can be made for targeting unemployed people and supporting them to move into paid employment as a health-promoting strategy.

Getting people into paid employment is a key national policy that is supported by many local initiatives. The approach is many pronged, and includes providing skills and training to enhance employability, helping people apply for jobs, supporting flexible hours through the provision of child care, and providing transport to enable people to get to work.

National policy addresses both health and safety in the workplace and unemployment issues. The Health and Safety at Work Act 1974 set out the employer's duty to protect the health, safety and welfare of employees and the wider public with regard to work processes. Dangerous substances used in the workplace are required to be satisfactorily controlled so that they pose no danger to the workforce and members of the public. Employees have a duty to take reasonable care with regard to health and safety issues, and to comply with any safety requirements. This Act also established the Health and Safety Executive and Health and Safety Commission, which are responsible for monitoring the workplace and ensuring that legal minimum requirements are met.

Locally the model of community-based occupational health centres, adapted from examples in Italy, Scandinavia and the USA, appears to be successful in tackling both the prevention and treatment of occupational ill health within a multidisciplinary and multiprofessional context. A pilot project was the Sheffield Occupational Health Advisory Service, the first of its kind in the UK. The service offers confidential advice sessions in 24 GP practices across the city (www.worksmart.org.uk accessed 7/8/03). Health Works, based in Newham, East London is also based in GP practices and offers specialist advice and signposting to further services as necessary. It also addresses homeworking hazards and workplace safety education for school leavers.

There are also many local interventions designed to assist people finding paid employment. For example, the Grimethorpe Jobshop, based in a community centre, offers help with CVs and applications and provides interview skills and further education for clients. Several other projects provide transport for workers and Northolt YWCA offers child care and work placements to enable mothers to take paid employment. Another strategy is to provide start-up loans to enable self-employment and the growth of small businesses. This approach was inspired by the example of the Grameen Bank in Bangladesh which has helped millions to set up their own businesses and has a default rate of less than 3%. Community projects offer the benefits of direct accessibility and the provision of services tailored to local needs.

Individually, health workers can try to be more rigorous in considering the impact of employment on health when seeing patients who are employees. Routinely documenting people's employment on their health records can be a first step. Monitoring and audit of records could then attempt to identify any patterns in illnesses related to workplaces.

CRIME

Crime is generally viewed as a social rather than a health issue. However, the known association of crime with inequalities, deprivation, social exclusion and marginalization suggests a health aspect. Violent crime is associated with income inequality. In the USA the greater the degree of income inequality, the higher the rates of homicide, robbery and assault.

Discussion point

How do crime and violence impact on individual and community health?

Crime may impact on health by its effects on:

- the physical health of victims
- the psychological health of victims and those who witness criminal acts
- the fear of crime in particular communities that reduces individual well-being and fractures community networks
- its impact on health services.

Box 9.3 Crime and health

- 10% of inner city residents are burgled more than once a year.
- 50% of people who are victims of crime are repeat victims.
- 25% of Black and ethnic minority residents in low income areas say racially motivated attacks are a big problem.
- 2002/3 British Crime Survey reports a reduction in most crimes including crimes against adults (2% reduction)
  - burglaries (39% fall since 1997)
  - robberies (14% reduction following the introduction of the street crime initiative in 10 forces)
  - vehicle-related thefts (5% reduction)
  - exceptions to this trend are violent crimes experienced by adults living in private households (no change), woundings and firearm offences (37% increase from previous year).
- 75% of the public believe that the national crime rate has been rising.

Source: Neighbourhood Renewal Unit (2002), Home Office (2003)

A public health approach to crime and crime prevention has seen much greater emphasis on community safety rather than policing. Such approaches to crime prevention reflect the importance of the focus on social conditions. Strategies to tackle crime include:

- crime prevention interventions, e.g. youth work to 'distract' young people from criminal activities, drug and alcohol initiatives such as the arrest referral schemes that refer users from police stations directly to rehabilitation programmes
- crime detection and prosecution strategies, e.g. closed circuit television (CCTV) and the witness protection scheme
- the identification and support for victims of crime, e.g. screening for domestic violence in primary care settings, victim support schemes
- treatment and rehabilitation of offenders, e.g. probation services.

Such varied activities require partnership working across professionals and agencies, and in particular the active involvement of communities. For example, the Crime and Disorder Act 1998 placed a responsibility on local authorities, the police and other agencies to work together to tackle crime and disorder.

A variety of strategies have been introduced to increase community safety including street wardens on housing estates, neighbourhood watch schemes and closed circuit television. Such schemes are often very popular although the evidence base to support the effectiveness of such measures is not solid.

Community safety measures

A variety of strategies have been introduced to reduce crime, including Neighbourhood Watch (NW) schemes and closed circuit television (CCTV)

CCTV

Evaluation of the effectiveness of CCTV is mixed. Several local studies report large reductions in crime. For example, the introduction of CCTV into a local authority in Darlington led to a 44% reduction in crime and very positive feedback from residents. However, a systematic review conducted by the Home Office found CCTV led to a non-sigificant reduction in crime of 6%. It has been argued that CCTV involves a number of different context-specific features that will impact on its effectiveness, e.g. deterrence, displacement of criminal activities elsewhere, greater public safety awareness leading to more defensive behaviour and informal surveillance, and more effective deployment of resources. Effectiveness measures should therefore include crime detection, conviction of criminals and fear of crime as well as crime reduction.

(Sources: Pawson & Tilley 1997; Welsh & Farrington 2002; www.crimereduction.gov.uk accessed 12/9/03.)

Neighbourhood Watch

Neighbourhood Watch (NW) schemes have grown in popularity and an estimated 27% of households were members of an NW scheme in 2000. However, membership was skewed towards more affluent households living in areas with low perceived crime rates. Approximately one-third of such households belonged to an NW scheme compared to approximately one-sixth of low income households in areas with high levels of perceived crime and disorder. Around three-quarters of all respondents thought that NW schemes were effective, and a similar proportion of non-members would join a scheme if it existed in their locality. However, there is no evidence that NW schemes actually reduce crime such as burglary, nor does membership significantly affect people's fear of crime.

(Source: Sims 2001)

Unlike crime, a neighbour dispute has no legally defined status and may include inconsiderate behaviour such as excessive noise to harassment and intimidation. Noise can undermine quality of life and although it does not necessarily translate into mental health problems it can lead to tension and irritability.

Noisy neighbours

People living next to noisy neighbours may suffer from sleep deprivation, increased aggression and a certain level of mental illness (CIEH 2001, London Health Commission 2003). Noisy neighbours are becoming a more common problem. In the 20 years between 1981 and 2001 the number of complaints about noisy neighbours made to UK local authorities rose more than seven-fold, from 764 per million of the population to 5540 per million of the population. Complaints about neighbours make up approximately 70% of all noise complaints. Approaches to tackling this problem include legal enforcement, education and community mediation. The Environment Protection Act 1990 (as amended) requires local authorities to investigate complaints about noisy neighbours. Where there is evidence of a nuisance, e.g. not merely a one-off incident, environmental health officers (EHOs) may serve a notice requiring

E *continued*

noise abatement. Enforcement of the Act can be difficult as an EHO needs to witness the noisy behaviour and this requirement may cause considerable time delays. Other strategies include diversionary activities targeted at young people playing loud music, and education targeted at young people excluded from schools to reduce noisy and antisocial behaviour.

(With thanks to Stephen Young)

Domestic violence is now recognized as a public health priority (WHO 1997). Domestic violence includes physical, sexual, psychological, emotional and economic abuse within the home. It results from a specific unequal power relationship and refers to the abuse of women at the hands of male partners or ex-partners. Other forms of intra-familial abuse exist, including the abuse of children and the elderly and, rarely, the abuse of men by women. Domestic violence is a common but often hidden problem, with one in four women experiencing domestic abuse at some point in their lives. The health effects of domestic abuse include poor physical health, chronic pain, mental health problems including depression, addiction and attempted suicide; and difficulties in pregnancy (McCartney 1999). Domestic violence often starts during pregnancy and may lead to maternal and fetal deaths, premature birth and low birth weight (Webster & Chandler 1996). The health services often miss the symptoms of domestic violence, and several programmes have been initiated that focus on training health staff to identify and intervene in cases of domestic violence.

Practitioner talking

Antenatal screening for domestic violence

I'm a midwife and I recently attended a programme on antenatal screening for domestic violence. This involved a taught study day where we practised and developed our skills in asking women about domestic violence and learnt more about interagency working and safety. I learnt about the five stages in antenatal screening for domestic violence:

- *Recognizing abuse as an issue – the wide range of indicators including late booking, repeated attendance in health care settings for minor injuries, physical injuries, mental health problems and emotional or behavioural patterns.*
- *Providing a quiet and private environment for consultation – ensuring privacy and communication, e.g. using an interpreter for deaf women or women with English as a second language.*
- *Identifying abuse and its effects – questioning women in an open and empathetic manner. Stating in advance that questions about domestic violence are routinely included in consultations is helpful, and both direct and indirect questions need to be used appropriately.*
- *Documenting the abuse – ensuring women's consent to any documentation and ensuring that information is confidential and cannot be accessed by the perpetrator, e.g. using a sealed envelope that is kept separately from women's hand held records.*
- *Providing information and on-going support to women – advising women of local agencies, liaising with local support services if women want to*

P *continued*

leave home and drawing up contingency plans if they decide to stay but might need to leave at very short notice.

The training has made me feel much more confident about asking women about abuse because now I know how to ask, and what to do if women disclose. It is also reassuring to know women feel it is an acceptable topic to broach with them. I know I can get support from other practitioners and agencies and won't be left on my own to deal with any problems that emerge.

(With thanks to Debra Salmon)

Commentary

Practitioners may need to withdraw and seek support if they feel personally threatened. Research has shown that although domestic violence is a very sensitive topic, women don't mind being asked about it as long as the questioning is done by a trained professional in a caring and non-judgemental manner and in a safe and confidential setting (Bacchus et al 2003). Several professional bodies support the introduction of routine antenatal enquiry into domestic violence nationwide (Bewley et al 1997, RCM 1997). There is a specific web site (www.northbristol.nhs.uk/midwives/domesticviolence).

The impact of crime and safety issues on health is increasingly being recognized as significant. Partnership working around such issues has the potential to promote the health of communities and individuals. At the individual level, greater awareness of violence and abuse can help practitioners to intervene effectively. Health practitioners working in the area of crime and safety is not unusual, and further networking of good practice examples and provision of appropriate training and support will help establish this topic as part of the health practitioner's remit.

HOUSING

There is a well documented association between housing status and health. Owner-occupiers enjoy better health status than people who rent their homes. Owner-occupiers report lower death rates and rates of long-term illness (Flakti & Fox 1995, Gould & Jones 1996). Usually this association is explained in terms of the links between income and housing status, with owner-occupiers enjoying higher income levels and socio-economic status than tenants. There is also a view that the link is due to psychological attributes such as perceived control and deferred gratification.

The pattern of housing tenure in the UK has shifted dramatically during the last 20 years. The most significant switch is from council tenancy to owner-occupier, fuelled by tenants' right to buy which was introduced in the 1980s. Housing tenure in 1998 was 68% home ownership, 10% privately rented, 5% housing associations and registered social landlords, and 17% council housing (Anderson & Barclay 2003).

There is evidence that housing quality impacts both directly and indirectly on health (Ellaway & Macintyre 1998, Macintyre et al 1998). Direct effects include:

- excess winter deaths due to fuel poverty (which affected 4.3 million people in 1996)
- home accidents (highest in temporary accommodation for the home-less)
- increases in infectious diseases such as tuberculosis, which are linked to overcrowding
- excess death rates (5 times the general population average for people living in houses with multiple occupation and 10 times the average for rough sleepers (Matthews 1999)).

Indirect effects are mediated by factors such as crowding, reduced access to amenities, and perception of low social capital in the neighbourhood and include health problems associated with crime, pollution and heavy traffic and problems for people living in deprived areas accessing health and welfare services. Figure 9.3 below illustrates possible pathways linking housing tenure and health status.

Figure 9.3 The relationship between housing tenure and individual health (from Macintyre S et al (2000) In Graham H (ed) Understanding health inequalities. Reproduced by permission of Open University Press)

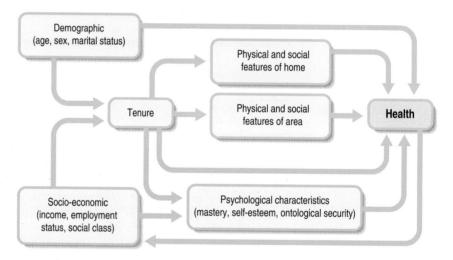

E**xample**

Keeping warm in winter

There are 40 000 excess winter deaths (deaths which would not be expected if the average death rate for the rest of the year applied in winter) each year in the UK. This level of excess mortality in the winter months is not seen in other countries that are much colder, such as Russia and the Scandinavian countries. Excess winter mortality is largely preventable if people keep warm. This depends on:

- energy efficiency in homes
- occupancy level (related to size of dwelling)
- income
- cost of fuel.

Over 50% of households in fuel poverty (i.e. spending more than 10% of household income on fuel) are composed of older people and most are owner-occupiers. The Health Homes Referral Scheme in Leicester is funded by a Health Action Zone. Nurses are trained to identify people at risk of ill health due to poor living conditions. They can then be offered a free home energy, security and hazard survey, advice on grants and a rapid response repairs service.

Source: Press (2003)

Unfit housing carries health risks for inhabitants. Unfit housing affected 6% of households in the UK in 2000 (Anderson & Barclay 2003). Unfit housing is most common in the private rented sector, and in the owner-occupier sector affects elderly owner-occupiers most. Disrepair is far more common, affecting almost one-third of homes in England. Poor heating and insulation is a significant problem, leading to 8000 extra deaths for each degree Celsius the temperature falls below average in winter months. Health problems related to unfit housing or housing of poor quality include:

1. Physical health problems, e.g.
   - respiratory diseases
   - hypothermia
   - ischaemic heart disease
   - gastroenteritis
   - dysentery
   - diarrhoea
   - infections and allergic responses.

2. Mental health problems, e.g.
   - stress and depression.

There is also a raised risk of accidents, fires and illnesses due to environmental toxins.

Although there is an obvious connection between housing and health, it is difficult to coordinate activity across the housing and health fields. This is due to many reasons, including the difficulty in isolating and quantifying the housing–health link and the historic separation of housing and health functions, professions and agencies, which makes joint working very challenging (Matthews 1999). Nationally what is needed is for housing to become integrated into the public health agenda at all levels. At present, housing standards are enforced by environmental health officers who are employed by local authorities and health professionals probably regard the provision of decent housing as outside the remit of the health services.

It is health professionals who see the effects of cold, damp housing. Housing and health are obviously linked at the strategic level, but there is also some scope to make links on the ground.

Reflection point

What opportunities are there in your work to address housing issues?

Example

Links between health and housing in practice

1. Strategic links between health and housing, e.g. the Director of Public Health's annual report and health commissioning plans can refer to local housing provision and need, and make explicit the link between housing and health.

2. The housing sector can take the lead in the use of health criteria to prioritize capital work, e.g. Bexley council, which targeted the council's housing association development programme to provide group homes and wheelchair-accessible housing. Bexley also used empty property to temporarily house high-rise residents experiencing emotional difficulties (Matthews 1999).

3. Practitioners linking health and housing in service delivery to vulnerable people: isolated, old people; those discharged from hospital; and those with mental health problems, e.g. district nurses who visit older people in their

E continued

homes should be alerted to the signs of fuel poverty in the home – for example, only one room heated or a cold, damp living room (Press 2003).

4. Single assessment, introduced as a central part of the Older People's National Service Framework, replaces multiple assessment of the same client by different health and social welfare agencies. The single assessment is shared between relevant agencies. Single assessment includes consideration of housing and the potential for accidents in the home.

Evaluating housing interventions is extremely difficult, due to the complex relationship between housing and other factors and health, and the practical and ethical problems of using experimental or quasi-experimental methods in this field. A recent systematic review of the health effects of housing improvement interventions concluded that whilst many studies showed health gains, the small study populations and number of confounding factors limits the generalizability of their findings (Thomson et al 2001).

REGENERATION AND NEIGHBOURHOOD RENEWAL

There is a large gap separating England's most deprived neighbourhoods and the rest. Four regions (the North West, North East, London and Yorkshire and Humberside) have particularly high concentrations of deprived neighbourhoods.

Box 9.4 The gap between deprived neighbourhoods and the rest (1998/99 statistics)

- In the 10% most deprived wards, twice as many people relied on means tested benefits compared with the national average (44% compared to 22%).
- In the 10% most deprived wards, over 60% of children lived in households that relied on means tested benefits.
- Only 11 of the 488 schools with more than 35% of pupils on free school meals attained the national average level of GCSE passes.
- 26% more people died from coronary heart disease in the 20% most deprived Health Authorities than in the country as a whole.
- In the 10% most deprived wards 43% of housing is not in a decent state (compared with 29% elsewhere) and 19% of homes suffer from disrepair, vacancy, dereliction or vandalism (compared with 5% of homes elsewhere).

Source: Social Exclusion Unit (2000)

Regeneration or neighbourhood renewal aims to improve disadvantaged urban areas and encompasses a wide range of activities including improved housing and recreation facilities, job creation, community safety interventions, and the active involvement and participation of local communities in these processes. As the government puts it, 'the goal is to break the vicious circle of deprivation and provide the foundation for sustainable regeneration and wealth creation' (DETR 1997, p. 3). Regeneration of urban areas has a history dating back more than 30 years. The current programme of regeneration is funded by the Department of the Environment,

Transport and the Regions (DETRA) through the Single Regeneration Budget (SRB). The SRB is allocated on the basis of need and competitive bidding. This seems to be effective in allocating resources to those most in need. Tyler et al (1998) found that 80% of SRB funding went to the 99 most deprived districts.

The rationale for regeneration is both economic (to increase local employment) and social (to build a future for local people). Tackling the disadvantage that includes lower standards of health involves partnership working with a wide range of organizations and agencies. A key feature of regeneration is the need to involve these partners and adopt an inter-agency approach. The health services have been identified as a key partner in renewal strategies. For example, health services are a major employer in communities and can thus have an impact on local economies through a commitment to provide training and education to local staff so that their careers can progress. In this way, communities become more self-sufficient, local job prospects are improved, and service providers are more in tune with the needs and wishes of service users. There is no definite evidence linking regeneration with health improvement, although the evidence linking poverty and social exclusion with health is extensive.

Discussion point

How might health professionals be involved in regeneration work?

Discussion point

Evaluating regeneration programmes

The objective of a regeneration programme is to tackle the broad determinants of health in an area. What would be the indicators of success of the programme for each of the following objectives:

- getting people into jobs?
- developing local businesses?
- promoting lifelong learning?
- developing a high quality living environment?
- developing a safer neighbourhood?
- promoting health?
- empowering communities?

Why might it be difficult to evaluate regeneration initiatives?

A variety of local indicators are already available via local councils, police forces and health trusts. However, there are problems with using these data to evaluate regeneration policies. Harrison (2000) identifies several factors that make such evaluation difficult including the political nature of urban policy, the complexity of interventions spanning many different policy arenas (such as employment, housing, education and crime reduction), the links between urban decline and national and global processes, the importance of the local context in determining processes and effects, the effect of displacement and migration (so that beneficiaries of regeneration may not be the originally targeted communities), and the need to measure processes as well as outcomes. Despite these confounding factors, there are some studies that show positive outcomes associated with urban regeneration. One example is Halpern's (1995) study which showed that mental health can be improved through environmental interventions – in this case the improvement of an unpopular new town estate. Equally it is important to recognize that there are aspects of regeneration that may be damaging to population and individual health:

- the process of decanting residents while housing improvements take place
- increased housing costs as a result of regeneration programmes
- the effect on populations outside the regeneration area through, for example, the displacement of drug dealing
- increased social divisions.

Regeneration and neighbourhood renewal are important health promoting strategies that directly impact on a variety of socio-economic and environmental determinants of health. Targeting the most deprived neighbourhoods is one means of tackling inequalities in health. Health practitioners have an important role to play as key partners in regeneration and renewal, and the experience of working with communities can also positively influence public involvement strategies used to plan health service provision. A challenge for regeneration is how to balance tackling the short-term and pressing needs of disadvantaged areas with the longer-term planning that is required.

TRANSPORT

Transport and health are linked in several ways:

- Adequate and appropriate transport increases people's mobility and access to a wide range of services, facilitating choice.
- The dominance of private car transport at the expense of public transport results in high rates of road accidents, air pollution, the loss of community networks and sedentary lifestyles.

Box 9.5 Transport and Health

- Road traffic accidents account for two-fifths of accidental deaths.
- Heavy traffic reduces physical and social activity, leading to:
  - isolation and the loss of community networks
  - reduced likelihood of people walking or cycling for short journeys
  - sedentary lifestyles and the growth in obesity.
- Pollution from traffic is the major cause of poor air quality in urban areas and contributes to respiratory and cardiac problems.
- In many areas of the UK, transport is the principal source of nitrogen dioxide and particulate matter (PM10) – two major air pollutants
- It is estimated that air pollution is responsible for the premature death of over 20 000 people each year across Europe, and serious ill health affecting many more thousands of people.
- Transport produces nearly one quarter of the UK's emission of carbon dioxide, which contributes to environmental damage and global warming.
- Noise pollution and stress from living and working in areas of heavy traffic contributes to mental health problems.

Sources: Kunzil et al (2000), McGrogan (1999)

Between 1986 and 2000 the number of cars registered in the UK increased from 17.4 million to 26.7 million. Today car journeys account for 82% of all journeys by mileage.

Public health action in the field of transport covers a variety of interventions including promoting physically active means of transport, such as cycling and walking to school and work; promoting the use of public transport to reduce traffic pollution; and measures to enhance the safety of roads, e.g. pedestrianization, traffic calming and speed cameras. Promoting physically active means of transport is discussed further in the Physical Activity section of Chapter 11. The most emotive issue, and hence the one likely to legitimize health practitioners' involvement, is probably the reduction of road traffic injuries and fatalities and this priority area is discussed further in Chapter 10. Child pedestrian injury arising from road accidents is the leading cause of accidental death in the UK. Social deprivation is strongly associated with child pedestrian injuries, with children from social class 5 being five times more likely to be killed in a road traffic collision than children from social class 1 (Liabo & Curtis 2003). Road accidents are estimated to cost Britain over £16 000 million per year. Involvement in such interventions could therefore be justified on the grounds of a concern with children's health, health inequalities and accident prevention.

> **R**eflection point
>
> How might you address transport issues within your work practice?

> **E**xample
>
> Traffic calming
>
> Traffic calming aims to reduce the volume of traffic using urban residential streets and traffic speeds. Traffic calming modifies the environment through, for example, introducing one-way systems, speed humps, narrowing roads, gateways at the entrances to areas and raised junctions. Evidence from systematic reviews shows that traffic calming can significantly reduce childhood injuries from road accidents by up to 15%. Introducing traffic calming to a local area is likely to be an effective measure in reducing inequalities in child health. In many consultations children themselves have called for safer streets.
>
> Source: Liabo & Curtis (2003)

Transport campaigns tend to be high profile and politicized, which may lead health practitioners to steer clear of them. The private car lobby is very powerful and influential, and has been linked to media campaigns that have tried to discredit road safety campaigns. These tensions are explored in the example of safety cameras below.

> **E**xample
>
> Safety cameras
>
> Excessive and inappropriate speed is the cause of over one-third of accidents on UK roads. By 2020 road accidents will have moved from ninth to third place in the world ranking of the burden of disease. In Britain around 3500 people are killed and 330 000 injured in road accidents each year. Research in Norway, Australia, Canada, New Zealand and the UK has shown that safety cameras affect driving speeds and improve safety. Results from a 2-year pilot scheme in 8 areas showed that the number of people killed or seriously injured fell by 35%. Average speed in the pilot areas fell by 10%. There has been a vigorous public media campaign against the introduction of safety cameras, claiming they are being used to raise revenue and are a punitive anti-motorist measure. However, the effectiveness of safety cameras in reducing accidents and injuries

E continued is indisputable, and has led to a major expansion of speed cameras. Local safety camera schemes are led by multi-agency Safety Camera Partnerships. A majority of the British public supports safety cameras.

Sources: Dept. of Transport News Release 11 Feb 2003, Pilkington (2003)

Road traffic accidents and fatalities are the most obvious and publicized aspect of the links between transport and health. However other issues, especially air and noise pollution, are also important, especially in the long term. The reliance in the UK on private cars for transport has led to increases in air and noise pollution. The Environment Act 1995 led to the development of a National Air Quality Strategy that sets targets for the reduction of eight major air pollutants known to affect human health by 2010. The aim is to ensure that everyone can breathe air in public places that poses no significant risk to health or quality of life. Local authorities are required to draw up their own Local Air Quality Management plans to achieve air quality objectives. Local Air Quality Management Areas (AQMAs) and action plans are declared if it is anticipated that targets will not be met. Following the first round of review and assessment, 129 local authorities declared AQMAs, 75% of these AQMAs were purely due to traffic. Local transport plans aim to reduce private car use and encourage other forms of transport such as walking, cycling and bus or shared car use. Other strategies include regulation to reduce vehicle emissions and improve fuels, tax incentives to use cleaner fuels and vehicles, and the development of an integrated transport strategy that supports sustainable development.

Evaluating transport interventions to promote health suffers from the problems of contamination with other variables and difficulty in isolating relevant factors. However research into this area does give grounds for optimism. A recent systematic review of the effectiveness of transport interventions in improving population health (Morrison et al 2003) concluded that the most effective interventions are health promotion campaigns (to prevent child accidents, to increase helmet use and promote the use of children's seats and seatbelt use), traffic calming, and specific legislation to ban drink-driving. This suggests that tackling transport does result in significant health benefits.

CONCLUSION

The social determinants of health have a profound impact on public health. This impact is both direct and indirect, and is often mediated by psychosocial factors such as self-efficacy and social capital. Because social determinants rarely fit the traditional medical disease model of pathogen–host–disease, their effect on health has not always been recognized. In addition, many of the social determinants of health are regulated and addressed by social and environmental services that have historically been separated from health services. However, there is now ample evidence and a general consensus that all the social determinants considered in this chapter – income, housing, crime, regeneration and neighbourhood renewal and transport – have a significant effect on health.

This chapter has provided a summary overview of some of the evidence linking social determinants to health, followed by examples of interventions designed to address determinants and promote health. Interventions are broad based and include regulation and legislation, community projects, and individually based work with clients. Although some of the most important interventions are at a macro policy level, practitioners have discovered a variety of innovative ways of supporting policies locally, enabling clients to address constraints, and supporting communities to overcome limitations. Successful work to tackle the social determinants of health is becoming integrated within health, social and environmental practitioners' workloads. Crucial to the continuing success of this work is effective partnership working and the involvement of communities. The growing evidence base for such work is also important in legitimizing and supporting this approach. There is a huge potential for such an approach to continue to promote and develop the public health.

FURTHER DISCUSSION

■ Consider how you might address a particular social determinant of health within your practice. What resources and skills would you need?

■ With reference to your practice, try to assess the impact of one particular determinant of health. What problems do you encounter? Are there ways in which you could collect relevant information routinely, or liaise more with other agencies, making such an assessment less problematic?

■ Consider your current networking and partnership work with other services and agencies. Can you identify ways in which this process could become more health promoting for the communities you serve?

Recommended reading

■ Griffiths S, Hunter D J (eds) (1999) Perspectives in public health. Abingdon, Radcliffe Medical Press.

An edited text with contributions from academics, practitioners and politicians on different social determinants of health. The book includes chapters on public health topics (such as housing, transport and food) as well as chapters on the contributions that can be made by different professional groups.

■ Russell H, Killoran A (2000) Public health and regeneration: making the links. London, Health Education Agency.

A short guide that summarizes some of the evidence linking issues such as community safety and housing with health.

■ Marmot M and Wilkinson R (1999) Social determinants of health. Oxford, Oxford University Press.

An accessible and thought-provoking book. The authors argue that addressing the social determinants of health is a more effective and more equitable strategy than working 'downstream' to provide health care services for the casualties. The book covers several different topics including work and employment, food, transport, and alcohol and drugs.

REFERENCES

Acheson D (1998) Independent inquiry into inequalities in health. London, The Stationery Office

Alcock P (2002) Anti-poverty strategies. In: Adam L, Amos M, Munro J (eds) Promoting health: politics and practice. London, Sage

Anderson I, Barclay A (2003) Housing and health. In: Watterson A (ed) Public health in practice. Basingstoke, Palgrave Macmillan.

Bacchus L, Mezey G, Bewley S (2003) Experiences of seeking help from health professionals in a sample of women who experienced domestic violence. Health and Social Care in the Community 11(1): 10–18

Benzeval M, Dilnot A, Judge K, Taylor J (2000) Income and health over the lifecourse: evidence and policy implications. In: Graham H (ed) Understanding health inequalities. Maidenhead, Open University Press, pp 96–113

Bewley S, Friend J, Mezey G (1997) Violence against women. London, Royal College of Obstetricians and Gynaecologists Press

Blackburn C (1993) Making poverty a practice issue. Health and Social Care 1: 297–304

Chartered Institute of Environmental Health (CIEH) (2001) Annual survey into local authority noise enforcement action. England and Wales: noise nuisance. London, CIEH

City of Toronto Community Health Information Section (1991) Health inequalities in the city of Toronto: summary report. Toronto, Department of Public Health

Dahlgren G, Whitehead M (1991) Policies and strategies to promote social equity in health. Stockholm, Institute of Future Studies

Department of the Environment, Transport and Regions (DETR) (1997) Regeneration – the way forward. DETR Regeneration website: www.roads.dtlr.gov.uk/roadsafety/strategy/tomorrow

Department of Health (DoH) (1999) Saving lives: our healthier nation. London, The Stationery Office

Department of Health (DoH) (2001) Valuing people: a new strategy for learning disability for the 21st century. A White Paper. Cm. 5086. London, The Stationery Office

Department for Work and Pensions (DWP) (2002) Opportunity for all: 4th annual report, Cm 5598. London, The Stationery Office

Ellaway A, Macintyre S (1998) Does housing tenure predict health in the UK because it exposes people to different levels of housing related hazards in the home or its surroundings? Health and Place 4: 141–50

Exworthy M, Stuart M, Blane D, Marmot M (2003) Tackling health inequalities since the Acheson Inquiry. Bristol, The Policy Press/Joseph Rowntree Foundation

Flakti H, Fox J (1995) Differences in mortality by housing tenure and by car access. Population Trends 81: 27–30

Gordon D, Pantazis C (eds) (1997) Breadline Britain in the 1990s. Aldershot, Ashgate

Gordon D, Middleton S, Bradshaw J R (2001) Millennium survey of poverty and social exclusion 1999. York, Joseph Rowntree Foundation

Gould M I, Jones K (1996) Housing as health capital: how health trajectories and housing interact. Cambridge, Polity Press

Halpern D (1995) Mental health and the built environment. London, Taylor & Francis

Harrison T (2000) Urban policy. In: Davies T O, Nutley S M, Smith P C (eds) What works? Evidence-based policy and practice in public services. Bristol, The Policy Press

Home Office (2003) British Crime Survey 2002/3. www.crimereduction.gov.uk/statistics accessed 12/12/03

Kunzil N, Kaiser R, Medina S et al (2000) Public health impact of outdoor and traffic-related air pollution: a European assessment. Lancet 356: 795–801

Liabo K, Curtis K (2003) Traffic calming schemes to reduce childhood injuries from road accidents and respond to children's own views of what is important. What Works for Children Group EvidenceNugget: www.evidencenetwork.org/

London Health Commission (2003) Noise and health: making the link. London, London Health Commission

McCartney S (1999) Domestic violence. In: Griffiths S, Hunter D J (1999) Perspectives in public health. Abingdon, Radcliffe Medical Press

McGrogan G (1999) Transport. In: Griffiths S, Hunter D J (eds) Perspectives in public health. Abingdon, Radcliffe Medical Press

Macintyre S, Hiscock R, Kearns A, Ellaway A (2000) Housing tenure and health inequalities: a three-dimensional perspective on people, homes and neighbourhoods. In: Graham H (ed) Understanding health inequalities. Maidenhead, Open University Press

Macintyre S, Ellaway A, Der G, Ford G, Hunt K (1998) Are housing tenure and car access simply markers of income or self esteem? A Scottish study. Journal of Epidemiology and Community Health 52: 657–664

Marmot M, Siegrist J, Theorell T, Feeney A (1999) Health and the psychosocial environment at work. In: Marmot M, Wilkinson R G (eds) Social determinants of health. New York: Oxford University Press, pp 105–132

Matthews G (1999) Why should public health include housing? In: Griffiths S, Hunter D J (1999) Perspectives in public health. Abingdon, Radcliffe Medical Press

Morrison D S, Petticrew M, Thomson H (2003) What are the most effective ways of improving population health through transport interventions? Evidence from systematic reviews. Journal of Epidemiology and Community Health 57(5): 327–333

Naidoo J, Wills J (2000) Health promotion: foundations for practice, 2nd edn. London, Baillière Tindall

Neighbourhood Renewal Unit (2002) Neighbourhood wardens and street wardens. Factsheet no. 5

Pawson R, Tilley N (1997) Realistic evaluation. London, Sage

Pilkington P (2003) Speed cameras under attack in the UK. Injury Prevention 9: 293–294

Press V (2003) Fuel poverty and health: a guide for primary care organizations and public health and primary care professionals. London, National Heart Forum/Faculty of Public Health

Royal College of Midwives (RCM) (1997) Domestic abuse in pregnancy. Position Paper No. 19. London, RCM

Shaw M, Dorling D, Gordon D, Davey Smith G (1999) The widening gap: health inequalities and policy in Britain. Bristol, Policy Press

Shibuya K, Hashimoto H, Yano E (2002) Individual income, income distribution, and self rated health in Japan: cross sectional analysis of nationally representative sample. British Medical Journal 324: 16

Sims L (2001) Neighbourhood Watch: findings from the 2000 British crime survey findings 150. London, Home Office

Social Exclusion Unit (2000) A new commitment to neighbourhood renewal. London, Cabinet Office

Steptoe A, Perkins-Porras L, McKay C, Rink E, Hilton S, Cappuccio F P (2003) Behavioural counselling to increase consumption of fruit and vegetables in low income adults: randomized trial. British Medical Journal 326: 855

Sturm R, Gresenz C R (2002) Income inequality and family income and their relationships to chronic medical conditions and mental health disorders. British Medical Journal 324: 20

Sutherland H, Sefton T, Piachaud D (2003) Poverty in Britain: the impact of government policy since 1997. York, Joseph Rowntree Foundation

Thomson H, Petticrew M, Morrison D (2001) Health effects of housing improvement: systematic review of intervention studies. British Medical Journal 323: 187–190

Townsend P (1979) Poverty in the UK. Harmondsworth, Penguin

Townsend P, Davidson N, Whitehead M (1988) Inequalities in health: the Black report and the health divide. Harmondsworth, Penguin

Tyler P, Rhodes J, Brennan A (1998) Discussion paper 91: the distribution of SRB challenge fund expenditure in relation to local areas needs in England. Cambridge, Department of Land Economy, University of Cambridge

Watterson A (2003) Occupational health. In: Watterson A (ed) Public health in practice. Basingstoke, Palgrave/Macmillan

Webster J, Chandler J, Battistutta D (1996) Pregnancy outcomes and health care use: effects of abuse. American Journal of Obstetrics and Gynecology 174: 760–766

Welsh B C, Farrington D P (2002) Crime prevention effects of closed circuit television: a systematic review. Home Office Research Study 252, Home Office Research Development and Statistics Directorate, homeoffice.gov.uk accessed 29/9/03

World Health Organization (WHO) (1997) Violence against women: a priority health issue. Geneva, Women's Health and Development, Family and Reproductive Health, WHO

10 The major causes of ill health

OVERVIEW

Over the last century there has been a big shift in the burden of disease – from the infectious diseases of the nineteenth and early twentieth centuries to chronic diseases in the twentieth century and now. Chronic diseases, such as coronary heart disease (CHD) and cancer are also strongly related to lifestyle factors such as smoking, poor diet, physical inactivity and alcohol consumption. Changes over time in the burden of disease have shifted the emphasis of public health from health protection measures to tackle infectious diseases, towards health promotion policy targeting individual behaviour and lifestyle risk factors, as well as the wider determinants of health, such as poverty and education. Health protection is nevertheless still an important strategy in the context of new, emerging and resurgent infectious diseases (such as HIV, Ebola virus, vCJD and tuberculosis), and with possible threats to health post-September 11th. New diagnostic technologies, including those based on genetics, could also play a role in improving population health. This chapter reviews two key strategies in disease prevention – immunization and screening – and goes on to discuss approaches to some of the major causes of ill health in the twenty-first century – coronary heart disease, cancers, accidents, mental illness and HIV.

Key Points

- Disease and national health strategy
- Approaches to disease prevention
  - Immunization
  - Screening
- Tackling the major causes of ill health
  - Cardiovascular disease
  - Cancers
  - Accidents
  - Mental illness
  - HIV

INTRODUCTION

Most international health strategies seek to secure improvements in health by increasing life expectancy and reducing premature death (adding years to life) and increasing the quality of life and minimizing illness (adding life to years). In England this is achieved by focusing on key health areas that:

- are a major cause of premature death or avoidable ill health
- are responsive to effective intervention
- are amenable to measurement and monitoring.

Saving Lives: Our Healthier Nation (DoH 1999a) identifies cancers, coronary heart disease and stroke, accidents and mental health as the priority areas. The focus of the strategy is on the prevention of specific diseases rather than the promotion of health in the community as a whole or improvements in the health of specific groups. Although other national strategies focus on risk factors that cause ill health such as smoking, alcohol and diet (e.g. Scottish Office 1998) the focus of the English strategy is on tackling the major killers.

This reflects the medical focus on individual or population health at the biological level rather than environmental or socio-economic issues.

The two most common causes of death in the UK are coronary heart disease (CHD) and cancers. Tackling these major causes of ill health is often driven by a medical model which focuses on early diagnosis and treatment of disease or its precursors such as hypertension or diabetes. The National Service Framework for Diabetes, for example, focuses on the identification of people with diabetes; clinical care; managing diabetic emergencies; the care of people with diabetes in hospital; diabetes and pregnancy and the detection and management of long-term complications. However, prevention of diseases requires addressing the risk factors which are common to many diseases:

- reducing smoking prevalence
- improving diet and nutrition
- increasing physical activity
- reducing overweight and obesity.

Chapter 11 discusses how these lifestyle changes are being addressed through health promotion interventions.

The most common way of assessing health improvement is through a reduction in mortality and morbidity. Practitioners may thus find it hard to move outside of this disease-focused framework and think about how they can tackle the major causes of health within a salutogenic approach. For example, the objective for the priority area of mental health is expressed as the promotion of health, but the setting of targets for achievement led to its expression as disease focused: 'To reduce the death rate from suicide and undetermined injury by at least a fifth by 2010' (DoH 1999a).

Disease prevention is only one strand of public health practice. The key purposes of public health identified in the standards for specialist public health practice are:

- to improve health and well-being in the population
- to prevent disease and minimize its consequences
- to prolong valued life
- to reduce inequalities in health.

One of the key areas of competence is the surveillance and assessment of the population's health and well-being. This chapter explores two different approaches to disease prevention: screening and immunization.

APPROACHES TO DISEASE PREVENTION

The central question in disease prevention is whether to adopt:

- the population approach in which the aim is to lower the average level of risk in the population
- the high-risk approach in which people at particular risk are identified and offered advice and treatment.

Because most conditions follow a roughly normal distribution in the population as a whole, there are many more people with a risk factor or condition in the main body of the population. The prevention paradox (Rose 1993) suggests that many people need to take protective action in order to prevent illness in a few. There would therefore be more improvement in population health if everyone reduces their risk (e.g. their cholesterol level) than if the few in the high-risk category reduced their cholesterol level to the mean.

Discussion point	What are the implications of the prevention paradox for health improvement?

This supports the whole population approach rather than a targeted approach, which might initially appear the more logical choice. Rose (1993) suggests that many interventions that aim to improve health have relatively small influences on the health of most people and therefore the purported benefits of population programmes are over-stressed to encourage people to take action. This section examines the concept of screening – the process of actively seeking to identify precursors to disease in those who are presumed to be healthy – as a means of preventing disease. Screening has been a recognized and accepted part of general health care but in recent years the cost-effectiveness, efficacy and acceptability of such mass programmes has been questioned.

Infectious diseases account for one-third of all deaths worldwide. Diarrhoea, measles, tuberculosis and malaria alone account for 10 million deaths every year (WHO 1999). *Getting Ahead of the Curve*, the UK strategy for combating infectious diseases (and other forms of health protection) (DoH 2002a), describes new threats to health:

- the re-emergence of diseases once thought to be conquered (e.g. tuberculosis, polio)
- the emergence of new diseases (e.g. most notably HIV but 2003 saw the emergence of SARS, an outbreak in China that rapidly spread to other countries)
- terrorism.

There are many reasons why infectious diseases have again become a major public health problem prompting the UK government to set up a Health Protection Agency in 2003 to review new and emerging infectious

Example The spread of tuberculosis (TB)	TB is an example of a disease where worsening social conditions enable the spread of infection. The WHO declared TB a global emergency in 1993 and in 1998 it estimated that one-third of the world's population is infected with mycobacterium tuberculosis. The UK saw a steady decline in TB notifications from 50 000 cases annually in the 1940s to about 5000 cases in the 1980s as a consequence of the introduction of BCG immunization and anti-tubercular therapies. Yet TB cases have risen by 73% in London since 1987 and the incidence in some London boroughs exceeds 50 per 100 000, the majority of these cases in people born in countries where the disease is endemic. The spread of HIV infection and emergence of multi-drug-resistance are contributing to the worsening impact of the disease worldwide. Source: British Thoracic Society (2000)

diseases and strengthen surveillance systems. One factor is the indiscriminate use of antibiotics to treat illnesses and to promote growth in animals which has led to increased microbial resistance. Other factors in the spread of such diseases include population movement, poverty and poor social conditions.

Immunization has been one of the major strategies to tackle infectious diseases. In Angola, for example, 10 million children were vaccinated against polio in three days in 2003. Yet the UK also saw the emergence of serious public concerns over the safety of the measles, mumps and rubella (MMR) vaccination programme that saw immunization rates in Lambeth in London drop to 55% in 2003 (www.lambethpct.nhs.uk). This section examines the dilemmas for practitioners posed by immunization and the challenges of assessing and communicating risk to the public.

Screening

The National Screening Committee define screening as:

> a public health service in which members of a defined population, who do not necessarily perceive they are at risk of, or are already affected by a disease or its complications, are asked a question or offered a test, to identify those individuals who are more likely to be helped than harmed by further tests or treatment to reduce the risk of a disease or its complications.

(www.nsc.nhs.uk)

There are several different types of screening in use:

- mass screening of whole population groups, e.g. breast and cervical screening
- selective screening of high-risk groups, e.g. the proposed testing of new arrivals for TB and HIV
- anonymous screening used to detect trends in public health, e.g. diabetic patients in general practice
- opportunistic screening when the opportunity is taken at a general consultation to ask about health-related behaviour
- health screening not linked to a particular disease, but looking at lifestyles in general, e.g. well woman clinics
- genetic screening investigating inheritable factors in order to assist parenting decisions, e.g. sickle cell screening
- routine screening in infancy and childhood.

Discussion point

What screening might take place in a primary care setting? What factors need to be taken into account to determine good practice?

There are particular ethical issues associated with screening and it is not unambiguously a good thing. It may move someone from presuming themselves to be healthy to a state of having an identified disease or condition, with the attendant anxiety and potentially invasive treatment for the patient. Its benefits, therefore, in terms of earlier diagnosis necessitating less radical treatment and reduced morbidity and mortality must outweigh the disadvantages or costs.

Table 10.1 Benefits and disadvantages of screening

Benefits	Disadvantages
Improved prognosis for some detected individuals	Over-treatment of insignificant or minor abnormalities, e.g. lumpectomy
Less radical treatment	Expensive
Reassurance for those with negative results	False reassurance for those with false-negative results
	Anxiety or unnecessary treatment for those with false-positive results
	Problems arising from the screening test itself

Source: Adapted from Chamberlain (1984)

The National Screening Committee has set out a framework for screening that elaborates on the guidelines and principles laid out by the World Health Organization in 1968 (Wilson Jungner 1968):

- The disease should be common and serious.
- The disease should have a recognized latent stage during which early symptoms can be detected.
- There should be a simple, safe, precise and validated screening test.
- The test should be acceptable to the population.
- There should be an effective treatment or intervention for patients identified through early detection, with evidence of early treatment leading to better outcomes than late treatment.
- The screening programme should be effective in reducing mortality or morbidity.
- The benefit from the screening programme should outweigh the physical and psychological harm (caused by the test, diagnostic procedures and treatment).
- The opportunity cost of the screening programme (including testing, diagnosis, treatment, administration, training and quality assurance) should be economically balanced in relation to expenditure on medical care as a whole (i.e. value for money).

Screening programmes may mean that less attention is given to understanding and tackling the causes of the disease. A range of risk factors have been identified as associated with cervical cancer and include smoking, use of oral contraceptives, age of first sexual intercourse, number of sexual partners (of women and their partners), lowered immune response and a range of viruses (especially Human Papillomavirus). An alternative to screening would be to focus on primary prevention such as increasing the use of barrier methods of contraception.

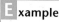xample

Screening for
prostate cancer

Prostate cancer is the second leading cause of cancer deaths in men. Each year 17 000 cases are diagnosed and there are over 9000 deaths (ONS 1999). Yet screening for prostate cancer is controversial. By the age of 80, approximately 50% of men will have some form of prostate cancer but more men will die with the disease than of it. Screening for prostate cancer involves the examination of asymptomatic men by blood test for prostate specific antigen (PSA). This may be followed by a digital rectal examination to detect enlargement or change in the prostate gland. Those that have the disease may be offered prostatectomy or radiotherapy and those with advanced disease may have hormone manipulation therapy to slow or shrink the tumour. These interventions carry risks of increased pain and varying levels of incontinence or impotence. An increased level of testing may lead to a dilemma of whether to treat any cancer aggressively or to adopt a more conservative approach of 'wait and see'. Screening for prostate cancer does not therefore currently satisfy the basic criteria for screening – that testing will improve the prognosis of those with the disease, improve quality of life and that there is an effective treatment available.

Because the accepted treatments may lead to impotence or urinary dysfunction and may not alter the progress of the disease, in 2001 the Department of Health set up a large randomized controlled trial to measure the effects of different treatment options on survival, disease progression and physical and psychological health. It will also provide information about the reliability of the PSA test. Current policy (DoH 2000c) states that any man considering a PSA test will be given detailed information to enable him to make an informed choice about whether to proceed with a test or not. Donovan et al (2001) cite several studies that show that decision aids such as videos result in higher levels of knowledge but have varying effects on the decisions themselves. They claim that at least 20 minutes is needed to provide accurate and understandable information. They also raise the problem of communicating risk to the public arguing that 'strong statements' are needed to explain the uncertainties of the benefits of early detection and treatment of localized prostate cancer.

Sources: www.prostatecancercharity.org.uk, www.menshealthforum.org.uk

Screening is a popular service and there is a constant demand for more screening from patients, pressure groups, the media and clinicians. Yet it is only worthwhile when there is an effective intervention or treatment that is more effective if delivered early on in the development of a disease condition. The national screening programmes for breast and cervical cancer highlight several issues about successful screening programmes in relation to these key principles outlined above. The first of these is whether there is evidence that it reduces mortality. Breast cancer is the largest cause of death in women aged under 65 and accounts for around 11 000 deaths each year (DoH 1999a). Cervical cancer occurs in 4000 women each year and over 1500 die from it, the majority of whom have never had a smear test (Austoker 1994). A number of trials were established to assess the effectiveness of a breast screening programme. The Forrest report in 1986 concluded that there was a case for mammography screening for women aged 50–64 (extended to 70 under the NHS Cancer Plan in 2004) and the programme started in 1988, centrally funded and with national quality assurance mechanisms. The cervical screening programme was established in 1964 but was not implemented consistently until the setting up of the computerized call/recall system for all women aged 20–64 (20–60 in

Scotland) in 1987. However, the relative contribution of both these programmes to any reduction in mortality is constantly questioned. The death rate from breast cancer has fallen from around 50 per 100 000 in 1990 to 44.2 per 100 000 in 1998. Some studies attribute this to the screening programme but as national coverage was not achieved until 1993 it is likely that the fall is due to improved treatment (see Baggott (2000) for an overview of radical critiques of the screening programmes).

Another criticism of national screening programmes is their quality. Media publicity about failings in the quality of the interpretation and reporting of smears at some laboratories (most notably Kent and Canterbury NHS Trust in 1990–1995 where the Trust eventually admitted liability for three deaths where high grade abnormalities had not been detected) has led to some women being recalled for further tests or unnecessary treatment and has damaged the credibility of the process. Concerns have also been expressed about breast cancer services particularly in the accurate reporting of results.

A key principle of screening is that the costs of testing, diagnosis and treatment should be balanced in relation to expenditure on care as a whole. The breast cancer screening programme was estimated to cost £8638 per life saved when it was set up (Clarke & Fraser 1991). Professor Michael Baum, a key figure in the setting up of the breast screening programme, has now called for it to be scrapped arguing that far more attention should be given to more effective treatment for those showing symptoms (Baum 1999).

Particular emphasis is placed on achieving high uptake rates of cervical smear tests through general practices that receive an incentive payment for achieving more than 80% of their eligible female population. The Calnan-Hine report (1995) in its review of cancer services recommended greater specialization in treatment units and that primary care teams should focus on better referral systems. Emphasis has been placed in the breast screening programme on systems that reduce the length of time that a woman has to wait for further tests or treatment (all urgent GP referrals should be seen within 14 days).

Discussion point

What health promotion interventions might improve the take-up of cervical screening?

- Targeting those never screened through careful checking of patient records and the Prior Notification List.
- Improving acceptability of the procedure through better training and health education information.
- More sensitivity to social and cultural factors.
- Restoring confidence in the service through improvements in laboratory service and liaison.

Another principle of screening is that the test should be socially and ethically acceptable and benefits should outweigh any physical or psychological harm that might arise from testing. Studies have however consistently shown that women do not like the smear test or mammography, finding them intrusive and painful. A study of the reasons given for non-attendance at a smear test included the following:

- unavailable – holidays, too busy, ill
- invulnerability – 'it won't happen to me'
- inconvenience of time or venue
- embarrassment or anxiety about the procedure
- 'forgot' (Howson 1999, Orbell & Sheeran 1993).

It is apparent that achieving good coverage of a national screening programme depends on understanding the psychological factors that may influence attendance and ensuring the accessibility and acceptability of the programme itself. Certain groups – working class women, lesbians and ethnic minorities – are much less likely to attend either mammography or for a smear test.

Immunization

Immunization has been a key strategy in the decline of infectious diseases over the last 100 years and one objective of the Alma Ata declaration (WHO 1978) was to immunize the populations of the world against the majority of infectious diseases. Vaccination works by introducing a small amount of the organism to stimulate the body's immune system to produce antibodies against that disease, resulting in immunity. The aim is to protect the individual against serious disease and to protect the community as a whole (herd immunity) – when members of a community who are not immune to a disease are still protected from it provided sufficient numbers of people in that community are immune. Achieving a high degree of herd immunity (e.g. for measles, 90% of the population needs to be immunized, see www.immunisation.nhs.uk) means that unprotected individuals are less likely to encounter the disease, and therefore both immunized and unimmunized individuals are protected.

The success of vaccination programmes against disease such as smallpox (declared eradicated by WHO) has meant that the introduction of other vaccinations such as influenza or meningitis has been less questioned. However, vaccines have been blamed for adverse health effects. For example, the whooping cough vaccine was linked to brain damage and in the late 1990s a major controversy arose in the UK over the measles, mumps and rubella (MMR) vaccine and a supposed link to autism and Crohn's disease. Public confidence in vaccine safety dropped and MMR uptake fell to 55% in some parts of London (see www.hpa.org.uk).

This concern led to the highlighting of major ethical concerns about immunization programmes. In June 2003 a High Court judge ruled that two girls aged 4 and 10 should be given the MMR vaccination according to their father's wishes and overruling their mother's objections. The judge's decision was not a move to compulsory vaccination but made in the interests of the children, where the separated parents could not agree.

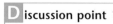

Discussion point

Should the UK introduce compulsory vaccination?

Refusing polio vaccination is illegal in Belgium. Vaccination is a condition of school entry in USA. In this way, individual freedom is curtailed to safeguard population health and all are exposed to the same risks and contribute to the herd immunity. Of course, the counter argument is that whilst there are reasonable grounds for doubt about vaccine safety, individuals should have the right to make their own competent and informed judgement. The challenge for practitioners is how they can enable parents to make informed decisions. The linking of doctor's payments to the number of children immunized may lead to a lack of trust by parents that any advice offered is disinterested.

There are many reasons in addition to current concerns about vaccine safety that explain why individuals may not be vaccinated and these are common to a range of diseases:

- low levels of knowledge about the disease, e.g. 17% of men who have sex with men do not know that hepatitis means inflammation of the liver and 25% do not know of the existence of a vaccine (Hickson et al 1999)
- low levels of perceived susceptibility
- lack of information about the vaccination process.

Different approaches have been taken to facilitate vaccination uptake including:

- social marketing campaigns promoting vaccination
- health care environments that enable disclosure and full discussion of risk assessment
- the use of peer educators.

Practitioners may find it challenging to negotiate the tension between meeting imposed targets and addressing clients' worries which may have been fuelled by negative media coverage. Arguments about the need to achieve a certain level of herd immunity are unlikely to persuade individual parents.

THE PREVENTION OF CORONARY HEART DISEASE AND STROKE

Discussion point

How should practitioners communicate risk when discussing immunizations?

Box 10.1 The scale of coronary heart disease

- The death rate from CHD continues to fall significantly (by 39% for men aged 35–74 between 1988 and 1998) but not as fast as in some countries (it fell by 49% in Denmark and 45% in Norway and Austria), and among developed countries only Finland and Ireland have higher death rates from CHD than the UK.
- There are over one million prescriptions of cholesterol lowering drugs – statins – dispensed in England every month and these now cost the NHS more than any other class of drug with over £440 million spent in 2001 (an increase of £113 million since 2000).
- Around 40% of men and women have raised blood pressure.
- Of the major risk factors for CHD, smoking levels remain static in the UK – 29% of men and 25% of women still smoke. Only 13% of men and 15% of women eat the recommended 5 portions of fruit and vegetables a day. Only just over a third (37%) of men and a quarter of women (25%) take the recommended 30 minutes of exercise five times a week. Obesity rates in men have tripled since the mid 1980s – with men now as likely to be obese as women. In the last ten years, the number of women drinking more than the weekly recommended levels of alcohol has risen by over 50% but remained stable in men.

Source: British Heart Foundation (www.bhf.org.uk/professionals)

Cardiovascular diseases, including coronary heart disease or ischaemic heart disease and cerebrovascular disease (stroke) and its precursors hypertension (high blood pressure) and angina, are common in the general population. In the Health Survey for England, in 1998 (Primatesta 1999) nearly 28% of the population reported a cardiovascular condition. Coronary heart disease (CHD) accounted for 110 000 deaths in England in 1998 including more than 41 000 deaths in people under 75 (DoH 2000a). *Saving Lives: Our Healthier Nation* (DoH 1999a) set a target to reduce the death rate from CHD, stroke and related conditions by 40% in those under 75 by 2010.

CHD is the most common cause of premature death in the UK. It is often thought of as a disease of affluence – the result of a diet high in fat, excessive alcohol and executive stress. In fact CHD like most other diseases is most common in deprived communities, death rates from CHD among unskilled men are three times higher than among professional men (Acheson 1998).

The National Service Framework (NSF) (DoH 2000a) identifies three levels of prevention:

- reducing heart disease in the population as a whole through reduction in the prevalence of risk factors
- prevention of CHD in high risk patients in primary care
- secondary prevention to reduce the risk of subsequent cardiac problems in patients admitted to hospital with CHD.

Whilst there is a recognition of the broader determinants of CHD, most interventions are underpinned by an individual behaviour change model of health promotion. There is an implicit assumption that it is lifestyle changes that will bring about a reduction in CHD and the NSF CHD (DoH 2000a) focuses specifically on smoking, physical activity and diet as modifiable risk factors. The incidence of CHD is, for example, highest in obese men and women, especially in those under 50 years old, yet little is done to control what the International Obesity Task Force call an 'obsogenic' environment.

As we have seen earlier, primary prevention can be developed in two ways: by using a whole population approach or through selective targeting of individuals deemed to be at higher risk. Large scale studies in the mid 1990s looked at the effectiveness of routine screening and lifestyle advice in primary care consultations by practice nurses (British Family Heart Study, Wood et al (1994), and OXCHECK study) and concluded such preventative checks were of little benefit. The NSF CHD requires that all practices have a systematic approach of identifying those at high risk using an appropriate protocol that would include smoking status, physical activity, body mass index, blood pressure, serum cholesterol and diabetes/plasma glucose. Those with high risk according to such indicators would then be offered tailored advice on how to reduce their risks.

In Chapter 12 we discuss the targeting of population groups for health promotion interventions and how this may mean a focus on lifestyle

---

D iscussion point

What are the main difficulties in taking a risk factor approach to the prevention of CHD?

E **xample**

Targeting South
Asians for CHD
prevention

It is a public health conundrum why the death rate from heart disease amongst
South Asian men is 38% higher, and amongst women 43% higher, than for the
general population. South Asians are a heterogeneous group yet most studies of
CHD treat Bangladeshis, Indians and Pakistanis as a single group. Indians probably have less CHD than Bangladeshis and Pakistanis. The risk factors for CHD
are common in South Asians:

- South Asian men smoke more than the general population. 42% of
  Bangladeshi men are smokers (compared to 29% in the general population).
  One fifth of Bangladeshi men and a quarter of women use chewing tobacco.
- Bangladeshi and Pakistani communities eat the least fruit and vegetables of
  all ethnic groups. Only 15% of Bangladeshi men and 16% of women consume fruit six or more times a week. Only 7% of Pakistani men and 11% of
  women eat vegetables on six or more days a week.
- South Asian men and women are less likely to participate in physical activity
  than the general population. Only 18% of Bangladeshi men and 7% of
  Bangladeshi women meet the current recommended physical activity levels
  (30 minutes of brisk walking, cycling or swimming at least five times each
  week).
- The prevalence of diagnosed diabetes is up to five times that of the general
  population in Pakistani and Bangladeshi men and women (diabetes
  increases the likelihood of developing CHD by around three times).

Source: British Heart Foundation (www.bhf.org.uk/professionals)

factors to the exclusion of basic structural factors such as education and
income. Chapter 9 discusses how successful health promotion means
tackling the broader determinants of health, and Chapter 11 examines
approaches to changing lifestyles and behaviour and notes that lifestyle
changes depend on more than information provision alone.

Whilst individually oriented programmes can help people choose
healthier lifestyles, a more effective approach is to introduce community
or society wide interventions, including health promoting policies, that
change the social determinants of health.

CANCER

Box 10.2 The scale of
cancers in England

- There are 200 000 new cases of cancer each year.
- Each year 18 000 men and 10 000 women die of lung cancer,
  approximately 25% of all cancer deaths.
- Each year 11 000 women die of breast cancer, approximately 30% of all
  cancer deaths. Survival rates are lower than the United States and lower
  than average for the European Union.
- Each year 14 000 people die of colorectal cancer.
- Death rates from some cancers are improving – the death rate from
  testicular cancer has fallen by 75% in the last 20 years.

Source: DoH (1999a)

The increase in the incidence of cancers has been thought to be the product of extended lifespans achieved as a result of the decline in infectious diseases. This is only partly true. While the incidence of cancers increases with age, most are associated with poverty, disadvantage and deprivation. For example, unskilled workers are twice as likely to die from cancer as professionals. In part, this reflects a higher incidence of risk factors such as smoking (linked to one-third of cancer deaths) and low consumption of fruit and vegetables (linked to one-quarter of cancer deaths). Survival rates are also lower in deprived areas, in part reflecting difficulties in gaining access to services and poorer service provision in such areas (DoH 1999a).

Cancer, despite being dreaded, is now also seen as a preventable disease in many cases. The NHS Cancer Plan (DoH 2000b), for example, has a chapter on improving prevention. This focuses on primary prevention (health education and support for behaviour changes particularly in relation to smoking and fruit and vegetable consumption) and secondary prevention (early detection and treatment of pre-cancerous cell changes through the national breast and cervical screening programmes and the possible development of programmes for colorectal, prostate and ovarian cancers). Environmental pollution, exposure to toxic materials and changes in the quality of food have all been linked to cancer but receive little attention in cancer prevention interventions.

Skin cancer is an example of a cancer whose incidence has risen steadily. Intense exposure to sunlight, especially in childhood, is the main cause of deaths. Wealthy lifestyles, with holidays abroad, mean that affluent people are more likely to be at risk, and skin cancer is one of the few cancers that shows rising incidence with rising socio-economic status. However, cheaper holidays overseas, and greater likelihood of outdoors work, mean that lower income groups, who tend to be less knowledgeable about the risks of skin cancer, are also at risk. Climate change and ozone depletion are likely to play an increasing role in the incidence of skin cancer, due to the time lag of 10 to 30 years in the development of the condition.

Figure 10.1
Improvements in cancer mortality from specific interventions
Source: Adapted from DoH (2001a) NHS Plan. Technical supplement on target setting for health improvement. Reproduced by permission of Prof. Nick Day, Institute of Public Health, Cambridge

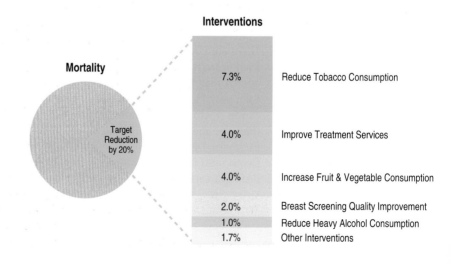

Discussion point

What elements would you include in a skin cancer prevention programme?

Tackling skin cancer illustrates the main approaches to cancer prevention:

- raising awareness
- environmental measures
- early detection.

In England the 'Sun Know How' programme, based on the Australian Sunsmart campaign in the State of Victoria, ran from 1994–2000. Australia has now recorded a downturn in melanoma mortality rates (see www.aihw.gov.au). Raising awareness has been largely achieved through mass media programmes and cues to sun protection such as routinely including UV forecasts in weather reports. Three key actions to halt the increased rates of skin cancer are:

- To increase the number of people who are aware of their own skin cancer risk factors.
- To persuade everyone, and especially people at high risk, to avoid excessive exposure to the sun and artificial sun lamps through the adoption of appropriate sun protection and sun safe behaviour (the 'Slip Slap Slop' campaign slogan referred to slipping on shirts, slapping on hats, and slopping on sun protection cream).
- To alter people's attitude to a tanned appearance.

The challenge for health promoters is that the message to reduce exposure to sunlight is at odds with the lay epidemiology and health beliefs and the behaviour of the public who believe that sunlight is beneficial (Frankel et al 1991). Whilst the focus of skin cancer prevention is on health education, attention has also been paid to environmental measures and enhancing access to shade is an important aspect of sun safe policies, especially in schools. Unlike other health issues, such as tobacco and alcohol, where there are strong industries with anti-health interests, the associated vested interests of cosmetic and sunscreen manufacturers are keen to sign up to skin cancer prevention programmes and promote reinforcing messages.

Discussion point

The following have been identified as signs of malignant melanoma:

- a mole with three or more shades of brown or black
- an existing mole getting bigger or developing an irregular outline
- a new mole growing quickly
- a mole that becomes inflamed or develops a reddish edge or that starts bleeding, oozing or crusting or starts to itch or becomes painful.

What problems might be associated with an effective skin cancer awareness campaign?

Skin cancer screening illustrates many of the problems common to all screening programmes (see pp. 206–210). Checklists of indicators lack specificity and do not exclude benign lesions or lesions that may not have progressed to invasive cancer if left alone. Screening always attracts those individuals who are more health conscious and least at risk.

Nevertheless screening programmes for skin cancer typically lead to earlier diagnosis and an increased percentage of skin tumours detected (HDA 2002).

Cancer is a condition that has attracted a great deal of scientific research. Cancer results from the interaction of many different variables, including genetic, behavioural and environmental factors. Yet cancer prevention programmes are skewed towards those that target individuals, and seek to increase knowledge, change behaviour and increase the uptake of screening services. As we have seen in this section, such an approach has limitations, and the potential of broader-based interventions that tackle some of the environmental factors linked to cancer is now being recognized and developed.

ACCIDENTS

Box 10.3 The scale of accidents in England

- In England 10 000 deaths each year are due to an accident.
- Accidental injury is the most common cause of death among children and young people in England, Europe and America.
- Across the whole population in 1997, 3559 people were killed, 42 967 were seriously injured and 280 978 were slightly injured in road traffic accidents.
- Each year in England nearly 180 children die and almost 4800 are injured as pedestrians or cyclists. England has one of the worst records in Europe for child pedestrian deaths.
- One third of all accidents to adults occur in the home. About half of all deaths among children under 5 happen in the home;

Source: DoH (1999a)

Discussion point

The basis of the national strategy on accidents is that they are predictable and therefore preventable. Do you agree?

Discussion point

What factors would you address in a campaign to reduce accidents in the home? What strategies would you use?

Risk has become the critical, determining concept in constructing strategies aimed at reducing the major causes of mortality, including accidental injury. Epidemiological research shows that certain factors are associated with an increased risk of accidental injury, so preventive activity addresses itself to removing or controlling those risk factors (e.g. traffic speed, see p. 197 in Ch. 9). At a population level, planned interventions to remove or control risk factors can successfully reduce rates of accidental injury. However, risk factor analysis can never tell us where and when or whom a particular accident will strike, because risk relates to people's perceptions and behaviours as well as to environmental factors. The complex interplay between people's behaviour and the external environment defies accurate prediction. As a unique event, an accident remains unpredictable (Green 1995) and, by implication, unavoidable.

Over the last 30 years, England has seen an overall downward trend in accidental deaths which can probably be attributed to successful preventive measures and to advances in emergency medical care in hospitals and at the scene of accidents.

Conventionally, accident prevention strategies are categorized as education, engineering or enforcement:

- **Education** involves raising awareness of hazards and how to avoid them. Examples include Junior Citizen schemes, Traffic Clubs and mass media campaigns as well as more traditional methods of imparting advice and information, such as leaflets, posters and safety counselling, e.g. community nurses' safety advice and education.
- **Engineering** refers to technical measures to increase the safety of the environment or product re-design. For example, the provision of cycle paths and pedestrian crossings, child-resistant packaging of medicines, smoke alarms in social housing, the use of fireguards and air-bags in cars.
- **Enforcement** is the use of legislation, regulations and standards to reduce accidents or control injury. For example, the compulsory wearing of seat-belts or motorcycle helmets, compliance with building regulations, product-testing for conformity with safety standards, e.g. fire-resistant furniture coverings.

The common theme to emerge from reviews of effective interventions is that engineering and enforcement can be effective, but more evidence is needed about the effectiveness of educational interventions (Towner et al 2001).

Children from lower socio-economic groups are more exposed to hazardous environments than children from higher socio-economic groups. For example, a key determinant of injuries to child pedestrians is the number of roads they cross and children of families in the lowest quarter of income cross 50% more roads than those of families in the highest quarter. Whilst accident prevention interventions may seek to modify environments, very few directly target social deprivation (Dowswell & Towner 2002).

There are a range of approaches to reduce inequalities and address the social determinants of health (see Chapter 9). In Table 10.2, Dowswell & Towner (2002) show how these may be employed to prevent injuries in house fires. Interventions that focus on environments tend to adopt a

Discussion point

How do you account for the pronounced inverse relationship between the accident mortality rate in childhood and social class? What health promotion interventions might be effective in reducing childhood accidents?

Table 10.2 The prevention of injuries in house fires
Source: Dowswell T & Towner E (2002) Social deprivation and the prevention of unintentional injury in childhood: a systematic review. Reproduced by permission of the authors and Oxford University Press

Strengthening individuals	Parent education on home hazards (knowledge/behaviour), child education on home hazards (knowledge/behaviour), education on developing escape plans (knowledge/behaviour), parent education on smoking (knowledge/behaviour), parent education on smoke alarms (knowledge/behaviour), installation and maintenance of smoke alarms (environmental change)
Strengthening neighbourhoods	Community-wide smoke alarm giveaway (environmental change), community-wide home inspections (environmental change)
Improving access to services	Developing professional knowledge/skills (knowledge/behaviour), strategies to improve the reach of health promotion activities targeting health promotion at those most at risk
Broad economic and cultural	Safe home design (environment/legislation), safe furniture design (environment/legislation), regulations on smoke alarms in all new/rented/other properties (environment/legislation)

universal approach, and may even end up reinforcing inequalities by making safe environments even safer. The other main approach, education and advice, implicitly views accident prevention as a matter of personal responsibility. Thus these types of interventions focus on pedestrian skills training, traffic clubs and cycling proficiency training.

The World Health Organization's *Targets for Health for All* challenged member states to use legislative, administrative and economic mechanisms to tackle a wide range of health issues, including accidents (WHO 1985). The *Ottawa Charter for Health Promotion* (WHO 1986) further reinforced the idea that health cannot be understood in isolation from social conditions and urged action to ensure safe products, public services and environments. Traffic calming schemes, remedial highway engineering, child-resistant packaging of drugs, and the compulsory use of seat-belts in cars and of helmets on motorcycles have all proved effective in reducing accidental death or injury (Towner et al 2001).

Most practitioners tend to see policy, legislative and enforcement approaches as remote from their everyday practice. There are exceptions – for example, environmental health officers have an enforcement role in relation to many aspects of the environment including food and water safety and occupational health and safety. Chapter 4 discusses in greater detail how practitioners can become involved in the lobbying process, and why an understanding of the policy process is vital to their health promoting and health improvement work.

R eflection point

As a practitioner, what role do you think you can have in promoting these kinds of interventions?

E xample

Data linkage of road traffic accidents

Highways departments and the police are concerned to reduce road casualties. Remedial highway engineering can significantly reduce road accidents but it is necessary to identify the sites with the worst records for accidents. Whilst police data record any road accident resulting in hospital admission as serious, hospital in-patient data provide more detail about the injuries sustained and outcome. Partnership working between the NHS and police in sharing information and linking data can provide the necessary detailed information to enable local highways departments to prioritize their work. The shared data can help identify and prioritize engineering work at sites associated with accidents resulting in the most severe injury.

D iscussion point

Why might it be important to understand lay explanations for the causes of accidents?

The popular definition of an accident is of an unpredictable chance event. Yet the incidence of accidents is patterned by socio-economic class, exposure to unsafe environments and hazards in the environment, as well as being linked to individual and group behaviours and attitudes. Successful accident prevention campaigns tend to focus on modifying environments, but winning over public opinion through educational campaigns is vital for building a consensus that allows further environmental modification via legislation, regulation or engineering to take place.

REDUCING MENTAL ILLNESS AND PROMOTING MENTAL HEALTH

There is increasing recognition of the need to address mental health as an integral part of improving overall health and well-being, and to focus on prevention and promotion in mental health (WHO 2002).

Box 10.4 Mental
health problems in
society

- 16% of adults living in private households in UK have a neurotic disorder (or common mental disorder) such as depression, anxiety or phobias (ONS 2000).
- Each year 5000 people take their own lives (DoH 2002b).
- Suicide is the most common cause of death in men under 35.
- Mental health problems account for the loss of 91 million working days each year and half of these are lost due to anxiety or stress conditions (Gray 2000).

See also Mind (2002) www.mind.org.uk/information/factsheets/statistics

Most strategies to promote mental health have in fact focused on mental illness, being concerned with conditions such as anxiety, depression or schizophrenia. Much less consideration has been given to issues relating to well-being such as isolation, loneliness or low self-esteem. The social environment in which individuals and communities live, and which impacts on people's health behaviours, is an important influence on their mental health.

Reflection point

How would you
define mental
health?

Mental health is often narrowly defined as the absence of mental illness, but mental health as a positive concept is complex and broad ranging. Mental health is more than the absence of metal illness or distress. It includes emotional health, mental functioning, self-determination, positive personal relationships and resilience (to manage and cope with the stresses and challenges of life). Given the diversity of concepts of mental health, it is not surprising that definitions of mental health promotion vary widely. Mental health promotion is essentially concerned with:

- how individuals, families, organizations and communities think and feel
- the factors which influence how we think and feel, individually and collectively
- the impact that this has on overall health and well-being (see www.mentality.org.uk or www.nelh.nhs.uk/nsf/mentalhealth/makeithappen).

Current national strategy includes a target to reduce the death rate from suicide and undetermined injury by at least a fifth by 2010 (DoH 1999b). The National Suicide Prevention Strategy (DoH 2002b) sets out the ways in which this might be achieved. In addition, the National Service Framework Standard One states that health and social services should:

- promote mental health for all, working with individuals and communities
- combat discrimination against individuals and groups with mental health problems, and promote their social inclusion (DoH 1999b).

The choice of suicide rates as an indicator of a reduction in mental health problems was widely criticized in the *Health of the Nation* strategy in 1992 but has persisted.

Discussion point

Why might there be criticism of a target to reduce suicide rates as part of a mental health strategy?

Whilst there has been particular concern at the rising trend in suicides amongst young men and in rural communities, the social factors that might explain this trend are largely ignored and suicide is seen as a psychological phenomenon requiring interventions to assist the individual. The *National Suicide Prevention Strategy* (DoH 2002b) focuses on targeting high-risk groups and reducing the opportunities for suicide. It identifies the following interventions:

- identifying mental illness and depression in primary and social care settings (50% of suicides have visited a doctor within a month of suicide and 25% during the week before death)
- assessment and support for those who have previously attempted suicide (people who have attempted suicide are at particular risk of another attempt in the first year)
- reducing access to methods of suicide, e.g. sale of paracetemol in blister packs, providing free helplines and environmental modification at suicide 'hot spots' such as bridges, increasing the use of catalytic convertors in cars.

The majority of mental health problems are managed within primary care and a high percentage of problems presented in primary care are psychosocial. Primary care therefore has a crucial role in promoting the mental well-being of people with mild or moderate levels of distress and managing those with severe or enduring mental health problems. A common response is to introduce training to identify early indicators of depression, but as Rogers et al point out 'despite the common assumption that GPs would be more effective if their psychiatric knowledge were increased and more emotional morbidity identified, from a service users' point of view ordinary relating and practical help may be more important' (1996, p. 42). A UK review of interventions to prevent and reduce depression in later life (HDA 2003) found little evidence of what works – whether primary care screening to ensure early diagnosis, psychosocial interventions, home visiting or crisis lines. Other initiatives such as 'walking for health' or benefit take up schemes (p. 102) may also be successful in tackling some of the wider causes of mental ill health and strengthening mental health within communities.

Discussion point

A target of the National Service Framework for Mental Health (DoH 1999b) is to 'promote mental health for all'. What might be the implications of such a target for mental health strategies?

MacDonald & O'Hara's (1996) model (see Figure 10.2) suggests that mental health for all can be promoted by enhancing those factors above the dotted line and by tackling those factors below it. Psychological protective factors for mental well-being include:

- feeling respected
- feeling valued and supported
- a feeling of hopefulness about the future.

Another important feature is the emphasis on three levels of action beyond the personal level:

1. Micro – the individual
2. Meso – groupings such as the family, workplace, peer groups, community groups and small neighbourhoods

Figure 10.2 The elements of mental health promotion Reprinted from Journal of Counselling and Development 72(2):115–123.©ACA. Reprinted with permission. No further reproduction authorized without written permission of the American Counseling Association

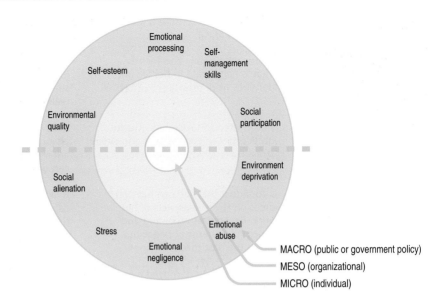

3. Macro – wider, larger systems that govern and shape many aspects of our lives such as government (local and national), large and influential companies and organizations like formal religions.

Interventions to strengthen protective factors thus need to take place at all levels and may include:

- **Micro** – strengthening psychosocial, life and coping skills of individuals through e.g. user empowerment, cognitive behaviour therapy, stress, anxiety or anger management, exercise.
- **Meso** – increasing social support as a buffer against adverse life events and reinforcing ways in which people can cooperate together, e.g. self-help and user-led initiatives, drop in centres for young people, family and parenting groups.
- **Macro** – increasing access to resources and services which protect mental well-being, e.g. employment and training opportunities, making mental health services more appropriate and accessible, anti-discrimination strategies.

Antonovsky (1987) described people's ability to cope positively with stressful events as a 'Sense of Coherence'. Those with a stronger sense of coherence have what Antonovsky terms 'generalized resistance resources', which include individual skills, social support and good social relationships, cultural stability and money. People with a strong sense of coherence share the following characteristics:

- better able to understand and explain the origins of their stress (comprehensibility)
- wish to address the stresses and respond proactively (meaningfulness)
- feel that they are able to respond effectively (manageability).

Table 10.3 The Sense of Coherence
Reprinted from Social Science and Medicine Vol 36, Antonovsky A, The structure and properties of the sense of coherence scale, pp 725–733. Copyright 1993, with permission from Elsevier

Anna (high SOC)	Barbara (low SOC)
– discuss with family and friends what is happening in her life and identifies work pressures as stressful.	– is so involved in coping with her stressful job that she hasn't identified its stress-inducing features. Blames herself for feeling tired and irritable all the time.
– is motivated to tackle her stressful job in order to cope with it and avoid 'stress leakage' into other areas of her life.	– believes there is nothing she can do to change her job; that this is the way things are and she is lucky to have a job. All she can do is try to cope and get on with it.
– is confident that she can have an effect on stressful aspects of her work. Recognizes repeating and unhelpful patterns of behaviour. Has in the past made changes to aspects of her life and circumstances (e.g. moved away from her home town).	– is lacking confidence that anything she can do will affect stress levels but hopes that something will turn up in the future.

The National Institute for Mental Health (2003) found that the level of mental health problems in children and young people is determined by low household income, coming from a lone parent household, being in institutional care and poor school performance. School is therefore a vital setting for promoting the mental health of children. Poor achievement and school performance are risk factors for conduct problems, involvement in crime and substance use (see www.nelh.nhs.uk/nsf/mentalhealth/whatworks/knowhow/schools-evidence.htm). Tilford et al (1997) in their effectiveness review of mental health promotion suggested a focus on generic lifeskills programmes that:

- develop self esteem, communication and problem solving skills
- encourage participation in outdoor pursuits
- develop coping skills and resilience in readiness for stressful situations
- tailor interventions for particular problems, e.g. bereaved children
- develop mentoring schemes that promote access to positive adult relationships

In common with strategies tackling other major causes of mortality and morbidity, the focus of mental health promotion has been to target high-risk groups rather than adopting population-based approaches. Young Black men are more at risk of developing mental health problems than their white counterparts. Socio-economic factors such as unemployment, deprivation and racism may contribute to this. There are also cultural differences in the way in which psychological distress is presented, perceived and interpreted and different cultures may develop different responses for coping with psychological distress.

Example

Mental health pro-
motion with young
Black men

Mellow (Men Emotionally Low Looking for Other Ways) is a project that seeks to address the complex range of factors which influence the mental health of young African and Caribbean men and their experience of mental health services. It aims to:

- raise the awareness of the extent and root causes of mental ill health amongst young African and Caribbean men
- find ways of reaching and engaging the target group so that they can obtain help earlier including school-based interventions
- develop alternative therapeutic models/approaches that will enhance mental well-being
- improve mental health services by developing user-led initiatives and raising awareness of the concerns of young Black men among practitioners and professionals.

Mellow uses music, arts, sport and drama to promote and raise awareness of mental health issues. There is some evidence that art and creative expression can improve the life of communities through the development of self expression and self-esteem as well as encouraging greater connectedness and improved local identity.

Promoting mental health and reducing mental illness is a complex task, not least because of the multiple meanings of mental health. One response, illustrated by national targets, is to target the most extreme manifestations of mental illness, such as suicide. An alternative, diffuse and longer-term strategy is to promote positive mental health and well-being through programmes aimed at enhancing people's self-esteem and personal relationships. Young people are a natural target group for these activities because they have high levels of suicide and self-harm, and also because strengthening their mental heath is a sound health investment for the future. The relationship between the organization of society and the mental health and well-being of the population is interdependent. Strategies to promote mental health and reduce mental illness must therefore take place at all levels: the modification of environments and products, adapting service provision to enhance sensitivity and hence access, community empowerment programmes that build and facilitate social networking and support, and education and skills training for both practitioners and the public. There is also a role for investing in social determinants that promote mental health and well-being, such as employment and good housing.

HIV AND AIDS

The scale of HIV in the UK is minimal compared to infection rates in Africa or Asia. An estimated 28.5 million people are infected with HIV in sub-Saharan Africa and 11 million children are orphaned by AIDS. The *Health of the Nation: a strategy for health in England* (DoH 1992) identified HIV/AIDS and sexual health as one of five priority areas: a decade later the number of cases has increased. Changes in sexual behaviour over the past ten years (decrease in the age of first intercourse, increase in lifetime and number of concurrent partners, and decrease in safer sex practices among

Box 10.5 The scale of HIV/AIDS in the UK

- An estimated 30 000 people are living with HIV in the UK, of whom a third are undiagnosed.
- 14 437 people have been recorded as dying from an AIDS related illness.
- The advent of antiretroviral drugs in 1995 has improved the lifespan of people living with HIV and this together with a growing number of new infections, means the number of people living with HIV is rising.
- The majority of cases of HIV infection and AIDS that have occurred in England have been amongst homosexual men, although new infections acquired through heterosexual sex have outnumbered those acquired through homosexual sex since 1999.
- About 75% of heterosexual infections are acquired abroad, mainly in Africa.
- In 2001, 0.5% of pregnant women delivering in London were infected with HIV. 87% of HIV infected pregnant women were diagnosed before they gave birth.

Source: DoH (2001b), Ellis et al (2003), Fenton (2002)

homosexual men) are likely to further increase infection rates (Second National Study of Sexual Behaviour and Lifestyles, NATSAL II (Erens et al 2001). Other factors including HIV testing, health service utilization and vertical (mother to child) transmission also influence the distribution of the disease. The sexual health and HIV strategy for England (DoH 2001b) includes a target to reduce by 25% the number of newly acquired cases of HIV infection by 2007, a reduction in undiagnosed HIV, and a reduction in HIV-related stigma.

In common with the other major causes of mortality and morbidity discussed in this chapter, HIV prevention work has targeted risk behaviours and target populations deemed at highest risk:

- **Risk behaviours**
  - by increasing the use of condoms
  - recommending a reduction in the number of partners and the number of concurrent partners
  - encouraging intercourse with people of the same HIV sero-status
- **Risk groups**
  - men who have sex with men (MSM)
  - injecting drug users
  - African communities
  - sex workers
  - prisoners.

Chapter 12 discusses how the categorization of groups into 'high risk' or 'low risk' is often an over-simplification and can lead to a focus on already marginalized groups. For example, there is little evidence of current HIV spread among injecting drug users in the UK and yet this is still deemed a high-risk group whereas those acquiring HIV heterosexually from a partner who acquired their infection heterosexually are increasing slowly and formed nearly 10% of new diagnoses of heterosexually acquired infections from 1997–2001 (Fenton 2002).

Interventions to reduce the spread of HIV can be categorized into those which seek to:

- reduce the risk of infection through information and education about safer sex
- reduce the risk of infection by increasing condom use
- reduce the number of sexual partners and increase safer sex practices through voluntary testing and counselling
- empower people through developing self-esteem and assertiveness skills so that they can negotiate safer sex
- strengthen particular communities (e.g. the gay community) so that safer sex norms, values and behaviours become accepted
- improve treatment for STIs which are thought to increase vulnerability to HIV infection.

Addressing risk behaviours may take place at different levels: individual, group, community or sociopolitical. Tackling social determinants of sexual health and ill health includes the use of legislation and policy, e.g. age of consent for gay sex, sex education in schools; and ensuring there is good access to appropriate information and services, e.g. provision and labelling of condoms including those for anal sex, provision of accessible services, advice and treatment for STIs. Community-based interventions have been successful in creating peer norms and support favouring safer sex and providing information or skills. In 1992 Rooney & Scott commented that 'The history of the last decade shows that there is a clear correlation between the widespread adoption of safer sex and the existence of a confident and supportive gay affirmative culture providing grassroots community education' (1992, p. 51). The attachment by gay men to an organised gay community is still one of the most significant factors in maintaining safer sex behaviour. Gay men remain, nevertheless, the group at highest risk of acquiring HIV in the UK (infections in those who have previously tested negative (seroconvertors), the under 25 age group who have only recently become sexually active and STIs in those diagnosed with HIV and the undiagnosed are all increasing).

Many interventions which seek to effect behavioural change at the individual level have been shown to increase knowledge but have had little effect on attitudes and behaviour, partly because perceptions of risk are low, especially amongst heterosexuals. Instead interventions need to address the personal and structural factors that give rise to risk behaviours such as:

- lack of skills in using condoms or negotiating safer sex
- availability of resources such as condoms or sexual health services
- the opinions of peers
- attitudes of society which affect access to services
- poverty, migrant labour and the disempowerment of women in poorer countries.

Reducing the rate of HIV/AIDS has been prioritized as a health target, although there are problems with addressing HIV/AIDS separately from sexual health in general. Chapter 11 includes a section looking at sexual behaviour as both a health risk and a health promoting factor. The narrower focus on HIV/AIDS discussed in this section has been linked to a variety of strategies, including legislative, community development, service development including screening services, and individual education and advice. Although recent rates of HIV infection amongst the gay community are lower than those predicted in the 1990s, demonstrating the effectiveness of community owned programmes, cases of HIV are rising.

CONCLUSION

This chapter has examined the four priority areas identified in the Our Healthier Nation strategy (DoH 1999a) and the additional priority of HIV/AIDS, separately identified in the National Sexual Health and HIV strategy (DoH 2001b). These issues represent a large burden of preventable disease and premature death; evidence exists of effective interventions and it is possible to set targets and monitor progress. Despite the recognition (reflected in Part 3 of this book) that a focus on diseases ignores the prerequisites for health such as adequate income, housing and employment and the needs of marginalized or vulnerable population groups, national health strategy has focused on the major causes of mortality and morbidity.

The sections in this chapter illustrate some of the challenges for practitioners in reaching the targets set for disease reduction. Cardiovascular disease, cancers and HIV/AIDS, for example, are diseases which are known to be linked to certain risk factors, some of which are modifiable by individual behaviour change. The key debate for practitioners is the nature of the identified risk factors and the relative emphasis on lifestyle versus structural changes. Accidents constitute a major cause of mortality but in this case, the notion of risk is debated and contested. Policy interventions have been shown to be most effective in reducing accidental injuries and yet this is an aspect of practice in which practitioners feel least able to effect change (see Ch. 4). By contrast, the key area of mental health poses immediate problems of definition and illustrates the way in which a focus on positive health can be skewed by a disease reduction target.

The sections in this chapter illustrate some of the challenges for practitioners in reaching the targets set for disease reduction. Four main approaches have been discussed:

- environmental modification through legislation and policy
- whole population health screening and immunization
- community development approaches to change risk factors relating to norms, beliefs and practices
- individually focused education, advice and counselling to change individual risk factors.

Health practitioners will probably feel most at ease with the second and fourth of these approaches, and examples have been given of effective strategies adopting these approaches. Lifestyle approaches are discussed further in Chapter 11. Screening and immunization, discussed earlier in this chapter, remain significant although contested strategies in the drive to reduce major diseases. As health service interventions they are subject to the inverse care law, and tend to be adopted most by those groups at least risk.

FURTHER DISCUSSION

- How do the key priority areas in this chapter illustrate the importance of partnership working?
- How appropriate is it to tackle disease reduction in these priority areas through a focus on individual risk factors?
- What can be learned from the examples in this chapter about the strengths and limitations of national screening programmes?
- What are the advantages and disadvantages of medically defined prevention targets?

Recommended reading

- Donaldson L J, Donaldson R J (2003) Essential public health, Oxford, Petroc Press.
- Pencheon D, Guest C, Melzer D, Muir Gray J A (eds) (2001) *Oxford handbook of public health practice*. Oxford, Oxford University Press.
- Detels R, McEwen J, Beaglehole R, Ytanaka H (eds) (2002) *Oxford textbook of public health*, 4th edn. Oxford, Oxford University Press.

These three textbooks examine public health issues and how they can be prevented and controlled as well as how to prioritize health issues, how to identify cost-effective strategies and how to mobilize the community through community involvement. The message of all three texts is that a comprehensive rather than an issue/disease oriented approach is necessary for public health problems.

REFERENCES

Acheson D (1998) Independent inquiry into inequalities in health. London, The Stationery Office

Antonovsky A (1987) Unravelling the mystery of health. San Francisco, Jossey Bass

Antonovsky A (1993) The structure and properties of the sense of coherence scale. Social Science and Medicine 36: 725–733

Antonovsky A (1996) The salutogenic model as a theory to guide health promotion. Health Promotion International 11: 11–18

Austoker J (1994) Screening for cervical cancer. British Medical Journal 309: 1611–1614

Baggott R (2000) Public health: policy and politics. Basingstoke, Macmillan

Baum M (1999) Money may be better spent on asymptomatic women. British Medical Journal 318: 398

British Thoracic Society (2000) Control and prevention of tuberculosis in the United Kingdom: code of practice 2000. Thorax 55: 887–890

Chamberlain J (1984) Which prescriptive screening programmes are worthwhile? Journal of Epidemiology and Community Health 38: 270–277

Clarke P R, Fraser N M (1991) Economic analysis of screening for breast cancer. Edinburgh, Scottish Home and Health Department

Department of Health (DoH) (1992) The health of the nation: a strategy for health in England. London, HMSO

Department of Health (DoH) (1999a) Saving lives: our healthier nation. London, The Stationery Office

Department of Health (DoH) (1999b) The national service framework: mental health. London, The Stationery Office

Department of Health (DoH) (2000a) The national service framework: coronary heart disease. London, The Stationery Office

Department of Health (DoH) (2000b) The NHS cancer plan. London, The Stationery Office

Department of Health (DoH) (2000c) The national prostate cancer plan. London, NHS Executive

Department of Health (DoH) (2001a) NHS Plan. Technical supplement on target setting for health improvement. The Stationery Office

Department of Health (DoH) (2001b) National strategy for sexual health and HIV. London, The Stationery Office

Department of Health (DoH) (2002a) Getting ahead of the curve: a strategy for combating infectious diseases. London, The Stationery Office

Department of Health (DoH) (2002b) National suicide prevention strategy. London, The Stationery Office

Donovan J L, Frankel S J, Neal D E, Handy F C (2001) Screening for prostate cancer in the UK. British Medical Journal 323: 763–764

Dowswell T, Towner E (2002) Social deprivation and the prevention of unintentional injury in childhood: a systematic review. Health Education Research 17(2): 221–237

Ellis S, Barnett-Page E, Morgan A, Taylor L, Walters R, Goodrich J (2003) HIV prevention: a review of reviews assessing the effectiveness of interventions to reduce the risk of sexual transmission. London, Health Development Agency

Erens B, McManus S, Field J, Korovessis C, Johnson A, Fenton K, Wellings K (2001) National Survey of Sexual Attitudes and Lifestyles II. London, National Centre for Social Research

Fenton K (2002) Sexual health in Britain: the changing epidemiology of high-risk sexual behaviours, STIs and HIV. Submission of evidence in support of the Health Select Committee review of GUM/HIV services

Frankel S J, Davison C, Davey Smith G (1991) Lay epidemiology and the rationality of responses to health educators. British Journal of General Practice 41: 428–430

Gray P (2000) Mental health in the workplace: tackling the effects of stress. London, Mental Health Foundation

Green J (1995) Accidents and the risk society: some problems with prevention. In: Bunton R,

Nettleton S, Burrows R (eds) The sociology of health promotion. London, Routledge

Health Development Agency (HDA) (2002) Cancer prevention: a resource to support local action in delivering the NHS cancer plan. London, Health Development Agency

Health Development Agency (HDA) (2003) Preventing and reducing depression in later life: evidence briefing. London, Health Development Agency

Hickson F, Weatherburn P, Reid D, Henderson L, Stephens M (1999) Evidence for change – findings from the National Gay Men's Sex Survey 1998. London, Sigma Research

Howson A (1999) Cervical screening, compliance and moral obligation. Sociology of Health and Illness 21(4): 401–425

MacDonald G, O'Hara K (1996) Ten elements of mental health, its promotion and demotion: implications for practice. Birmingham, Society for Health Education/Promotion Specialists

Mind (2002) Mental health statistics: how common is mental distress? London, Mind www.mind.org.uk/information/factsheets/statistics

National Institute for Mental Health (2003) Inside outside: improving mental health services for Black and minority ethnic communities in England. London, Department of Health

Office for National Statistics (ONS) (1999) 1993 Cancer statistics: registration. London, The Stationery Office

Office for National Statistics (ONS) (2000) Psychiatric morbidity among adults living in private households in GB. London, The Stationery Office

Orbell S, Sheeran P (1993) Health psychology and the uptake of preventive health services – a review of thirty years research on cervical screening. Psychology and Health 8(6): 417–433

Primatesta P (1999) The health survey for England 1998. London, The Stationery Office

Rogers A, Pilgrim D with Latham M (1996) Understanding and promoting mental health. London, Health Education Authority

Rooney M, Scott P (1992) Working where the risks are: health promotion interventions for men who have sex with men. In: Evans B, Sandberg S, Watson S (eds) Working where the risks are: issues in HIV prevention. London, Health Education Authority

Rose G (1993) The strategy of preventive medicine. Oxford, Oxford University Press

Scottish Office (1998) Working together for a healthier Scotland. London, The Stationery Office

Tilford S, Delaney F, Vogels M (1997) Effectiveness of mental health promotion interventions: a review. London, Health Education Authority

Towner E, Dowswell T, Mackreth C, Jarvis S (2001) What works in preventing unintentional injuries in children and young adolescents? An updated systematic review. London, Health Development Agency

Wells J, Barlow J, Stewart-Brown S (2001) A systematic review of universal approaches to mental health promotion in schools. Health Services Research Unit, University of Oxford, Institute of Health Sciences (www.hsru.ac.uk)

West Midlands Public Health Observatory (2002) West Midlands Health Issues: Cancers. Birmingham, WMPHO (www.wmpho.org.uk)

Wilson J M G, Jungner G (1968) Principles and practice of screening for disease. Geneva, WHO

Wood D A, Kinmouth A, Pyke S D M, Thompson SG (1994) Randomized controlled trial evaluating cardiovascular screening and intervention in general practice: principal results of British family heart study. British Medical Journal 308: 313–320

World Health Organization (WHO) (1978) Report on the international conference on primary health care, Alma Ata, 6–12 September. Geneva, WHO

World Health Organization (WHO) (1985) Targets for health for all. Copenhagen, WHO

World Health Organization (WHO) (1986) Ottawa charter for health promotion. Copenhagen, WHO

World Health Organization (WHO) (1999) World health report 1998: life in the 21st century: a vision for all. Geneva, WHO

World Health Organization (WHO) (2002) Prevention and promotion of mental health. Department of Mental Health and Substance Dependence, Geneva, WHO

11 Lifestyles and behaviours

Key Points

- Social construction of risky behaviours and risk perception
- Approaches to changing lifestyles
  - Educational interventions
  - Mass media campaigns
- Smoking
- Diet
- Exercise and physical activity
- Alcohol and drug use
- Sexual health

OVERVIEW

The shift in disease patterns in developed countries, from communicable diseases to chronic diseases, has highlighted the importance of lifestyles and behaviours as potential contributors to disease or health. Behavioural lifestyle choices, such as diet, exercise and the use of recreational drugs, are major factors in determining health status. A single lifestyle behaviour, such as diet, can affect the likelihood of developing a range of conditions including life-threatening illnesses such as cancers of the digestive system, severe chronic conditions such as diabetes and many more minor conditions such as irritable bowel syndrome and dental decay. It has therefore become a common strategy in public health and health promotion to target behaviours. This approach aims to persuade people to change unhealthy behaviours and adopt health promoting behaviours. This chapter explores approaches to behaviour change and their popularity. It then goes on to examine in more depth five key areas where behaviours impact significantly on people's health – diet, exercise, smoking, drugs and alcohol use, and sexual behaviour. The dilemmas of targeting behavioural choices are identified and illustrated.

INTRODUCTION

Certain behaviours have become labelled as 'risky behaviours' associated with negative health outcomes. Such behaviours include smoking, excessive use of alcohol and other recreational drugs, unsafe sex, poor diet (high fat and high sugar diet) and sedentary lifestyles. These have all been the subject of UK national health strategies. Risky behaviours are often linked to a range of illnesses and conditions. For example, smoking is linked to lung cancer, coronary heart disease, chronic obstructive lung disease and asthma. Lifestyle risk behaviours have been associated with most of the common chronic diseases in developed countries. These conditions (e.g. diabetes, coronary heart disease and cancers) represent a significant disease burden and are very costly to manage and treat. The Coronary Heart Disease National Service Framework (NSF) (DoH 2000a) highlighted the importance of tackling smoking, healthy eating, physical activity and overweight and obesity as a means towards reducing the incidence of coronary heart disease. As discussed in Chapter 10, most research into the prevention of risk factors for disease has focused on 'downstream' interventions, that aim to affect the lifestyle and behaviour of individuals, rather than 'upstream' interventions such as policies that seek to influence the broader determinants of health. This has led to greater evidence for individually focused interventions than for social policy interventions. Targeting lifestyles has therefore been viewed as both an effective and an efficient strategy to promote health.

Targeting lifestyles has a long history: 'The way in which people live and the lifestyles they adopt can have profound effects on subsequent health. Health education initiatives should continue to ensure that individuals are able to exercise informed choice when selecting the lifestyles which they adopt' (DoH 1992, p. 11). The lifestyles approach is popular because it is focused on individuals and can therefore be integrated into one-to-one contacts between practitioners and their clients. It also reinforces the popular concept of individual freedom and autonomy in lifestyle choices. However, it has also been criticized for taking behaviours out of their social context and ignoring the structural constraints (such as income) on behavioural choices. The lifestyles approach also assumes that people make rational choices based on weighing up the pros and cons of adopting a specific behaviour, and this too has been criticized for failing to take into account custom, habit, identity and the meaning of behaviours within people's lives. Behavioural change models, such as the Stages of Change model, that assume individual autonomy and choice have been seen as unrealistic. These critiques of the behavioural change approach are discussed in greater detail in Chapter 11 of *Health Promotion: Foundations for Practice* (Naidoo & Wills 2000).

The construction of certain behaviours as risky is, however, problematic. In particular, there is a gap between epidemiological and lay perceptions of risk. Epidemiological risks are scientifically calculated and presented as statistical probabilities. However, people interpret epidemiological risks within their own behavioural landscape, according to their own circumstances and priorities (Lupton 1999). For example, someone may have unsafe sex, and underestimate the risks of so doing, because they want sex to be spontaneous and not negotiated.

Lupton (1995, p. 9) argues that risk has replaced the notion of sin. Taking risks is attributed to lack of will power and moral weakness and as a result people do not seek advice because they fear they will be 'told off'. Research suggests that health risk behaviours should not be perceived as 'wrong' lifestyle choices, but as rational coping strategies adopted in the context of the demands of caring and the constraints of poverty (Graham 1993). People have very different constructions of risk, and people's personal 'landscapes of risk' vary according to their social situation and status. For example, smoking is a high-risk behaviour but its risk may be downplayed and offset against its positive role, for example as a stress management and coping tool, within people's lives. In this way epidemiological risk factors such as smoking or poor diet may be overridden by more immediate risks and more urgent problems. The link between unhealthy lifestyles and poverty has been recognized in official government documents:

The key lifestyle risk factors, shared by coronary heart disease and stroke, are smoking, poor nutrition, obesity, physical inactivity and high blood pressure. Excess alcohol intake is an important additional risk factor for stroke. Many of these risk factors are unevenly spread across society, with poorer people often exposed to the highest risks.

(DoH 1999, p. 74)

Reflection point

Do you engage in any behaviour that might be deemed to carry a risk?
(If yes) How do you justify continuing with these behaviours?

Risk perception is also influenced by role models. 'Candidates' for premature death who in fact lived to a ripe old age (e.g. 'grandad smoked 40 a day and lived to 93'), and 'victims' who lived healthily but died prematurely (e.g. 'my aunt never smoked, ate healthily all her life, and then died of breast cancer aged 48') are referred to as reasons for treating epidemiological risk assessments sceptically (Davison et al 1992). In our first book, *Health Promotion: Foundations for Practice*, the sociopsychological models of behaviour that explain health related decision making are discussed in depth (Naidoo & Wills 2000). Lay perceptions of risk are also affected by social and cultural norms. If for example one's peer group values a risky behaviour, e.g. binge drinking among young women, its risk is likely to be underestimated or offset against other immediate benefits, such as belonging and peer approval. Illegal behaviours are also likely to be assessed as much more risky than legal behaviours, regardless of the evidence. For example, the use of the illegal drug ecstasy is generally viewed as more risky than the use of alcohol, although alcohol represents a much more significant health risk.

APPROACHES TO CHANGING LIFESTYLES

There are three main approaches to changing lifestyles:

- changing individual behaviour through the provision of information or motivational messages
- empowering individuals to make healthy choices
- addressing socio-economic and environmental factors to enable healthier choices to be made.

The potential of policy interventions and their impact on health has already been considered in Chapter 4. Educational approaches focus on enabling voluntary behaviour change that is achieved by providing education, information and advice. This approach prioritizes the ability of people to make their own choices. The persuasive approach seeks to maximize opportunities for achieving behavioural change even if these embody elements of manipulation and persuasion. The use of mass media campaigns is an example of the persuasive approach. Its advocates justify this approach by citing equally persuasive techniques used to get people to adopt unhealthy behaviours (see Ch. 8 for further discussion of social marketing techniques).

Educational interventions

Educational interventions take place in a variety of settings including schools, primary care settings and the voluntary sector. The intervention may be undertaken by a practitioner, a teacher, or members of a peer group. The relationship between knowledge, attitudes and behaviour has been explored in social cognition models. These models suggest that decision making is based on individual assessments of costs and benefits. For a more detailed discussion of behavioural change models, see Chapter 11 in *Health Promotion: Foundations for Practice* (Naidoo & Wills 2000). Interventions may provide specific inputs, such as accurate risk assessment, or an available substitute behaviour. Barriers to the change process, such as having an external locus of control, or lack of self-efficacy, whereby someone does not believe they are capable of initiating and sustaining change, may also be targeted. Maintenance of the desired behaviour change has been less of a focus although there are indications that this deserves more attention. For example, high relapse rates for behavioural changes are common, and sustained change is much more difficult to achieve than attempted change. Prochaska & diClemente's (1984) Stages of Change model includes maintenance and relapse as separate stages, but more work needs to be done on how to successfully achieve maintenance of change.

Educational interventions are valued and popular with practitioners because they:

- empower people, enabling them to make desired changes and increase their control over their health
- involve working directly with people, enabling communication and feedback that in turn can be used to fine-tune the intervention, enhancing its effectiveness.

Educational and behaviour change approaches have been criticized for:

- failing to take sufficient account of the social and environmental context in which behavioural choices are made
- reinforcing health inequalities because educational and motivational messages are more likely to be acted upon by those with the most resources, who already enjoy better health due to their more advantaged circumstances
- being 'victim-blaming' – holding people responsible for their lifestyles when change is very difficult or even impossible to achieve has been viewed as unethical because it blames people for circumstances beyond their control
- assuming a link between knowledge, attitudes and behaviour
- encouraging state intervention and interference in people's private lives.

Practitioners will often need to discuss behavioural lifestyle changes with their patients or clients. This may be in the form of information, advice or a more structured and client-led examination of opportunities for change.

People may reject education or advice because it runs counter to their intuitive understanding, their life experience, or the example of significant others. However, even when a message is understood and accepted, it may still not be acted upon. Being exposed to behavioural

> **Discussion point**
>
> Many practitioners will suggest education as a strategy to improve health. Why are educational interventions so popular?

> **Discussion point**
>
> What factors might enable a client to take more control over their health? What role does information and/or advice play?

R eflection point

Think of a patient or client you regarded as 'difficult' because they resisted or didn't follow your advice. Can you identify why they may have been like this?

D iscussion point

Should practitioners encourage clients to change their lifestyles?

change messages that are accepted but impossible to achieve is likely to lead to loss of self-esteem and feelings of inadequacy. The alternative is to reject or deny such messages.

Another criticism of the lifestyles approach is that it interferes with people's private lives. This argument holds that people freely choose their lifestyles and behaviours, and that unless this impacts negatively on the quality of others' lives, it concerns no one but themselves. This is an example of individualism, a highly valued concept in modern developed countries, which stresses the autonomy and freedom of individual people. The former Conservative Prime Minister Margaret Thatcher once remarked that 'there is no such thing as society, just individuals' and attacked the welfare state as a 'nanny state'. The degree to which individual lifestyles impact on others is hard to determine.

It is arguable whether lifestyles are a matter of choice. In addition to the constraints on choice imposed by the socio-economic context some behaviours, e.g. smoking and excessive alcohol use, are addictive and therefore not freely chosen. This is supported by the 70% of smokers claiming to wish to quit at any one time. People may not have all the relevant facts to hand when making behavioural choices, and access to more information may change their choices. The behaviour of significant others has an impact on lifestyles, and advertising and marketing are also significant factors determining individual behavioural choices. Recognition of the persuasive effect of mass media techniques has led health promoters and public health practitioners to adopt such techniques to try to achieve healthy lifestyle changes (see Ch. 8 for further discussion of this topic).

Mass media interventions

Lifestyle behaviour campaigns often use the mass media to try to get persuasive messages accepted by the target audience. The use of the mass media in health promotion is discussed in detail in Chapter 12 of *Health Promotion: Foundations for Practice* (Naidoo & Wills 2000). Mass media campaigns have become increasingly sophisticated in terms of targeting (see Ch. 8, this volume). Messages are now tailor-made with specific population groups in mind, and are pre-tested to ensure their acceptability. Nevertheless efforts to target may appear tokenistic (e.g. one Black face in a crowd) or scapegoating (e.g. suggesting Black Africans are disproportionately responsible for HIV). Campaigns recognize the complexity of behaviour change and may:

- provide knowledge
- change attitudes or beliefs
- advocate specific behaviour change
- reinforce behaviour changes that have been made.

Long-running campaigns may be planned with different aims at different times (e.g. road safety campaigns may focus on drink-driving, seat-belt use or driving speeds). One problem with the use of mass media interventions is that health promotion and public health budgets for such campaigns are tiny in comparison to the budgets used to promote anti-health products such as junk food. Their effect is correspondingly diluted when compared with the effect of commercial marketing. This has led to calls for legislation and regulation of the marketing of unhealthy products.

Example	There is a mounting campaign to ban the advertising of junk food, much of which is targeted at children and young people. Taking the successful campaign to ban tobacco advertising and promotion as its model, a coalition of nearly 90 organizations (including the National Consumer Council, the Community Practitioners and Health Visitors Association, the National Union of Teachers, the British Dietetic Association and the Women's Institute) have signed up to the Sustain (the alliance for better food and farming) campaign to ban the advertising of junk food to children. In particular, the use of sports personalities who promote junk food, the BBC's franchising of the Tweenies characters to McDonalds, and Cadbury's vouchers for sports equipment campaign have been criticized. Sustain's campaign has been spurred on by concern about the rise of obesity, especially amongst children, noted by the Chief Medical Officer in his 2002 annual report on the state of the nation's health. A parliamentary health committee inquiry into obesity set up in 2003 includes consideration of the effect of advertising and marketing of junk food. Worldwide, the World Health Organization (WHO) has launched a major consultation into diet-related disease. WHO has noted the link between high levels of consumption of high calorie, low-nutrient foods and sugar-sweetened drinks and heavily marketed processed foods and fast-food outlets. A Food Standards Agency (Hastings et al 2003) review of evidence linking food promotion and children's eating behaviour concluded that food promotion does affect children's preferences, purchasing behaviour and consumption. The report found that this effect is independent of other factors and operates at both a brand and category level. The sum effect is to persuade children to eat less healthy foods. It now looks increasingly likely that legislation to ban the advertising and marketing of junk food to children will be passed in the UK, following the example of Sweden where advertising of junk food on children's TV has been banned.
Campaign to ban the advertising of junk food	

Source: Hastings et al (2003),
www.foodstandards.gov.uk/news/pressreleases/foodtochildren accessed 16/12/03

Individually focused educational and persuasive approaches have been used to try to change many behaviours. In addition many other approaches have been used, including legislation and regulation, policy formation and implementation, and community development. The following sections examine a range of strategies addressing smoking, diet, exercise, alcohol and drug use and sexual health. Within each section, the contribution of this behaviour to ill health is first outlined, followed by a discussion of approaches used in practice and evidence as to their effectiveness.

SMOKING

Although the detrimental effects of smoking on health have been known for half a century, smoking remains a common habit that significantly affects the health of the population, both in the UK and worldwide.

Box 11.1 Smoking and health

- Smoking tobacco is the single most important preventable cause of ill health and premature death.
- More than 120 000 people a year in the UK die from smoking.
- A third of all cancer deaths are caused by smoking.
- Smoking is also linked to coronary heart disease, chronic obstructive lung disease and a host of other conditions.
- A lifetime non-smoker is 60% less likely than a current smoker to have coronary heart disease and 30% less likely to suffer a stroke.
- One in two smokers will die prematurely due to their smoking habit.
- Passive smoking, or exposure to the tobacco smoke of others, affects the health of non-smokers including children.
- Children who are passive smokers due to parental or carers' smoking are at increased risk of respiratory disease, asthma, glue ear, sudden infant death syndrome and school absences.
- Each year several hundred passive smokers die from lung cancer.
- Smoking is estimated to cost the NHS £1.7 billion each year.

Sources: Department of Health (1998), Royal College of Physicians (1992)

In 2001, the General Household Survey showed that 27% of adults aged 16 and over (28% of men and 26% of women) were current cigarette smokers (Walker et al 2002). Cigarette smoking was most common among younger age groups (37% of 20–24-year-olds and 34% of those aged 25–34 were current smokers) and least likely amongst those aged 60 and over (17% were current cigarette smokers). The General Household Survey has consistently shown a strong social class gradient in smoking, with cigarette smoking being considerably more prevalent among those in manual groups (33%) than among those in non-manual groups (19% for managerial and professional households). In households on income support, 55% of lone mothers and 70% of two parent households buy cigarettes. Smoking has been identified as one of the greatest causes of the health divide between rich and poor (www.hda-online.org.uk/evidence). Due to its expense, smoking also has a significant financial impact on low-income households, and money spent on cigarettes may lead to shortages in essential items such as food, heating and clothing.

The evidence relating to the harmful health effects of tobacco has been well documented for over half a century, dating back to Doll and Hill's (1950) original work, published in the British Medical Journal in 1950, which demonstrated the link between smoking and lung cancer. The 1963 Report by the Royal College of Physicians, which led to the setting up of the pressure group ASH (Action on Smoking and Health) and the Froggatt Report on passive smoking published in 1988, summarized the available evidence and made the case for stronger controls on smoking in public places and the advertising and promotion of tobacco. The government finally acted on this evidence base and in 1998 published the White Paper *Smoking Kills* (DoH 1998), followed in 2002 by the UK Tobacco Advertising and Promotion Act that banned all tobacco advertising, with international sports sponsorship by tobacco companies to be finally banned by 2005. *Smoking Kills* targeted three groups in particular:

- young people under 16 who smoke
- disadvantaged adults who smoke
- pregnant women who want to stop smoking.

Smoking is a global health issue affecting all countries. The WHO global burden of disease study (Ezzati et al 2002) found that in developed countries tobacco is the leading cause of disability adjusted life years (DALYs), and tobacco remains a significant cause of disability and a major health risk factor in developing countries. WHO has recognized the global impact of tobacco in its Framework Convention on Tobacco Control (WHO 2003). The Framework Convention is a legal instrument based on evidence that is intended to be incorporated in law and implemented in different countries.

Box 11.2 WHO Framework Convention on Tobacco Control (2003)

1. Measures relating to reducing demand for tobacco:
   - price and tax measures
   - protection from exposure to environmental tobacco smoke
   - regulation and disclosure of the contents of tobacco products
   - packaging and labelling
   - education, communication, training and public awareness
   - comprehensive ban and restriction on tobacco advertising, promotion and sponsorship
   - tobacco dependence and cessation measures.
2. Measures relating to reducing the supply of tobacco:
   - elimination of the illicit trade of tobacco products
   - restriction of sales to and by minors
   - support for economically viable alternatives for growers.

Reflection point

Which of the measures in Box 11.2 do you think has most impact on smoking rates?

WHO report that the most cost-effective option in all countries is taxation on tobacco products, followed by comprehensive bans on advertising tobacco. Together, it is calculated that these two measures could reduce the global burden of tobacco by 60%. In countries such as the UK, where these two measures are already in place, additional measures such as education and smoking cessation interventions become cost-effective. A comprehensive approach is the most effective, combining community wide interventions with economic and regulatory measures and educational and clinical approaches targeted at individuals (HDA 2001). Nicotine Replacement Therapy with cessation support is very effective in increasing quit rates (NHS Centre for Reviews and Dissemination 1998):

- Smoking cessation services are now available under the NHS, including counselling, support and access to nicotine replacement therapy (NRT) and buproprion (Zyban) on prescription.
- Around 5% of smokers will quit if they receive opportunistic advice from GPs (HDA 2001).
- Around 120 000 people had successfully quit smoking at the four week stage during April 2001 to March 2002 (www.nice.org.uk).

Most of the recent decline in smoking rates is due to people quitting rather than a reduced number of young people starting to smoke. This suggests that education and interventions targeted at young people have not been very successful (HDA 2001). By the age of 15, just over one in five young people is smoking. Although peer pressure is undoubtedly an influence, parental smoking has also been shown to increase the likelihood of teenagers smoking.

Tobacco use is unique in that its effects are unequivocally negative, both for the immediate user and others exposed to tobacco smoke. Strategies to reduce tobacco use are correspondingly well advanced and multi-pronged, including legislation to ban tobacco advertising and promoting access to nicotine replacement drugs on prescription. The WHO Framework Convention demonstrates the potential for global strategies to change unhealthy behaviours. A range of strategies is necessary because the addictive nature of tobacco means that education and advice alone are insufficient. However the use of complementary strategies at different levels (individual, community, national, global) has been shown to be effective in reducing tobacco use.

DIET

Diet is a crucial factor contributing to health. Diets in Western developed countries have changed rapidly, alongside changes in farming, cooking habits, processing and the availability of prepared and packaged food. Unhealthy diets, characterized as high fat, high sugar and high calorie diets, are linked to the rise in obesity, which itself is implicated in a host of diseases and illnesses including diabetes, coronary heart disease and some cancers. The prevalence of overweight and obesity has increased rapidly over the past two decades in developed countries.

Box 11.3 Obesity in the UK

- Obesity has nearly trebled in the UK since 1980 and is still increasing.
- In 2001 nearly two-thirds of men and over half of women were either overweight or obese (for the same year, 8.5% of six-year-olds and 15% of fifteen-year-olds were obese).
- Obesity is linked to social disadvantage and poverty, with higher rates for overweight and obesity amongst Asian groups, lower social classes, and people living in Wales and Scotland.
- In England in 1998 an estimated £2.6 billion was spent on sickness attributed to obesity. On current trends, this is set to rise to £3.6 billion by 2010.

Sources: Joint Health Surveys Unit (2002), Mulvihill and Quigley (2003)

Substantial evidence shows how poverty affects food choice:

- People in lower socio-economic groups have higher intakes of saturated fats and lower intakes of antioxidants, vitamins and some minerals (DoH 2000b).
- The consumption of fresh fruit and vegetables rises with increasing income. People on benefits eat fewer portions of fruit and vegetables each day and adults and children in the lowest income groups eat up

to 50% less fruit and vegetables than those in the highest income groups (DoH 2003).

D iscussion point

Is the '5-a-day', message to eat five portions of fruit and vegetables a day relevant and realistic for families on a low income?

- People living in the most deprived neighbourhoods are unlikely to have access to a car, and local shops charge almost a quarter more than supermarkets for basic foods including fruit and vegetables (DoH 2003).

For low income families whose budgets only just cover basic food requirements, experimenting with unfamiliar fruits and vegetables in the family diet may not be a feasible option. To make '5-a-day' a viable option for all families, attention needs to be paid to the availability, accessibility and price of fruit and vegetables. Reducing the price of fruit, or ensuring it is available daily in school meals, may be far more effective than educational advice on the nutritional benefits of fruit. The policy context therefore needs to be included in any discussion about lifestyles and behaviours. (For a more detailed discussion of the policy context see Ch. 4). The 5-a-day programme has taken these factors into consideration. Included in the programme is the national school fruit scheme, which aims to offer a free piece of fruit to all 4–6 year olds at nursery and school by 2004 (DoH 2000c). The nutritional standards for school meals introduced in 2001 states that fresh fruit and vegetables should be available each day as part of the school meal. Catering outlets also need to be targeted, as 10% of people's total food intake is now eaten outside the home (Office for National Statistics 2000).

Since the first Committee on the Medical Aspects of Food in 1984, the focus of government interventions on nutrition has been dietary recommendations. However it is difficult to get widespread changes in dietary patterns because diet is determined by a number of different interweaving factors. Figure 11.1 below illustrates this.

A review (HEA 1997) of effective interventions promoting healthy eating found the following factors were associated with effectiveness:

R eflection point

Is the message of '5-a-day' clear? E.g. what is a portion of fruit or vegetables? Does a glass of fruit juice contribute to the five daily portions?

- a focus on diet or diet and physical activity
- using behaviour change approaches to set clear goals
- giving feedback to participants about behaviour change and risk factors
- personal and sustained contact with participants
- promoting changes in the local environment, e.g. food access and availability.

Improving knowledge about diet does not necessarily lead to changes in consumption. Healthy foods need to be accessible and available and people need the skills and confidence to prepare these foods.

E xample

Food Dudes

Food Dudes is a programme designed to encourage children to eat more fruit and vegetables. Bangor Food Research Unit developed the Food Dudes programme using three main psychological techniques: taste exposure, modelling and rewards. Food Dudes consists of two key elements: short video programmes featuring the Food Dudes who enjoy eating fruit and vegetables and provide effective social models for children to copy, and small rewards such as stickers,

Figure 11.1
Determinants of food
and nutrition
consumption
Source: DoH Nutrition
Task Force 1996, p. 4

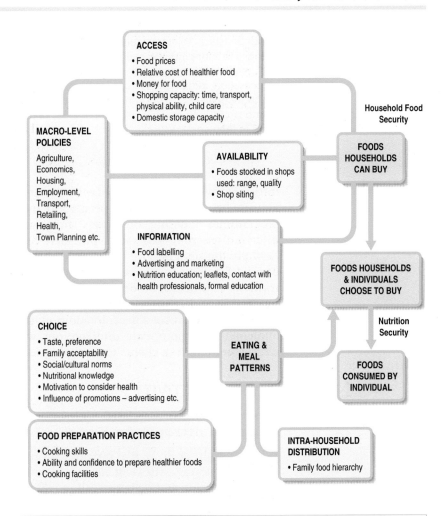

ACCESS
• Food prices
• Relative cost of healthier food
• Money for food
• Shopping capacity: time, transport, physical ability, child care
• Domestic storage capacity

MACRO-LEVEL POLICIES
Agriculture,
Economics,
Housing,
Employment,
Transport,
Retailing,
Health,
Town Planning etc.

AVAILABILITY
• Foods stocked in shops used: range, quality
• Shop siting

Household Food Security

FOODS HOUSEHOLDS CAN BUY

INFORMATION
• Food labelling
• Advertising and marketing
• Nutrition education; leaflets, contact with health professionals, formal education

FOODS HOUSEHOLDS & INDIVIDUALS CHOOSE TO BUY

Nutrition Security

CHOICE
• Taste, preference
• Family acceptability
• Social/cultural norms
• Nutritional knowledge
• Motivation to consider health
• Influence of promotions – advertising etc.

EATING & MEAL PATTERNS

FOODS CONSUMED BY INDIVIDUAL

FOOD PREPARATION PRACTICES
• Cooking skills
• Ability and confidence to prepare healthier foods
• Cooking facilities

INTRA-HOUSEHOLD DISTRIBUTION
• Family food hierarchy

E *continued*

pens and rulers to ensure children begin to taste and consume fruit and vegetables. Evaluation of the programme shows that it leads to major and lasting increases in children's consumption of fruit and vegetables. This is especially true for children living in deprived areas. For example, children in Salford increased their lunchtime consumption of fruit by 150% and vegetables by 315% following the Food Dudes programme.

Source: www.fooddudes.co.uk

The rise of fast food, takeout meals and the loss of practical food preparation skills in schools' curricula has led to a focus on providing cooking skills. Cooking skills programmes seek to encourage people to practise food preparation in a safe environment and stimulate home cooking using fresh foods.

E **xample**

Cooking skills

Local food projects tend to be evaluated in relation to their contribution to improved nutritional knowledge and eating behaviour. They can also improve access to food and enhance cooking skills. There are clear social gains for individuals and communities that are intrinsic to projects achieving nutritional and

E *continued*

health benefits. Projects should be evaluated on the increase in skills, confidence, changes to shopping and eating behaviour, as well as on longer term nutritional and health outcomes. Food projects are often funded short term as part of regeneration initiatives but can only make a slight contribution to reducing health inequalities. They do not provide comprehensive coverage or integrated solutions but may provide opportunities for practitioners to work with communities in innovative ways.

Source: McGlone et al (1999)

Integrated programmes that adopt a variety of strategies including individually based education and persuasion and community based structural programmes focusing on access and availability are most effective. Interventions may also target providers further up the food chain, for example the sourcing of locally grown produce sold in farmers' markets, or food labelling to ensure consumers can easily compare fat and sugar contents of processed foods. Practitioners can play an important role in supporting and reinforcing such programmes through the provision of dietary education and advice. In addition, practitioners can take a lead in implementing appropriate interventions within the health care service setting and referring clients to local programmes.

PHYSICAL ACTIVITY

Physical activity is associated with positive health benefits as well as reducing the risk of coronary heart disease:

Keeping physically active provides strong protection against coronary heart disease and stroke. It also has beneficial effects on weight control, blood pressure and diabetes – all of which are risk factors in their own right; protects against brittle bones and maintains muscle power; and increases people's general sense of well-being.

DoH 1999, p. 76

The Health Survey of England (Erens & Primatesta 1999) found that around six out of ten men and seven out of ten women are not active enough to benefit their health. The British Heart Foundation (2003) estimates that 37% of deaths from coronary heart disease could be attributed to inactivity. The degree of risk of inactivity is comparable to the relative risk associated with the three main risk factors for coronary heart disease, e.g. smoking, high blood pressure and high cholesterol. Inactivity is the biggest risk factor for the population as a whole and has one of the largest potentials for improvement. The recommended minimum is 30 minutes of moderate exercise five times a week.

A review of the effectiveness of physical activity intervention studies among the general public (Hillsdon et al 1999) found that those interventions that were effective in attracting and sustaining high levels of participation had the following features in common:

- home-based activity, rather than structured programmes based in a special facility or centre

- informal and unsupervised exercise
- frequent professional contact for encouragement, either by telephone or home visit
- interventions that encourage walking
- interventions aimed at modifying the environment such as signs posted to increase stair walking.

The focus of most work on physical activity has been on the individual making behavioural changes, yet the barriers facing different population groups vary considerably. Asian women surveyed in Bristol for example cited the following as barriers to increasing their activity levels (Pilgrim et al 1993):

- burden of other duties
- fear of racism (including when out walking)
- language difficulties
- inappropriateness of facilities including dress code, male/female provision, high cost.

Effort is needed to ensure that physical activity interventions address the needs of lower socio-economic and other marginalized groups. The following example illustrates how this can be done.

Example The Exercise on Referral scheme	This scheme, which operates in Leicestershire and Rutland, aims to provide sedentary members of the local community with the opportunity to undertake a programme of exercise under the guidance of qualified instructors. A range of health care professionals have the opportunity to refer people who have a health condition that can be ameliorated through physical activity and who are largely inactive. The scheme aims to provide participants with the knowledge and confidence to become independent exercisers so that they remain physically active after the programme ends. The exercise is mainly located within local authority leisure centres and includes some local community venues. Activities include exercise using gym equipment and exercise classes such as aerobics and aquaerobics, and home-based exercise, walking and environmentally based activity such as conservation work are also planned. Source: www.exercisealliance.org.uk accessed 17/11/03

Exercise referral schemes do show evidence of short-term increases in physical activity levels although there is no evidence of sustained long-term change. A national quality assurance framework for GP exercise referral schemes has been published and evidence suggests that the effectiveness of such schemes is enhanced when:

- staff are trained in behaviour change strategies
- practitioner–patient ratios are adequate, enabling quality supervision
- there is good liaison between health and leisure service staff
- community based networks build on and sustain the original intervention (HDA 2001, DoH 2001c).

Discussion point

Who would you target for interventions to increase physical activity, and why?

Children are a particular target group for increased physical activity. The rise in passive hobbies and leisure pursuits, such as using the computer or watching TV, together with fears about road safety and the loss of sports activities in school (driven out partly by the demands of the national curriculum) have all combined to reduce the physical activity patterns of a whole generation. Behavioural patterns established in childhood exert an influence on later adult behaviour and cardiovascular risk factors have their origins in childhood. Positive changes within a school setting are associated with the following characteristics (HDA 2001):

- appropriately designed, delivered and supported physical activity curriculum
- access to suitable and accessible facilities and opportunities for physical activity
- the involvement of young people in planning the programmes.

There are clear gender differences, with young women less likely to be physically active. Professional education to enhance teacher skills, community involvement and support, and provision of appropriate activities to meet religious and cultural needs of people from minority ethnic groups, are also important factors associated with effective schemes (HDA 2001).

Example	Safe Routes to School is a project coordinated by the voluntary organization Sustrans that aims to encourage children to walk and cycle to school. Safe Routes to School projects cite a variety of health and environmental benefits including increased activity levels, alertness at school and interest in the local neighbourhood, and reduced pollution from traffic. Cycling can be encouraged through the creation of safe cycle paths that are separated from road traffic and secure cycle parking spaces and lockers within school grounds. Walking buses operate with parent volunteers, with a 'driver' at the front and a 'conductor' at the back. The walking bus follows an agreed route to school with set pick-up points.
Safe Routes to School	

Source: www.saferoutestoschool.org.uk

Health promotion and public health interventions to promote physical activity have focused on targeted interventions that reduce barriers to exercise rather than persuasive mass media campaigns. Often a settings approach is used, as in the school setting in the example above. User and community involvement enhance the effects of an intervention. A targeted focus on a particular group in a particular setting, that enables appropriate and accessible interventions, appears to be a successful strategy, and one that could be transferred to other groups and settings.

ALCOHOL AND DRUGS

Alcohol and drug use is associated with many health and social problems including violence, burglary, hazardous driving and public disorder in addition to physical and mental health problems. The links with criminal justice tend to receive a higher profile than the health issues. This is illustrated by the public focus on drugs, especially illegal drugs, rather than alcohol, although alcohol poses a more serious risk to the public health. This is reflected in government spending patterns, with £500 million per year allocated to drugs programmes and only £95 million per year allocated to alcohol services (McCurry 2003).

Discussion point

What accounts for the low profile of alcohol policy?

There is considerable ambivalence in the UK about tackling alcohol. On the one hand there is evidence of alcohol abuse and a recognition that reducing consumption is a legitimate policy aim. On the other hand the UK alcohol industry employs more than one million people and is the fourth largest producer of spirits and the sixth largest producer of beer in the world. Alcohol constitutes over 3% of total tax revenue.

Health messages relating to alcohol may be ambiguous and confusing because a limited intake of alcohol is associated with reduced risk of coronary heart disease. However, excessive use of alcohol is linked to a variety of health and social problems.

Box 11.4 Alcohol and health

- Alcohol is directly responsible for over 5000 deaths and is implicated in a further 33 000 deaths per year in England and Wales.
- Alcohol is ranked the third highest risk to health in developed countries by WHO.
- Alcohol is a factor in 20–30% of all accidents.
- Excessive use of alcohol is linked to many health problems including raised blood pressure, certain types of cancers, strokes, fertility problems, gastritis, pancreatitis, liver disease, mental health problems, accidents and suicides.
- Excessive use of alcohol is also linked to social problems such as violence and crime.
- Alcohol has been estimated to cost the NHS up to £3 billion a year.
- 1 in 4 acute male admissions is alcohol related.

Sources: www.alcoholconcern.org.uk, WHO (2002), Department of Health (2001a)

Discussion point

Most interventions have focused on an approach based on self regulation and personal responsibility through the provision of information on the effects of alcohol. There has also been limited legislative activity focused on drinking hours, drink-driving and public order offences. What other policies and interventions might be effective?

The rise in alcohol-related health and social problems has been fuelled by increases in alcohol consumption, especially amongst young people and women. The recommended maximum intakes are 21 units per week for men and 14 units per week for women. A unit of alcohol is equivalent to half a pint of beer, a glass of wine or a measure of spirits. The General Household Survey shows that in 2001, as in previous years, men were almost twice as likely as women to have exceeded the recommended daily alcohol limits at least once during the week prior to interview (more than four units of alcohol for men and three for women) – 39% of men compared with 22% of women had done so. 'Heavy' drinking (6 plus units per day for women; 8 plus units per day for men) showed the same pattern, with 10% of women and 21% of men having had at least one episode of heavy drinking in the week before interview (Walker et al 2002). For women only, heavy drinking showed a positive association with managerial and professional class.

Alcohol misuse has very significant economic costs. A recent report estimated that for 2001/2, in addition to costs to the NHS, alcohol misuse was responsible for workplace and wider economy costs in the region of £2.2 billion and alcohol-related crime costs were around £12 billion (Cabinet Office Strategy Unit 2003). A national alcohol strategy for England is planned to be implemented by 2004, aimed at tackling the problems of alcohol misuse and reducing its economic, social and health costs.

An evidence briefing summary produced by the Health Development Agency (Waller et al 2002) found that systematic review level evidence showed the following types of interventions were associated with reduced alcohol intakes:

- Peer-led programmes in schools rather than teacher led programmes.
- Interactive programmes that foster the development of interpersonal skills in schools reduce alcohol use.
- Intensive training of the staff who serve drinks plus managerial support reduces the level of intoxication in patrons/drinkers.
- Alcohol screening and interventions in hospital accident and emergency departments reduces risky drinking.
- Extended brief interventions in primary health care settings targeted at heavy drinkers reduces alcohol consumption.
- Very brief interventions delivered opportunistically by health care professionals to non-treatment seeking populations.

There was weak evidence for other kinds of interventions including workplace and community programmes and programmes targeting young people. Some of the strongest evidence supported the use of laws lowering the drink-drive limit of blood alcohol concentration and enforcing minimum legal drinking age laws in reducing alcohol-related driving accidents, injuries and fatalities.

Drugs

The use of illegal drugs has been linked to many health and social problems, including crime and family break-ups. It is estimated that there are around 250 000 problematic drug users in England and Wales and that drug misuse costs between £10 and £18 billion a year in social and economic costs (Home Office 2002). The updated National Drug Strategy (Home Office 2002) focuses on four key areas:

1. **Young People** – preventing today's young people from becoming tomorrow's problematic drug users.
2. **Reducing supply** – reducing the supply of illegal drugs.
3. **Communities** – reducing drug-related crime and its impact on communities.
4. **Treatment** and harm minimization – reducing drug use and drug-related offending through the provision of effective treatment and rehabilitation services.

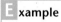 **xample**

The FRANK campaign

Caught between media hysteria, adult denial and anecodotal stories from peers, young people can find it hard to get the plain facts about drugs. As part of the national drug strategy, the FRANK campaign, including a telephone helpline and a new interactive website, www.talktofrank.com, has been launched. FRANK is aimed at both young people and their parents and carers. FRANK aims to provide young people with credible and reliable information to understand the risks

E continued

associated with drug use. FRANK also aims to give parents and carers the skills and confidence to communicate with their children about drugs. The website offers honest and impartial information and advice about drugs, and individual queries can be e-mailed. A number of sources of help are signposted from this website. The FRANK campaign is jointly funded by the Home Office and the Department of Health, working closely with the Department for Education and Skills and has an advertising budget of £3 million for the first year. FRANK is already handling 1200 calls a day and has received over 320 000 hits to his website.

Source: www.talktofrank.com

Local communities bear the brunt of drug-related disorder and crime. Coordinated action between local people and agencies and local police can have a dramatic effect on the local availability of drugs and associated problems. Lambeth in London was facing a major problem with crack cocaine in 2002. Open crack markets and crack houses had led to open street prostitution and gun use. Following a meeting between politicians and services, Lambeth launched a multi-agency initiative against drugs. Swift and decisive police action led to raids on crack houses, removal of abandoned vehicles and arrests of people suspected of drug dealing and of prostitutes, who were referred for treatment. Since the start of the initiative, robberies have been reduced by a third.

Treatment is a crucial part of the overall strategy. Treatment is both effective and cost-effective – for every £1 spent, an estimated £3 is saved in criminal justice costs alone (Home Office 2002). The National Treatment Agency oversees treatment services that are locally coordinated and provided by Drug Action Teams. Services range from in-patient detoxification and prescribing to structured counselling and residential rehabilitation. The aim is to provide a positive route out of addiction and crime for drug users.

Harm minimization is another important aspect of strategy. Changing the approach from a simple 'just say no' message to providing the information and skills to enable people to reduce their risks is a complex and challenging transition. Some practitioners may find such an approach difficult because it acknowledges people's right to make unhealthy or illegal decisions. For some, this may be an unethical stance and one they cannot endorse. For others, using such an approach can provide a useful way to contribute effectively to reducing risks without having to adopt an unrealistic 'all or nothing' approach.

Alcohol and drug use present law and order challenges as well as health problems. The most effective approaches combine the use of different strategies targeting different aspects of the problem. The use of legislation, regulation and the criminal justice system is an important adjunct to the individual health screening, education, advice and medication provided by practitioners. The evidence demonstrates that specific targeted interventions by health practitioners are effective and contribute to the reduction of the disease burden caused by alcohol and drug use.

R eflection point

How easy and ethical is it for practitioners to adopt a harm minimization approach?

D iscussion point

Why do you think there are separate national strategies for alcohol, tobacco and drugs?

SEXUAL HEALTH

The term sexual health has many contrasting definitions that are influenced by beliefs about concepts such as health and sex. Definitions may range from a focus on the clinical causes of ill health, such as infections, to a celebration of pleasure.

Reflection point

How would you define sexual health? Does your definition impact equally on men and women? On heterosexual and homosexual people?

Sexual health has been defined in various ways. Whilst there is often a focus in service provision on sexual ill health and disease, most definitions refer to a holistic positive concept of sexual health. For example, the World Health Organization refers to 'the integration of the physical, emotional, intellectual and social aspects of sexual being, in ways that are enriching and that enhance personality, communication and love' (WHO 1974, quoted in HEA 1994, p. 4). More recently, the Department of Health reinforces the holistic concept of sexual health whilst acknowledging the need to avoid unintended consequences of sexual activity including disease.

Sexual health is an important part of physical and mental health. It is a key part of our identity as human beings together with the fundamental human rights to privacy, a family life and living free from discrimination. Essential elements of good sexual health are equitable relationships and sexual fulfilment with access to information and services to avoid the risk of unintended pregnancy, illness or disease.

(DoH 2001b, p. 7)

Gender is an important factor affecting sexual health. 'The differential power of men and women is evident in most sexual intercourse as it is in the wider context of male–female relations' (Doyal, 1995, p. 62). Women's capacity to enjoy and express their sexuality is limited by the fundamentally unequal relationship between men and women. Women may have to negotiate their concerns about fertility and safer sex and may be threatened with violence, harassment or abuse from their partners. A survey of young women's sexual attitudes concludes that 'For a young woman to insist on the use of a condom for her own safety requires resisting the constraints and opposing the construction of intercourse as a man's natural pleasure and a woman's natural duty' (Thomson & Holland 1994, p. 24). Homosexuality remains a less socially valued and more discriminated against sexual identity, compared to heterosexuality. Activities that heterosexuals take for granted, such as public recognition and acceptance of their sexual partners, can be problematic for homosexuals. The rights of homosexuals are proscribed by law, e.g. the age of consent for homosexuals is 18 compared to 16 for heterosexuals.

The element of sexual health that is defined as being free from sexually transmitted infections (STIs) has declined in recent years. All STIs have increased in the past 5 years, especially gonorrhoea (78% increase), chlamydia (73% increase) and syphilis (374% increase) (Adler 2003). Teenage pregnancy rates have remained unchanged over the last 10 years and cases of HIV are expected to double between 1997 and 2005. These statistics are driven by changes in sexual behaviour including:

- a decrease in the age of first intercourse
- an increase in lifetime partners and concurrent relationships

- a decrease in safe sex practices among homosexual men (Johnson et al 2001 and Wellings et al 2001, cited in Ellis et al 2003).

The findings of a Parliamentary Health Select Committee on Sexual Health report in 2003 (www.parliament.the-stationary-office.co.uk accessed 29/11/03) were that sexual health was in crisis and was a significant public health issue that demanded immediate attention. Sexual health services were inferior to those provided 10 years earlier, with longer waiting times, under-resourced clinics and demoralized staff. NHS contraceptive and abortion services were fragmented and of variable quality and availability in different geographical regions of the country. Sexual health services remain underfunded and relatively invisible, tainted with the stigma still associated with STIs. Nevertheless the work of GUM services is changing from a simple provision of screening and information within a medical model to a broader promotion of sexual health as part of a more person-centred approach.

A national strategy for sexual health and HIV in England was announced in 2001 (DoH 2001b). The focus of the strategy is on tackling HIV, sexually transmitted infections (STIs) and unintended pregnancies and improving the relevant health and social care services. The strategy has been allocated £47.5 million for the next two years – a sum that critics argue is manifestly insufficient. The strategy aims to:

- reduce the transmission of HIV and STIs
- reduce the prevalence of undiagnosed HIV and STIs
- reduce unintended pregnancy rates
- improve health and social care for people living with HIV
- reduce the stigma associated with HIV and STIs.

The strategy intends to use a variety of methods and approaches but focuses on service improvements especially for young people (such as one-stop clinics and dedicated services) and increasing access to GUM services. HIV testing, chlamydia testing and the hepatitis B vaccine are all to be offered more widely.

England's teenage pregnancy strategy published in 1999 has two aims:

- to halve the under 18 conception rate by 2010
- to reduce social exclusion by increasing the participation of teenage mothers in work, training or education by 60% by 2010.

The teenage pregnancy strategy includes a mass media advertising campaign targeted at more deprived and less well educated young people. Key campaign messages have focused on choices, responsibility, resisting peer pressure and using contraception and used the slogan, 'Sex, are you thinking about it enough?' Evaluation of the campaign shows the most commonly recalled message was the need to use contraception. Evaluation also demonstrates the continued misconceptions surrounding the subject of sex. For example, more than half of the target group believe most young people have had sex before the age of 16 (in reality only a third have done so – a key campaign message); 10% believe having sex for the first time, standing up or washing immediately after sex prevents conception; and 40% were not aware that free condoms are available from family planning clinics (UCL, LSHTM, BMRB Int. 2002).

R eflection point

Why do sexual health services remain the Cinderella of the NHS – under-funded, under-staffed and relatively invisible?

D iscussion point

What are the advantages and limitations of linking HIV prevention to the overall task of reducing STIs?

D iscussion point

What do you think should be the role of abstinence-centred approaches and safer sex approaches in a sexual health and teenage pregnancy strategy?

Abstinence-centred approaches have been unpopular in the UK, partly because it has been claimed that they are ineffective. This claim is now being challenged, as the example below demonstrates. However, abstinence is still viewed with suspicion by many, who see it as an attempt to disempower young people and impose on them moral values that they may not share. Others see abstinence education as ineffectual when set against current trends in youth culture.

Example Saved Sex – the abstinence-centred approach	There is substantial accumulating evidence from the USA, Uganda, Zambia and Jamaica that abstinence education delays the onset of intercourse by up to three years and reduces both STI rates and unplanned pregnancies. The 'Not Me, Not Now' programme in Monroe County, New York reports the following results from an abstinence programme: ▪ The percentage of students who felt they were ready to deal with the consequences of sexual activity fell from 34% to 22%. ▪ Students having sexual intercourse by the age of 15 fell from 47% to 32%. ▪ Teenage pregnancy rates reduced from 63.4 per 1000 in 1993 to 49.5 per 1000 in 1996. Source: Doniger et al (2001)

By contrast, much work on reducing HIV infection has targeted risk groups (men who have sex with men, African communities, sex workers, prisoners) with information and education about safer sex. The simple message to use a condom has been replaced by a more complex empowerment approach aimed at increasing decision making skills and feelings of control.

Example Gay Men Fighting AIDS (GMFA)	Gay Men Fighting AIDS runs mass media campaigns offering information, advice and support to gay men in London. The campaigns are developed by volunteers and health promotion professionals and are pre-tested with the target group, gay men on the scene, and partnership agencies. Campaign advertising is placed in the gay and HIV positive press. GMFA also works with the media to provide supportive editorial coverage alongside their campaigns. GMFA campaigns acknowledge the complexity of decisions around reducing the risk of HIV and the many relevant factors, including whether the man is in a relationship; whether that relationship is monogamous; their HIV status and that of their partner/s. Campaigns to date include: ▪ Relationships – focusing on issues around testing, telling and listening. ▪ You can't spot them all – focusing on the fact that although gay men think they may be able to guess the HIV status of others (just as they can guess whether someone is heterosexual or gay), they will not always be correct. ▪ Enjoy fucking – focusing on harm reduction through the practice of safer sex including the use of condoms, water-based lubricants and withdrawal before ejaculation. Source: www.metromate.org.uk accessed 18/11/03

Health promotion and public health interventions aimed at changing sexual behaviour face particular challenges due to the sensitive nature of the subject and the power of gender and sexual orientation in shaping people's perceptions and attitudes. Sexual health is also a complex area and includes both fertility and STIs. The focus of the national strategy is on increasing access, availability and acceptability of NHS sexual health services. This may involve practitioners developing more client-centred, flexible approaches to service delivery. The priorities remain, however, more focused on sexual ill health – to reduce STIs and HIV, and also to reduce the teenage pregnancy rate.

CONCLUSION

Lifestyles and individual behavioural choices have a long history of being targeted for change by health promoters. The significance of behaviours such as diet, exercise, smoking, alcohol and drug use, and sexual activity in affecting or even determining health outcomes is widely accepted. What is disputed is the effectiveness of different kinds of approaches to changing lifestyles and whether they are ethically defensible. Lifestyles are generally viewed as an individual choice that should be respected unless they directly infringe someone else's freedom to choose. The impact on others is generally easier to appreciate when it involves aspects such as safety and crime (linked to alcohol and drug use) rather than aspects such as health (linked to smoking). However, the counter case may be made; that the government has a duty to protect people from known health risks especially when these are socially patterned and linked to socio-economic inequalities. When behaviours directly impact on others, it is much easier to get support for legislation and regulation to control such behaviours. When the effects are more diffuse the case for legislation is correspondingly more difficult. This can be demonstrated by comparing the existence of laws regulating drunkenness in public places and whilst in charge of vehicles with the long battle to legislate to ban the advertising and promotion of tobacco products. Whilst smoking causes ill health and distress to passive smokers as well as to smokers, it is not associated with visible antisocial behaviour. The campaign to ban tobacco advertising therefore took a long time to build the evidence and win support. Even now comprehensive bans on smoking in public places are not seen as realistic, although the Big Smoke Debate (an online survey of attitudes to smoking in public places in London) is challenging this, and smoking in public is now banned in Ireland, and Brighton and Sheffield in England.

Whilst legislation and regulation may be the most effective means of changing lifestyles, in many cases they are seen as inappropriate because of the right to individual freedom and liberty. In these cases, education and persuasion through the use of mass media campaigns may be the appropriate strategy. Health practitioners have an important role to play in using educational and motivational strategies with individual clients, and also with groups and local communities if the opportunity arises. These techniques seek to change people's behaviour voluntarily as a result of education, information, support and advice. An evidence base on effective techniques to use in educational and motivational interventions is growing. A combination of different strategies that includes legislation and regulation, is the most effective means of achieving behavioural changes.

FURTHER DISCUSSION

▪ Identify the opportunities and barriers to working with individual clients to change one of the behaviours discussed in this chapter.

▪ How (if at all) can you justify seeking to change people's behavioural choices as long as these are legal?

▪ Discuss the relative contribution of individual education and advice, mass media campaigns and legislation in achieving behavioural change.

Recommended reading

▪ Rollnick S, Mason P, Butler C (1999) Health behaviour change: a guide for practitioners. London, Churchill Livingstone.

A practical guide to support practitioners working with clients to change behaviours.

▪ Marks D F, Murray M, Evans B, Willig C (2000) Health psychology: theory, research and practice. London, Sage.

A psychology textbook that looks at health behaviours and how psychological theory can help to develop appropriate interventions.

▪ The Health Development Agency produces a range of Evidence Briefing Summaries. Each Evidence Briefing Summary presents an overview of the findings and recommendations from a review of recent selected systematic and other reviews and meta-analyses. Evidence Briefing Summaries include:

▪ Ellis S, Barnett-Page E, Morgan A et al (2003) HIV prevention: a review of reviews assessing the effectiveness of interventions to reduce the risk of sexual transmission. London, HDA.

▪ Mulvihill C, Quigley R (2003) The management of obesity and overweight: an analysis of reviews of diet, physical activity and behavioural approaches. Evidence Briefing Summary. London, HDA.

▪ Waller S, Naidoo B, Thom B (2002) Prevention and reduction of alcohol misuse: review of reviews. Evidence Briefing Summary. London, HDA.

REFERENCES

Adler M W (2003) Sexual health – health of the nation. Sexually Transmitted Infections 79: 84–85

British Heart Foundation (2003) Coronary disease statistics. London, BHF

Cabinet Office Strategy Unit (2003) Alcohol misuse: how much does it cost? London, COSU

Davison C, Frankel S, Davey Smith G (1992) The limits to lifestyle: reassessing 'fatalism' in the popular culture of illness prevention. Social Science and Medicine 34(6): 675–685

Department of Health (DoH) (1992) The health of the nation: a strategy for health in England. London, HMSO.

Department of Health (DoH) Nutrition Task Force (1996) Low income, food, nutrition and health: Strategies for improvement. London, HMSO

Department of Health (DoH) (1998) White paper: smoking kills, Cm 4177. London, The Stationery Office

Department of Health (DoH) (1999) Saving lives: our healthier nation. London, The Stationery Office

Department of Health (DoH) (2000a) National service framework: coronary heart disease. London, The Stationery Office

Department of Health (DoH) (2000b) National diet and nutrition survey. London, The Stationery Office

Department of Health (DoH) (2000c) The NHS plan: a plan for investment, a plan for reform. London, The Stationery Office

Department of Health (DoH) (2001a) Statistical bulletin: statistics on alcohol – England, 1978 onwards. London, The Stationery Office

Department of Health (DoH) (2001b) The national strategy for sexual health and HIV – consultation. London, The Stationery Office

Department of Health (DoH) (2001c) Exercise referral schemes: a national quality assurance framework. London, The Stationery Office

Department of Health (DoH) (2003) A local 5 a day initiative: increasing fruit and vegetable consumption – improving health. Booklet 1. London, DoH

Doll R, Hill A B (1950) Smoking and carcinoma of the lung: preliminary report. British Medical Journal 143: 329–336

Doniger A S, Adams E, Riley J S, Utter C A (2001) Impact evaluation of the 'Not Me, Not Now' abstinence-oriented, adolescent pregnancy prevention communications program, Monroe County, New York. Journal of Health Communication 6: 45–60

Doyal L (1995) What makes women sick?: gender and the political economy of health. Basingstoke, Macmillan

Ellis S, Barnett-Page E, Morgan A et al (2003) HIV prevention: a review of reviews assessing the effectiveness of interventions to reduce the risk of sexual transmission. London, HDA

Erens B, Primatesta P (eds) (1999) Health survey for England: cardiovascular 1998. London, The Stationery Office

Ezzati M, Lopez A D, Rodgers R, Vander Hoorn S, Murray C J L (2002) Selected major risk factors and global and regional burden of disease. Lancet 360(9343): 1347–1362

Froggatt P (1988) 4th Report of the Independent Scientific Committee on smoking and health. London, HMSO

Graham H (1993) When life's a drag: women, smoking and disadvantage. London, HMSO

Hastings G, Stead M, McDermott L, Forsyth A, MacKintosh A, Rayner M, Godfey C, Caraher M, Angus K (2003) Review of research on the effects of food promotion to children. Final report prepared for the Food Standards Agency. Strathclyde, University of Strathclyde

Health Development Agency (HDA) (2001) Coronary heart disease: guidance for implementing the preventive aspects of the national service framework. London, HDA

Health Education Authority (1994) Update no. 4 sexual health. London, Health Education Authority

Health Education Authority (1997) Health promotion interventions to promote healthy eating in the general population – a review. London, Health Education Authority

Hillsdon M, Thorogood M, Foster C (1999) A systematic review of strategies to promote physical activity. In: MacAuley D (ed) Benefits and hazards of exercise, Vol. 1. London, BMJ Publications

Home Office (2002) Updated drug strategy. Available at www.drugs.gov.uk/Reports and Publications/NationalStrategy, accessed 30/11/03

Joint Health Surveys Unit on behalf of the Department of Health (2002) Health survey for England 2001. London, The Stationary Office

Lupton D (1995) The imperative of health. Public health and the regulated body. London, Sage

Lupton D (1999) Risk. London, Routledge

McCurry P (2003) Last orders. Guardian Society 29 April

McGlone P, Dobson B, Dowler E, Nelson M (1999) Food projects and how they work. York, Joseph Rowntree Foundation

Mulvihill C, Quigley R (2003) The management of obesity and overweight: an analysis of reviews of diet, physical activity and behavioural approaches. Evidence Briefing Summary. London, Health Development Agency

Naidoo J, Wills J (2000) Health promotion: foundations for practice, 2nd edn. London, Baillierè Tindall

NHS Centre for Reviews and Dissemination (1998) Smoking cessation: what the health service can do. Effectiveness Matters 3(1)

Office for National Statistics (2000) National food survey 1999. London, The Stationery Office

Pilgrim S with Fenton S, Hughes T, Hine C, Tibbs N (1993) The Bristol Black and ethnic minorities survey. Bristol, University of Bristol

Prochaska J O, diClemente C (1984) The transtheoretical approach: crossing traditional foundations of change. Harnewood, IL, Don Jones/Irwin

Royal College of Physicians (1992) Smoking and the young. London, RCP

Thomson R, Holland J (1994) Young women and safer sex: context, constraints and strategies. In: Kitzinger C, Wilkinson S (eds) Women and health: feminist perspectives. London, Falmer

University College London, London School of Tropical Hygiene and Tropical Medicine, British Market Research Bureau International (2002)

Evaluation of the teenage pregnancy strategy. Annual Synthesis Report No. 1, 2001 available at www.teenagepregnancyunit.gov.uk accessed 18/11/03

Waller S, Naidoo B, Thom B (2002) Prevention and reduction of alcohol misuse: review of reviews. Evidence briefing summary. London, Health Development Agency

Walker A, O'Brien M, Traynor J, Fox K, Goddard E, and Foster K (2002) Living in Britain: results from the 2001 General Household Survey. London, The Stationery Office

World Health Organization (WHO) (2003) Framework convention on tobacco control A56/8. Geneva, WHO

World Health Organization (WHO) (2002) The world health report 2002: reducing risks, promoting health life. Geneva, WHO

12 Population groups

OVERVIEW

Targeting interventions towards specific groups such as Black and ethnic minorities or young people is often advocated as a means of achieving equity. By directing activities to groups in need, practitioners seek to address health inequalities. This chapter reviews the arguments for targeting particular groups because of their health risks and needs and attempting to create more flexible and responsive services. It discusses different approaches to working with population groups from targeting resources to particular groups to interventions to improve opportunities or strengthen communities. The chapter outlines the health needs of older people, children, Black and ethnic minority groups, refugees and asylum seekers and then discusses some examples of effective interventions or projects that work with these groups to illustrate a range of health promoting or health developing activities.

INTRODUCTION

The establishment of Britain's NHS as a universal service for everyone, available according to need and free at the point of delivery, has been heralded as one of the great health achievements of the twentieth century. The NHS has enjoyed unparalleled public support, and its achievements in providing high quality care at relatively low cost are undeniable. There have, however, been some criticisms of this universalist model of provision. Whilst it appears equitable, in that the same service is available for all, in reality certain groups fare better than others. This has been evident in the debate around the 'postcode lottery' whereby certain geographical areas provide better services and manage to recruit and retain staff more easily than other more disadvantaged areas. In general this reflects the socio-economic makeup of the local population, with poorer areas receiving poorer services. Many commentators have argued that the NHS perpetuates sexist, ageist and racist stereotypes and fails to adequately meet the needs of particular population groups (Doyal 1998). In order to meet the needs of specific marginalized, 'hard to reach' groups, targeting has been suggested as an appropriate strategy.

Targeting means identifying particular needs and creating more flexible services in order to meet those needs. Targeting has been proposed as both a more equitable and efficient means of meeting health needs. Opponents argue that targeting involves additional resources being directed at small

Reflection point

What do you understand by targeting? How do you target programmes/services in your practice?

communities or groups, and that this is inequitable. This fails to take account of the fact that any universal service will appeal more to certain groups than others, and also that certain groups have much greater levels of need than others. Proponents of targeting also argue that linking provision to needs should be done for all groups, and that flexibility is a hallmark of high quality services.

The targeting of population groups has three rationales:

1. an ethical rationale based on equity
2. a scientific rationale based on the notion of risk
3. an economic rationale based on cost-effectiveness.

The ethical rationale argues that on the grounds of equity, targeting is needed to supplement a universal service if the needs of all population groups are to be met equally. For example, homeless people without a fixed address are unable to register with a GP and are therefore denied access to a range of community services. Innovative strategies to meet the needs of homeless people include using public addresses such as park benches in order to register homeless people, and employing staff with a specific remit for this group.

The economic rationale argues that it is more cost-effective to provide resources to meet needs effectively rather than have to spend resources later addressing the multiple social effects (e.g. crime, unemployment, acute and chronic ill health) resulting from a failure to meet needs. The broad argument that prevention is cheaper than cure has been recognized; it merely needs to be reinforced for specific groups.

The scientific rationale rests on a notion of risk. Epidemiological evidence identifies these groups on the basis of their behavioural risk factors (see Ch. 11) or their health outcomes (ill health or premature death), access to care and services or in relation to particular characteristics such as low income, housing or work (see Ch. 9). For example:

- the prison population suffers high rates of mental illness
- life expectancy among street homeless is mid forties
- infant mortality in social class 5 is double that of social class 1.

Traditionally, analysis of modern society has seen it as divided by class, gender, sexuality and ethnicity and this social stratification as shaping experience and opportunities. Targeted population groups are normally those who share one of these characteristics and are deemed to have special health needs such as men/women, older people/children, homeless, teenage mothers, minority ethnic groups, gay men and lesbians.

A report by the Health Education Authority on the needs of the homeless provides a common argument for the explicit targeting of a population group 'due to the wide range of health-related problems that affect homeless people, and their particular living environment and lifestyle, interventions should be targeted to their specific needs, rather than relying only on those aimed at the general population' (HEA 1999, p. 30). Simply, blanket approaches cannot cater for everyone.

The term 'vulnerable groups' has been widely adopted (DoH 1999) to indicate those in need of particular provision. This could be because they have greater health needs; because their health needs are not being adequately addressed; or because they are at risk of social exclusion.

Groups such as people with learning disabilities and looked after children might then be seen as vulnerable.

D iscussion point

What are the problems of defining groups in this way?

The use of this term has been criticised for projecting a view of such groups as helpless or dependent. Defining groups as vulnerable ignores the fact that most needs are met privately, and that vulnerable groups in fact possess valuable resources for meeting needs. Recognizing what groups have to offer, rather than seeing them solely as recipients of services, is a more health promoting strategy that builds community self-esteem.

'Social exclusion' is a relatively new term used to describe groups of people who are marginalized and on the outside of society usually because of their lack of access to material and social resources but also because of their isolation from social interactions. The UK government has defined social exclusion as 'what can happen when people or areas suffer from a combination of linked problems such as unemployment, poor skills, low incomes, poor housing, high crime, bad health and family breakdown' (Social Exclusion Unit, www.socialexclusionunit.gov.uk). Refugees and asylum seekers are an example of a group that is seriously threatened with problems of social exclusion. A disproportionate number of refugees become long-term unemployed, no matter what qualifications and experience of work they bring with them and most have problems of housing and community settlement.

D iscussion point

How useful is the term 'social exclu-sion' in identifying target population groups?

Social exclusion, unlike poverty, includes several dimensions of deprivation and participation and draws attention to the ways in which people's position in society may change over time (Hills et al 2002). It changes the focus of interventions from those to take people out of poverty or ameliorate its effects (see Chs 5 and 9) to those that focus on involvement and engagement.

APPROACHES TO WORKING WITH POPULATION GROUPS

Targeting risk groups can seem an attractive proposition. Resources may be directed towards groups with the highest level of health needs, which should prove effective and equitable. As discussed in *Health Promotion: Foundations for Practice* (Naidoo & Wills 2000), needs assessment is intended to look at unmet need for services and to provide information that will allow services to be tailored to local populations.

Target groups can be distinguished in two ways:

- geographical groups bound together by locality
- social groups bound together by some other attribute, such as age.

Within any target group such as older people (60 or more years of age) there are some people who have more needs than others, e.g.:

- those over 80 years of age (mainly women)
- those who live on their own
- those who belong to ethnic minority groups.

Targeting any group is thus problematic. Groups are often assumed to be homogenous for policy interventions when they may share important characteristics such as income or gender. Whilst this is important, behaviour is not simply a matter of following a social script and nor do individuals who share one characteristic such as their age group necessarily form one homogenous group. For example, the experience of older women is very different to that of older men (Arber & Ginn 1999).

Understanding health disadvantage is often within a medical model that identifies physical health needs and barriers to accessing primary care services. Homeless people for example, have marked health needs (see Box 12.1).

Box 12.1 Homelessness and health

- People sleeping rough have a rate of physical health problems that is two or three times greater than in the general population.
- The rate of tuberculosis among rough sleepers and hostel residents is 200 times that of the known rate among the general population.
- Rough sleepers aged between 45 and 64 have a death rate 25 times that of the general population.
- Of people sleeping rough, 30 to 50% suffer from mental health problems.
- About half of people sleeping rough are heavy drinkers and about one in seven is a drug addict.

Source: HEA (1999)

D iscussion point

What difficulties do marginalized groups face in accessing primary care?

Marginalized groups can have considerable difficulties accessing health services which may be:

- intimidating
- stigmatizing
- inaccessible.

Interventions targeted to homeless people's health needs thus tend, in acknowledging the wide range of health problems they face, to focus on improving access to primary care services. Many homeless are not registered with a GP and most will go to an A&E department as a consequence. Attempts to improve access to primary care tend to take the following forms:

- outreach workers
- NHS walk-in centres
- Satellite clinics, mobile services, home visits, drop-ins.

This example shows how services can exclude population groups but also the importance at practitioner level, of raising awareness of the nature of that exclusion. A key aspect of work with the homeless is values-training with practitioners – to tackle the attitudes of primary care workers that make access difficult such as views about the deserving and undeserving patient, the perception that homeless patients are violent and the reluctance to treat because of the perception that they are migrant.

R eflection point

Have you come across views on the 'deserving' and 'undeserving' patient?

Being homeless also encompasses other aspects of health including isolation, insecurity and poverty and one of the problems of targeting a population group is that these interconnecting needs that are pathways or barriers to health also need to be addressed. This requires partnership working across professional and organizational boundaries, so that social and health needs are met. It also means working *with* (rather than for) homeless people as partners, listening to their views, and acknowledging their areas of expertise. For more discussion of issues relating to partnership working, see Chapter 7.

Carers are an example of a population group (estimated at 5.7 million in the UK) that has only recently been recognized as having specific health needs in common. The role of caring itself has meant that carers have been invisible in society and the National Carers' Strategy (DoH 1998) urges recognition of carers as individuals in their own right separate from those they care for and as a group with distinct needs:

- A large proportion of carers are over 60 and therefore more likely to suffer physical injury such as back injuries.
- Around a third of carers feel their health is affected by caring.
- Around two-thirds report stress.
- Around half of carers have periods of depression (DoH 1998, Henwood 1998).

Strengthening the community of carers may mean providing emotional support or help and advice from a support group. Mental and emotional well-being can also result from feeling in control of the situation – which means, for carers, having the information and resources to help them to care. Birmingham Carers has set up a befrienders project to support isolated carers who have become inactive within the community due to their caring role. The role of the befriender is to provide company either in the carer's home or on social outings and to offer support that is reliable, consistent and dependable. This example shows how a significant mental health issue may remain largely invisible unless a specific population group is targeted. By targeting carers, they become part of the mainstream health agenda.

The example of HIV/AIDS illustrates some of the dilemmas associated with both targeting specific groups for health education and services, and adopting a universal approach. Gay men and intravenous drug users were the initial target of HIV health education messages in the early 1980s. Alongside some success of this approach in reducing the HIV infection rate amongst gay men were the negative effects such as the maintenance of heterosexuals' illusion of invulnerability and a homophobic backlash. Predictions in the later 1980s of a heterosexual epidemic led to a change in emphasis and by 1990 the message was 'it's not who you are but what you do', i.e. targeting risk behaviours not risk groups. This was accompanied by a shift in funding from gay projects to professionally led initiatives aimed at the heterosexual population. Whilst this has meant more mainstream funding, the 'de-gaying' of HIV also led to a shift of attention from the group most at risk. Health authorities and health boards are unwilling to risk public and media criticism by working with gay men unless there is strong central pressure to do so. The linking of HIV to broader sexual health issues (see Chs 10 and 11) means that prevention funds are mostly used to support generic health promotion activities, drugs treatment and sexual health promotion aimed only at heterosexuals.

D iscussion point

What are the advantages and disadvantages of targeting versus a universalist approach?

National patterns of HIV incidence, however, and what is known of the existence of priority groups in local communities, would suggest that interventions targeting gay men and African communities should take precedence over interventions targeting groups who are easier to access but at little risk of HIV such as 'the general public'.

This chapter considers four different population groups – older people, children, Black and minority ethnic groups (BMEG) and refugees and asylum seekers – in more detail. For each population group, their specific health needs are outlined, followed by examples of different kinds of strategies and interventions targeted at the group to meet their needs.

OLDER PEOPLE

Box 12.2 Inequalities in health: older people

- Older people are more likely to live in poverty, in poorer and older accommodation and as such are at risk of fuel poverty and accidents.
- Access to transport is difficult which limits access to goods and services and social contacts; which is reflected in a decline in psychosocial health in some older people, especially widows.
- Poverty in older people particularly affects women as there are 3 times as many women as men aged 85 and over and most of these live alone – only 38% of older women live with a partner/husband.

The developed world talks of a demographic time bomb in the twenty-first century. The UK census of 2001 has revealed that for the first time there are more people aged over 60 than there are under 16. Sixty-plus year olds have risen from 16% of the whole of the population in 1951 to 21% in 2001. There are also over 1 million people aged over 85. This poses major problems for the care and costs to the state of supporting an ageing population. Reducing mortality and life expectancy is also not seen as an unmitigated public health success. The quality of life is also important. Although chronological age is not synonymous with disease and ill health, nevertheless there is an increase in frailty, chronic illness and greater use of health and social care services with increasing age.

Any targeting of a population group marks that group as distinctive and 'a problem'. Whilst this can be helpful in drawing attention to marked inequalities, it can also be a source of discrimination. The use of the term 'elderly' has been abandoned in health discourse because it marks out people as different rather than merely relatively older to others. Old age is not in itself a problem although in public and professional discourse it is seen as a time of decline, physical and economic dependency and separation from everyday life.

Organizations such as Age Concern (1999) have consistently highlighted incidences of lower quality care and rationing of services based on age and not individual need. This has been of sufficient concern for the first standard of the National Service Framework for Older People (DoH 1999) to be 'Rooting out age discrimination'.

The health of older people does decline with age although there may be little association between chronology and physiological age. Degenerative

R eflection point

How is old age framed in your practice? What language is used?

D iscussion point

Ageism can be defined as 'legitimating the use of chronological age to mark out classes of people who are systematically denied opportunities that others enjoy' (Bytheway 1995). Are there examples of ageism in health and social care?

conditions such as weaker muscles, loss of flexibility in joints, poor vision and hearing may occur in the 'young old' of 60–70 or the 'old old' of 85 plus or not at all. Health problems tend to be related to a number of limited diseases for which the risk factors are well known – coronary heart disease (CHD) and stroke, cancers, respiratory illness and osteoporosis. Dementia affects 1 in 5 people over 85 although its severity varies. Although it is clear that as men and women reach very late life their activities become more circumscribed, as Jarvis et al (1996) argue, in earlier late life their mobility and task capacity are unimpaired and they are well able to be involved beyond their home and household, in work, care giving, sport and recreations. A longer life does not necessarily mean worsening health. As people live longer, most morbidity gets compressed into the later years of life and many people reach 'natural death' without ill health. A review of health status in 1994 found it impossible to conclude whether the health status of the older population had improved, deteriorated or remained the same over the preceding decades of mortality decline (MRC 1994). Although health spending is higher for older age groups (40% of the NHS budget), the economic argument to prioritize older people because of their greater consumption of services and health needs is not the only, or most convincing argument. An alternative argument is a rights-based one – to tackle age-based inequalities.

Standard 8 of the UK National Service Framework for Older People aims to 'extend the healthy life expectancy of older people'. For most older people this means their independence, autonomy and maintaining functional capacity. Yet disability as measured in relation to activities of daily life tends to rise in those over 70 and is mostly related to locomotor function. A survey in North London cited by Howse and Prophet (2000) found that 40% of people aged over 70 could not walk 400 m or climb the stairs normally. Falls and fractures are associated with high morbidity, mortality and substantial costs. In 1999, there were over 3000 deaths and over 85 000 serious injuries as a result of falls in older people (DoH 2001). Hip fracture is the most common serious injury and this can precipitate admission to long-term care. Even those falls that do not result in injury may have psychological consequences of loss of confidence and fear (of a future fall), decreased activity, social isolation and depression.

R eflection point

What does quality of life in older age mean to you?

E xample

Falls prevention

Many epidemiological studies have explored the causes of falls and over 400 variables have been investigated (National Centre for Reviews and Dissemination 1996). These include nutritional status, environmental hazards such as lighting or loose carpets, medication and its effect on balance and inactivity. A consistent feature of falls is that the person is likely to be less mobile, in poorer health and more overweight. A systematic review of interventions for preventing falls in older people (Gillespie et al 2002) concludes that interventions likely to be beneficial are:

- muscle strengthening programmes and balance retraining carried out at home by a trained health professional
- Tai Chi – a programme of at least 15-weeks' duration
- home hazard assessment and modification for people with a history of falling including personal alarms and hip protectors
- gradual withdrawal of psychotropic medication.

E continued

The relative importance of different strategies is not known – vision screening and home hazard management, for example, are not markedly effective as single interventions but add value when combined with an exercise programme.

In the acute settings, practice development initiatives have focused on developing best practice guidelines and assessment tools for those at risk of falls and integrated care pathways for fractured neck of femur which is the most common injury.

Encouraging older people to remain physically active is a major priority. This means action in broader areas – ensuring the maintenance of pavements, better lighting in streets and parks, restricting traffic in residential and shopping areas and improving town centres, as well as developing affordable and accessible public transport through concessionary fares and mobility buses and tackling community safety so that older people feel safe in public areas.

In this section we have examined some of the arguments for targeting a population group for specific health promotion interventions. Improving quality of life for an ageing population is important in terms of health improvement and to reduce some of the strain on services.

CHILDREN

Box 12.3 Inequalities in health: children

- A child from social class 5 (8.1 per 1000 births) is twice as likely to die before 15 as a child in social class 1. Infant mortality among babies of mothers born in Pakistan is 12.2 per 1000 live births.
- Babies with fathers in social classes 4 and 5 have a birthweight that is on average 130 grams lower than babies with fathers in social classes 1 and 2.
- Children in poorer families are more likely to experience illness especially respiratory infections, gastroenteritis, *Helicobacter pylori*, TB.
- A child from social class 5 is five times as likely to die from injury or poisoning as a child from social class 1.

Source: Roberts (2000), Northern and Yorkshire Public Health Observatory (2001)

In 1943, following the publication of Richard Titmuss' *Birth, Poverty and Wealth*, newspapers reported that 'poor folks' babies stand less chance'. More than half a century later, this headline is still true. Evidence shows this is not inevitable, but can be addressed by social and health policies. Parental poverty triggers a chain of social risk which is transmitted to the next generation. Children are therefore identified as a population group as having specific health needs that should be targeted. The reasons relate to a commitment to reduce health inequalities whose origins are said to lie in childhood and to provide the basis for health in later years. Intervening in childhood is seen as a key strategy to break the cycle of social disadvantage.

Childhood is a critical stage in health when many diseases such as cardiovascular disease and diabetes have their origin and economic and social circumstances can have lasting effects. Despite the existence of a welfare state in the UK for 50 years, there are still 3 million children living in poverty, a higher proportion of the population than any other developed country apart from the USA (Smith 2001). The British government has committed itself to eradicating child poverty and one of the national inequalities targets is to reduce the gap in infant mortality between the least well off and the population as a whole.

Although infant mortality is falling, there has been a dramatic increase in morbidity as measured by self-reported illness. Just over a quarter of boys and just under a quarter of girls aged 2–15 years reported a long-standing illness with 10% indicating that it limited their activities in some way (Prescott-Clarke & Primatesta 1998). Psychological disorders in children show similar increases.

There are two arguments why it is important to focus on children in social policy interventions:

1. the biological rationale
2. the social rationale.

The biological explanation suggests that events such as malnutrition and exposure to smoking, alcohol or infections in utero may 'programme' an individual's risk before they encounter other risk factors. For example, infants whose mothers are obese are at greater risk of developing coronary heart disease. Those small at birth have a greater risk of developing non-insulin dependent diabetes.

The social explanation is that low birthweight and delayed growth are merely markers for social disadvantages. Socio-economic differences in adult life can be explained by these earlier life processes. Michael Wadsworth (1999) has analysed birth cohorts and shown that family circumstances influence later health status. The cycle of deprivation includes poor physical development and low educational attainment which leads to a raised risk of unemployment or low status/low control jobs and perceived social marginality. Roberts (1997) argues that family structure, whether lone, reconstituted or intact, has less influence on health status than family centredness (time spent in family activities). Conflict between young people and their parents is related to poor health and social outcomes such as smoking and alcohol consumption, delinquency and contact with the police.

One element of policy interventions may focus on the protective factors for childhood – optimizing growth before birth and early education interventions. Policy interventions also need to be safety nets to prevent the accumulation of further disadvantage, be springboards to help young families onto a more advantageous trajectory and need to occur at critical social transition points such as the early years and starting secondary school (Arblaster et al 1998).

Tackling childhood disadvantage has tended to be through early intervention programmes offering social and emotional support and interventions to improve health status. Roberts (2000) looks at evidence of effective interventions providing social and emotional support; early detection of postnatal depression; policies to increase the initiation and maintenance of breastfeeding; policies which improve the health and nutrition of women of childbearing age and their children; and preschool education.

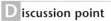

Discussion point

What types of policy intervention may follow from this analysis?

Box 12.4 Young people and social disadvantage

- One in five children in UK grows up in a workless household.
- One in 16 young people leaves school with no qualifications each year and the numbers of excluded pupils is rising (2000 in London in 1996–7), disproportionately affecting Black children.
- One in six 16–24-year-olds is the victim of a violent offence each year. Five in 100 teenagers in London have been accused of a crime (theft 37%, drugs 11%, criminal damage 11%).
- 10% of children under 18 lived at a different address one year before the 1991 census.

Source: Acheson (1998)

Example

Food supplementation

Addressing the nutritional health of pregnant women is a priority in tackling health inequalities. In many countries this is tackled through food supplementation programmes. In the USA, for example, the Special Supplementation Programme for Women, Infants and Children (WIC) is a huge federally funded nutrition programme targeted at low income women who are pregnant or who have just had a baby and children up to five years old. A cheque or food token is issued which allows the purchase of foods (e.g. cereals, milk, cheese, eggs, peanut butter, fruit or vegetable juice, carrots, tuna and pulses). The WIC programme has shown increases in birthweight and fewer pre-term deliveries but what isn't clear from the evidence is whether it is the addition of the food supplements, nutrition education or contact with health and social care professionals that makes a difference.

In the UK a welfare foods scheme has been in place since 1940, originally providing cod liver oil and orange juice. In its current form, it provides guaranteed quantities of milk or infant formula (7 pints each week up to the age of five) and includes 23% of the population aged 0–4 (DoH 2003). Proposals for 'Healthy Start', the new scheme, include widening its nutritional basis to include fruit, vegetables and cereal-based foods as well as liquid milk or formula. Initiatives such as this bring families into contact with the NHS in the early years of life and can link with other schemes aimed at improving food access such as food co-ops and community kitchens.

Sure Start is a programme targeted at preschool children and their families in disadvantaged areas of England. Over £450m was allocated for spending between 1999 and 2002 and there were 250 local programmes covering 150 000 children. The objectives are to:

- improve social and emotional development
- improve health
- improve the ability to learn
- strengthen families and communities (DfEE 1999).

Sure Start was developed following evidence from the United States High Scope programme, a preschool intervention based on child initiated learning. It started 30 years ago in Michigan and has been comprehensively evaluated. By the age of 19, those who took part in the programme were more likely to have completed their schooling, be in paid employment and girls were less likely to have become pregnant. At 27 years, participants had higher monthly earnings, were more likely to own their own home, and were less likely to have been arrested for crimes including drug taking or dealing.

The competitive tendering for funding means some areas will miss out on funding. The money is time limited so it is hard to build sustainability and continuity into programmes. Because it is area-based, Sure Start funding goes to many families who are not poor but live in a poor area, and misses many poor families who live in more affluent areas and may therefore be even more marginalized. The evaluation of Sure Start focuses on specific outcomes such as a 5% reduction in low birthweight babies that may be difficult to achieve.

In this section we have seen a different response to the targeting of a population group that includes a rounded approach to child health which encompasses anti-poverty and social exclusion strategies. Early intervention programmes provide education and care and improved nutrition. Supporting education and tackling 'the poverty of expectation' is a major plank of UK policy. As Wilkinson has pointed out 'The problems being experienced by families today are rooted in economic stress and in family disintegration. Any progressive family policy must address both these issues' (1998).

BLACK AND MINORITY ETHNIC GROUPS

Ethnic minority disadvantage cuts across all aspects of deprivation. Taken as a whole, ethnic minority groups are more likely than the rest of the population to live in poor areas, be unemployed, have low incomes, live in poor housing, have poor health and be the victims of crime.

(Social Exclusion Unit 1998, 1.26)

The term Black and minority ethnic groups (BMEGs) is an attempt to move away from the medicalized concept of 'race' referring to biological and physical differences between human groups, such as skin colour. This concept of 'race' has now become discredited, due to the lack of significant separation of biological characteristics between different 'racial' groups, and its association with racism, or discrimination based on 'racial' attributes. The concept of BMEGs prioritizes notions of culture rather than race, and highlights the importance of social rather than biological characteristics. Ethnicity refers to a shared cultural heritage including language, religion, history and customs, and as such can be applied to the majority White population in Britain as well as minority groups. The term BMEGs includes a number of very different ethnic groups with different experiences of health, education, employment and income. However, there is a unity due to a common experience of being discriminated against and overall there is evidence of higher than average health and social care needs (Gill et al 2003, Nazroo 1997).

There is a substantial body of evidence demonstrating differences in health status between ethnic groups and a complex picture of high or low

Discussion point

Do early intervention programmes improve health?

Discussion point

'Joined up thinking' is a familiar phrase in UK government policy but to what extent is it evident in tackling childhood poverty? What needs to be addressed?

Reflection point

Do you use the term 'Black and ethnic minority groups' in your practice? Why do you think this term has been adopted?

rates of specific conditions among ethnic groups. South Asians have high mortality rates from diabetes and coronary heart disease. Caribbean people have low death rates from coronary heart disease but a relatively high mortality from stroke, linked to high prevalence of diabetes and hypertension. There is a higher than average infant mortality for most BMEGs, and a particularly high rate among babies of Pakistan-born mothers. People from Pakistani, Bangladeshi and Caribbean communities perceive their health to be significantly poorer than does the average population. On the plus side, there is generally lower than average mortality due to breast and lung cancer amongst people from BMEGs, although there is some evidence that these patterns may be changing.

The diversity of health experience between different BMEGs may be caused by several different factors, or a combination of these factors:

- Different causes of poor health, especially social and environmental factors but also cultural and genetic factors, e.g. low income, sickle cell disease.
- Different susceptibility to poor health caused by social factors, e.g. social isolation, stress due to migration, and experiences of racism.
- Reduced access to health and social services due to institutional and/or individual racism.

Discussion point

What is the main focus of health promotion interventions targeted at Black and minority ethnic groups?

Whilst many health promotion programmes targeting BMEGs have focused on cultural differences, often using stereotyping rather than concrete evidence, it seems likely that, just as with social class inequalities, it is material factors that are most significant in causing excess ill health and mortality. However, cultural norms of religion, diet and recreational activities continue to be blamed for the health deficit suffered by BMEGs. Examples of this are a focus on high fat diets, and the alleged prohibition on physical activity especially for women, which are perceived to be cultural norms amongst people from Asian communities. The Stop Rickets campaign of the early 1980s, targeted at the Asian population, was criticized for focusing on lifestyle changes such as dietary change and exposure to sunlight. The alternative strategy of adopting a structural approach, such as dietary supplementation (e.g. adding vitamin D to a basic food such as chapatti flour), had proved successful amongst the majority White population in the 1940s.

Discussion point

Is it appropriate to focus on culture as the key to tackling BMEG health inequalities?

Cultural essentialism, or a focus on cultural norms as the key to health inequalities, has been a feature of much of the activity directed towards improving the health of people from BMEGs. Culture is assumed to affect health through health-related behaviours (such as smoking, exercise, diet, sexual behaviour) and the organization of families affecting child rearing and gender roles. Cultural practices in ethnic minority groups are compared to the ethnic majority. Frequently these are seen as accounting for health inequalities and thus viewed as 'problematic'. Cultural essentialism is a form of victim blaming at the community level, and has strong parallels with victim blaming at the individual level. In both cases, universalist and structural strategies which would affect health, such as higher incomes through employment or benefits, are overlooked in favour of targeted campaigns advocating lifestyle changes.

Positive features of the lifestyles of people from BMEGs, such as the low rates of women smoking amongst Asian women, and the generally low levels of alcohol consumption for men and women from BMEGs, tend to be ignored. There is much to be learnt from BMEGs about how people from disadvantaged communities cope without recourse to recreational drugs, but the stereotyping of minority cultures as problematic and the pathogenic focus of health promotion means that what keeps people healthy often fails to be articulated.

The focus on health care for a diverse society has tended to concentrate on improving access, removing language barriers and providing culturally sensitive information.

Access to appropriate and available services is often perceived to be a problem for BMEGs rather than service providers. For example, the low rates of referral of BMEGs to services such as respite care, social care and community care are often explained away by referring to the desire of people from BMEGs to provide care from within extended families. Research demonstrates that this is not the case, but it continues to be used to exonerate service providers from being proactive about providing flexible, appropriate services for everyone within their areas.

Discussion point

What are the main barriers for BMEGs in accessing and using primary care?

Reflection point

Consider the following quote. What would be your response?

'Equal opportunities is not an issue here. There are very few people from BMEGs living locally. We provide a "colour-blind" service that is the same for everyone irrespective of their colour or culture.'

This is a common response from service providers, even in areas with large communities of people from BMEGs. Whilst on one level it encapsulates an ideal, in reality holding this view is likely to be associated with providing a relatively poorer service for people from BMEGs. This is because factors that are taken for granted within the majority White population, such as easy communication and a broad consensus on cultural norms, may be problematic for people from BMEGs.

Example

Young Asian women and suicide

Making assumptions and stereotyping BMEGs is common. A study in Newham, an area of London with a large Asian population, found that service providers believed that the main reason for self harm was culture conflict (balancing family traditions against influences of Western culture). Young Asian women, however, identified lack of information about mental health services and not being understood by primary care professionals. A focus on culture conflict meant that health services did not examine the scope for other interventions or service improvements.

Source: Arora et al (2000)

The desire to reflect a multicultural society in service provision has led to an emphasis on practitioners being more 'culturally aware', understanding the customs, traditions and religious beliefs of different ethnic communities. Increasingly, the term 'cultural competence' is used to describe an organization that has a clear understanding of how it addresses issues of diversity.

Reflection point

Have you attended any training on the cultural practices of ethnic minority groups? What is your reaction to such training?

The targeting of any population group assumes a homogeneity of the group. The beliefs associated with any ethnic group will be adhered to with varying degrees and 'they are constantly refashioned within a culture, especially after migration when people have access to the resources of two different cultures' (Davey Smith et al 2000, p. 400).

Separate interventions targeting Black and minority ethnic groups inevitably risks marginalizing minority ethnic issues. It also implies that the health problems in minority ethnic groups are different from those in the ethnic majority, with different causes and different solutions, whereas in fact the similarities are greater than the differences. However, unless specific consideration is given to minority ethnic issues, interventions may unintentionally favour the ethnic majority. Thus policies to consider inequalities in health should include consideration of the application of these policies to minority ethnic groups as a matter of course, including ways of ensuring that racial prejudice and harassment are overcome. This requires that the structures and processes of policy making are sensitive to the position and needs of people from minority ethnic groups. One way of ensuring that the needs of Black and minority ethnic groups are integral to programme planning and policy making is to ensure that minority ethnic groups are represented, consulted and involved in planning and delivery. As with all excluded groups, their visibility can help to reduce the sense of exclusion.

REFUGEES AND ASYLUM SEEKERS

Refugees and asylum seekers are an example of a population group that may be targeted for interventions because they have specific health needs and can be amongst the most vulnerable and excluded groups in society, facing poverty and lack of cohesive social support.

Discussion point

What is the difference between a refugee and an asylum seeker?

The UN convention of 1951 defines a 'refugee' as someone who 'owing to a well founded fear of being persecuted for reasons of race, religion, nationality, membership of a social group or political opinion is outside the country of his nationality and is unable, or owing to such fear, is unwilling to avail himself of the protection of that country; or who, not having a nationality and being outside the country of his former habitual residence, as a result of such events is unable to or owing to such fear, is unwilling to return to it'. Asylum seekers are those who have applied for refugee status. In order to be admitted to countries such as the UK it is necessary to have first applied for asylum.

There are 21 million refugees worldwide with a further 25 million people displaced within their own countries. The vast majority of refugees remain in countries close to their own. Asylum applications have been rising in the UK but it ranks ninth among EU countries in terms of asylum seekers per head of the population with 1.7 asylum seekers/1000 population (www.homeoffice.gov.uk; www.refugeecouncil.org.uk).

As we have seen in this chapter, targeting any population group means assuming a degree of homogeneity. Refugees and asylum seekers like older people or people from Black and minority ethnic groups are not a homogenous group and may come from a wide range of countries, ethnic groups, social backgrounds and have different histories. War, conflict and

Discussion point

What are the likely
health problems of
refugees on arrival?

Discussion point

Health problems may
even worsen after
arrival. Why might
this be?

economic poverty have resulted in rising numbers of refugees across Europe, often leading to negative media reports and racist attacks. Of the 12 million refugees worldwide, 86% originate from developing countries and 72% remain in a developing country.

For most refugees immediate concerns are safety, food and shelter. Some may have experienced war, rape, torture and other traumatic events as well as displacement and a difficult journey to a new country resulting in complex mental health needs (trauma, stress and depression). Most will have experienced anxiety or depression but do not have a mental illness. Those fleeing for safety may arrive with physical disabilities such as amputations. Most refugees arriving in the UK are young and physically fit and the health problems experienced are similar to those of deprived groups and excluded groups who are isolated and unable to feel part of a community.

The practice of dispersal, accommodation in poor housing and public hostility in some areas exacerbate isolation. Current regulations in the UK mean asylum seekers cannot be employed and are only eligible for 70% rate of income support benefits. Asylum seekers therefore have reduced access to many of the basic determinants of health such as good housing or an adequate income.

The health needs of refugees, in common with homeless people, have been seen within a medical model that prioritizes physical health. Burnett & Peel suggest that 'refugee health in many areas of Britain has become the responsibility of communicable disease departments, giving the impression that refugees are vectors of infection, but refugees with infectious diseases needing care and treatment are the minority' (2001, p. 544). On arrival many refugees may have untreated conditions but screening on arrival seems more to protect the host population than benefiting the health of the refugee. HIV prevalence mirrors the country of origin and TB, although rising in areas with high numbers of refugees such as some London boroughs, is not common in new arrivals. A Home Office pilot scheme in Kent screened 5000 refugees for TB but all tested negative according to a report in the *Guardian* newspaper on 7 February 2003. Because refugees live in poor, overcrowded conditions the possibility of infection developing and then spreading is likely.

Whilst the health needs of refugees and asylum seekers are similar to those of the host population, many experience difficulties accessing health care. Many refugees have problems registering with a GP either because the patient list is closed or sometimes, because of a lack of awareness by primary care staff about the rights and entitlements of refugees. Asylum seekers may be refused registration due to fears about language problems resulting in lengthy consultations and a reputation for high mobility (Fassil 2000, Jones & Gill 1998). Refugees then tend to either accept temporary registration which restricts their access to other services, or cluster on the lists of a few practices which puts a strain on those services due to the time-consuming nature of most refugee health issues. Language difficulties, in both personal contact with practitioners and in filling out forms, is another barrier for many refugees and asylum seekers. The onus is nevertheless on the refugee to use services but for many, health problems are not a priority and remain untreated until they become chronic or an emergency.

Interventions to meet refugee health needs have focused on:

- developing networks of support
- using link workers to provide better integration with mainstream services
- providing interpreters and advocates to ensure available services are accessed
- providing better information on arrival
- offering specialist locality-based services on mental health, women's services, TB screening.

Many health professionals have difficulty working with marginalized groups, seeing them as an excessive burden on the NHS or adopting stereotyped attitudes. Many areas have produced information packs for practitioners working with refugees that provide basic information on:

- understanding refugee support needs
- exile and identity
- cultural differences
- communication in health care
- issues of women (sexual health, possible survivors of rape and as main health care provider in families)
- working with survivors of torture and rape.

Communication is essential to the delivery of services. There are three broad categories of interventions used to improve communication (Sanders 2000):

1. A linguistic model that assumes the barrier to communication is language and uses interpreters or telephone language link.

2. A professional-centred model that attempts to build service teams with knowledge and understanding of target communities. They may use link workers or bilingual workers as 'intercultural mediators' and focus on developing culturally appropriate materials.

3. A client-centred or advocacy model that focuses on the client, communicates their wishes, and acts as an advocate to ensure needs are met in an appropriate and accessible manner.

Example	An East London Primary Care Trust (PCT) has tried to improve the access to primary care of refugees and BMEGs by providing independent bilingual health advocates who educate primary care staff about the culture and socio-economic conditions of different groups; support patients in consultations and provide feedback on services to the PCT. Patients may need rapid access to a professional interpreter and a telephone interpreting service was set up that could also cope with several languages (www.languageline.co.uk). Sessional advocates were offered for smaller minority ethnic communities.
Good practice in increasing access to primary care	
	Source: Baylav and Fuller (2003), Levinson & Gillam (1998)

In this section we have seen how health promotion may target a population group on the basis of specific health needs but this can be problematic. The laudable attempts to meet those needs can appear stigmatizing with the singling out of particular conditions whilst the health needs that are shared with the rest of the population may be ignored.

CONCLUSION

Targeting health promotion at specific population groups is based on several different rationales, including a scientific notion of risk, an ethical notion of equity, and an economic notion of cost-effectiveness. The scientific notion of risk is problematic in practice, focusing on biological, genetic or lifestyle factors that have less impact on health status than basic structural factors such as education and income. In addition, this notion of risk can very easily become victim blaming, assuming that the responsibility for poor health lies with the individual or group and their chosen lifestyles. For BMEGs in particular, this ignores the importance for overall health of following cultural and religious norms, and also the reality of a mixed cultural heritage for second generation migrants. Using a notion of risk also focuses on what are perceived to be problematic behaviours and neglects the health promoting aspects of the lifestyles of people from BMEGs.

Targeting is more strongly based on ethical notions of equity. Certain marginalized groups in society have both high levels of health need and low access to services. In order to provide an equal service for all, such groups need specific targeted services to enable them to have the same access as the general population. Examples of such groups are homeless people and people from BMEGs. Other groups, such as mothers and children, are targeted because they are pivotal in breaking the cycle of disadvantage that perpetuates inequalities from one generation to the next. Groups such as older people and people with learning disabilities are targeted because society in general, including health and social care provision, is often guilty of discrimination due to reduced expectations of the health potential of people in these groups. Without specific targeting these groups are likely to have problems accessing relevant services and reaching their full health potential.

There is also an economic rationale for targeting. Providing additional resources to proactively meet the health needs of marginalized groups is likely to be far more cost-effective than waiting to meet the costs of a range of health and social needs resulting from increased marginalization and corresponding ill health and social exclusion.

There are therefore sound reasons for targeting specific groups as a public health and health promotion strategy. However, there are also problems and challenges attached to using targeting as a strategy. Targeting may reinforce, instead of challenging, stereotypes by labelling specific groups as dependent and problematic. Targeting is often used as a substitute for universalism and may become a means of avoiding, instead of supplementing, mainstream provision. People with learning disabilities for example, may have particular health needs (higher incidence of sensory impairment and epilepsy), but in many other ways their needs are the same yet they experience poor access to services and limited social and economic opportunities.

Identifying groups with unmet health needs is a key aspect of reducing health inequalities but is not always the most effective way to achieve equity. Targeting groups may be linked to short-term funding and limited resourcing, leading to uncertainty and an inability to plan ahead.

FURTHER DISCUSSION

■ How might health promotion interventions targeted at specific population groups avoid falling into the traps of cultural essentialism and stereotyping?

■ Is targeting population groups an effective way to achieve equity?

■ Who stands to gain most from targeting specific population groups – organizations, clients or practitioners?

Recommended reading

■ Department of Health (DoH) (2002) Addressing inequalities – reaching the hard to reach groups. National Service Frameworks: a practical aid to implementation in primary care. London, DoH.

A resource pack providing guidance for reaching 'hard to reach' groups together with case studies of good practice.

■ Kai J (2003) Ethnicity, health and primary care. Oxford, Oxford University Press.

A practical guide to some of the challenges of providing health care in the diverse ethnic communities in the UK.

■ Health Education Authority. Promoting the health of vulnerable groups series including: refugees (1998); teenage and lone mothers (1999); homeless (1999); older people (2000).

A series of short reports that examine the evidence on the health needs of vulnerable population groups and discusses existing interventions and their effectiveness.

REFERENCES

Acheson D (1988) Independent inquiry into inequalities in health. London, The Stationery Office.

Age Concern (1999) Turning your back on us: older people and the NHS. London, Age Concern

Arber S, Ginn J (1999) Gender differences in health in later life: the new paradox? Social Science and Medicine 48(1): 61–76

Arblaster L, Entwistle V, Fullerton D, Forster M, Lambert M, Sheldon T (1998) Review of the effectiveness of health promotion interventions aimed at reducing inequalities in health. York, NHS Centre for Reviews and Dissemination

Arora S, Coker N, Gillam S, Ismail H (2000) Improving the health of black and minority ethnic groups: a guide for PCGs. London, King's Fund

Baylav A, Fuller J (2003) Working with link workers and advocates. In: Kai J (ed) Ethnicity, health and primary care. Oxford, Oxford University Press

Burnett A, Peel M (2001) Health needs of refugees and asylum seekers. British Medical Journal 322: 544–547

Bytheway W (1995) Ageism. Maidenhead, Open University Press

Davey Smith G, Chaturvedi N, Harding S, Nazroo J, Williams R (2000) Ethnic inequalities in health: a review of UK epidemiological evidence. Critical Public Health 10(4): 375–408

Department for Education and Employment (1999) Sure Start: making a difference for children and families. London, DfEE

Department of Health (DoH) (1998) National carers' strategy. London, DoH

Department of Health (DoH) (1999) Saving lives: our healthier nation. London, The Stationery Office

Department of Health (DoH) (2001) Accidental injury task force working group: priorities for prevention. London, DoH

Department of Health (2003) Healthy start: proposals for reform of the welfare foods scheme. London, DoH, www.doh.gov.uk/healthystart.htm

Doyal L (1998) Women and health services: an agenda for change. Maidenhead, Open University Press

Fassil Y (2000) Looking after the health of refugees. British Medical Journal 321: 59

Gill P S, Kai J, Bhopal R S, Wild S (2003) Health care needs assessment of black and minority ethnic groups in NHS health needs assessment, the fourth series of epidemiologically based reviews. Oxford, Radcliffe, www.hcna.radcliffe-oxford.com/bmegframe.htm

Gillespie L D, Gillespie W J, Robertson M C, Lamb S E, Cumming R G, Rowe B H (2002) Interventions for preventing falls in elderly people (Cochrane Review), Issue 3. Oxford

Health Education Authority (HEA) (1998) Promoting the health of refugees. London, HEA

Health Education Authority (HEA) (1999) Promoting the health of the homeless. London, HEA

Henwood M (1998) Ignored and invisible? Carers' experience of the NHS. London, Carers' National Association

Hills J, Le Grand J, Piachaud D (2002) Understanding social exclusion. Oxford, Oxford University Press

Howse K, Prophet H (2000) Improving the health of older Londoners: reviewing the evidence. London, CPA Publications

Jarvis C, Hancock R, Askham J, Tinker A (1996) Getting around after 60: a profile of Britain's older population. London, HMSO

Jones D, Gill P S (1998) Refugees and primary care: tackling the inequalities. British Medical Journal 317: 1444–1446

Levinson R, Gillam S (1998) Linkworkers in primary care. London, King's Fund

Medical Research Council (MRC) (1994) The health of the UK's elderly people. London, MRC

Naidoo J, Wills J (2000) Health promotion: foundations for practice, 2nd edn. London, Baillière Tindall

Nazroo J (1997) The health of Britain's ethnic minorities: findings from a national survey. London, Policy Studies Institute

National Centre for Reviews and Dissemination (1996) Effective health care: preventing falls and subsequent injury in older people. York, NCRD

Northern and Yorkshire Public Health Observatory (2001) Inequalities in the health of children and young people. Occasional Paper No. 3 at www.nypho.org.uk

O'Leary J (1997) Beyond help. London, National Housing Alliance

Prescott-Clarke P, Primatesta P (1998) Health survey for England: the health of young people 1995–97. Dept Epidemiology and Public Health, University College London, The Stationery Office

Roberts H (1997) Socio-economic determinants of health: children, inequalities and health. British Medical Journal 314: 1122–1129

Roberts H (2000) What works in reducing inequalities in child health. London, Barnardo's

Sanders M (2000) As good as your word: a guide to interpreting and translation services. London, Maternity Alliance

Smith R (2001) Countering child poverty. British Medical Journal 322: 1137–1138

Social Exclusion Unit (1998) Rough sleeping. London, Cabinet Office

Wadsworth M (1999) Early life. In: Marmot M, Wilkinson R G (eds) Social determinants of health. Oxford, Oxford University Press

Wilkinson H (1998) The family way: navigating a third way in family policy. In: Hargreaves I, Christie I (eds) Tomorrow's politics: the third way and beyond. London, Demos

Index

Note: In order to save space in the index the following abbreviations have been used. GMFA – Gay Men Fighting Aids; IEC Strategy – Information, education, communication strategy.

Page numbers in *italics* refer to figures.